CHILD
TRAUMA I
Issues & Research

Garland Reference Library of
the Social Sciences (Vol. 739)

CHILD TRAUMA I
Issues & Research

Ann Wolbert Burgess, Editor

Garland Publishing, Inc.
New York & London
1992

Library of Congress Cataloging-in-Publication Data
Child Trauma I: issues and research / edited by Ann
Wolbert Burgess.
    p. cm. — (Garland reference library of the social
sciences: vol. 739)
        ISBN 0-8153-0036-0
    1. Children—United States—Crimes against. 2.
Sexually abused children—United States. 3. Child
molesters—United States.
    I. Burgess, Ann Wolbert. II. Title: Child trauma
one. III. Series: Garland reference library of social
science; v. 739.
HV6250.4.048C45   1992   92–7875
362.7'6'0973—dc20   CIP

Printed on acid-free, 250-year-life paper
Manufactured in the United States of America

TABLE OF CONTENTS

CONTRIBUTORS

Judith V. Becker, Ph.D.
Department of Psychiatry
University of Arizona
Tucson, Ariz.

Eugene Borgida, Ph.D.
Department of Psychology
University of Minnesota
Minneapolis, Minn.

Margaret Bull Kovera, M.A.
Department of Psychology
University of Minnesota
Minneapolis, Minn.

Allen G. Burgess, D.B.A.
School of Management
Northeastern University
Boston, Mass.

Ann Wolbert Burgess, R.N.,
  D.N.Sc.
van Ameringen Professor of
  Psychiatric Nursing
University of Pennsylvania
Philadelphia, Penn.

Elizabeth Burgess Dowdell,
  R.N., M.S.
Doctoral Candidate
University of Pennsylvania
Philadelphia, Penn.

John Campbell, M.S.
Unit Chief, Behavioral Science
  Unit
FBI Academy
Quantico, Va.

Jon R. Conte, Ph.D.
School of Social Work
University of Washington
Seattle, Wash.

David L. Corwin, M.D.
Department of Psychiatry
Washington University
  School of Medicine
St. Louis, Mo.

Margaret Cotroneo, R.N.,
  Ph.D.
School of Nursing
University of Pennsylvania
Philadelphia, Penn.

Thomas F. Curran, M.S.W., J.D.
Executive Director
Children's Advocacy Center
Philadelphia, Penn.

Theresa A. Delaney
Director of Publications
National Center for Missing and Exploited Children
Arlington, Va.

John W. Fantuzzo, Ph.D.
School of Education
University of Pennsylvania
Philadelphia, Penn.

Linda Fogarty, M.A.
Doctoral Student
School of Public Health
The Johns Hopkins University
Baltimore, Md.

The Hon. Charles D. Gill
Superior Court Judge
Hartford, Conn.

Evelina Giobbe
Project Director, WHISPER
Minneapolis, Minn.

Christine A. Grant, R.N., Ph.D.
School of Nursing
Widenor University
Chester, Penn.

Ellen B. Gray, Ph.D.
Center for Applied Social Science Research
Allegheny College
Meadville, Penn.

April W. Gresham
Department of Psychology
University of Minnesota
Minneapolis, Minn.

Laura T. Gutman, M.D.
Department of Pediatrics
Duke University Medical Center
Durham, N.C.

Carol R. Hartman, R.N., D.N.Sc.
School of Nursing
Boston College
Chestnut Hill, Mass.

Robert R. Hazelwood, M.S.
Supervisory Special Agent
FBI Academy
Behavioral Science Unit
Quantico, Va.

Robert O. Heck
Program Manager
U.S. Department of Justice
Washington, D.C.

Marcia E. Herman-Giddens,
  P.A., M.P.H.
Department of Pediatrics
Duke University Medical
  Center
Durham, N.C.

Anne Holland
School of Education
University of Pennsylvania
Philadelphia, Penn.

Meg S. Kaplan, Ph.D.
Department of Psychiatry
College of Physicians and
  Surgeons
Columbia University
New York, N.Y.

Susan J. Kelley, R.N., Ph.D.
School of Nursing
Boston College
Chestnut Hill, Mass.

Raymond Knight, Ph.D.
Professor of Psychology
Brandeis University
Waltham, Mass.

Barbara A. Lane, M.S.N.
Department of Pediatrics
Duke University Medical
  Center
Durham, N.C.

Kenneth V. Lanning, M.S.
Supervisory Special Agent
FBI Academy
Quantico, Va.

Garrett J. McAvoy, B.A.
University of West Virginia
School of Law
Morgantown, W.V.

Arlene McCormack
Professor of Sociology
Lowell University
Lowell, Mass.

Gloria MacFarland, M.S.
Assistant Director of Classifi-
  cation and Movement
New York State Division for
  Youth
Albany, N.Y.

Ross E. McKinney, Jr., M.D.
Department of Pediatrics
Duke University Medical
  Center
Durham, N.C.

Helene Moriarty, R.N., Ph.D.
School of Nursing
Villanova University
Philadelphia, Penn.

Jeanne G. Niemeyer, M.S.W.
Department of Pediatrics
Duke University Medical
  Center
Durham, N.C.

Robert A. Prentky, Ph.D.
Director of Research
Massachusetts Treatment
  Center
Bridgewater, Mass.

John B. Rabun, Jr., A.C.S.W.
Vice-President
National Center for Missing
  and Exploited Children
Arlington, Va.

Pamela C. Regan
Department of Psychology
University of Minnesota
Minneapolis, Minn.

Robert K. Ressler, M.S., FBI
  (Ret.)
Forensic Behavioral Services
Spotsylvania, Va.

Frances E. Rokous
Doctoral Candidate
Yale University
New Haven, Conn.

Edward R. Shaw, Ph.D.
Director of the Bureau of
  Mental Health Services
New York State Division for
  Youth
Albany, N.Y.

Karen St. Claire, M.D.
Department of Pediatrics
Duke University Medical
  Center
Durham, N.C.

Chris Weedy, M.S.W.
Department of Pediatrics
Duke University Medical
  Center
Durham, N.C.

INTRODUCTION

Child trauma has been a social issue and problem throughout civilization. It seems that in the United States each generation has increasing difficulty dealing with it. Currently there are strong social forces giving child trauma heightened perspective.

In the decade of the 1980s the sexual exploitation of children was identified as a major public health and criminal justice problem. Tremendous strides have been made in shifting the traditional balance of the criminal justice system in the United States from an offender orientation focusing on the apprehension, prosecution, punishment, and rehabilitation of wrongdoers to concerns of victims, witnesses, and their extended families. Although previously it was acknowledged that the justice system could not function without the assistance and cooperation of victims and witnesses, little recognition was given to their rights and little effort was made to assist them in overcoming the frustrations and economic sacrifices that involvement in the criminal proceedings caused. This attitude began to change in the past decade with the emergence of a strong national victim and witness assistance movement, which achieved success in establishing programs to assist victims and witnesses and in increasing the public's awareness of their problems and rights. At the national level, President Ronald Reagan appointed a Task Force on Victims of Crime in 1982; the Congress enacted the Federal Victim and Witness Protection Act of 1982 and the Victims of Crime Act in 1984.

When the President's Task Force on Victims of Crime studied the experience of crime victims in America, it recognized that family violence is often much more complex in causes and solutions than are crimes committed by unknown attackers. Because of this realization, the Task Force recommended a separate study be undertaken and thus the Attorney General's Task Force on Family Violence was appointed in 1983. Important outcomes in the form of recommendations from this Task Force included:

- O Judges to consider treating incest and molestation as serious criminal offenses,
- O Judges to adopt special court rules and procedures for child victims such as the use of hearsay evidence at preliminary hearings, the appointment of a special volunteer advocate for children when appropriate, the presumption that children are competent to testify, allowing children's trial testimony to be presented on videotape with agreement of counsel, flexible court room settings and procedures, and carefully managed press coverage,
- O Development of more effective prosecution techniques in order to minimize additional trauma for the victim created by court procedures,
- O Development of law enforcement techniques to investigate sex crimes against children,
- O Research on how child molesters select victims, what strategies they use to entice victims to cooperate, and what circumstances they consider favorable for proceeding with an assault.

In 1984, a national symposium on child molestation was sponsored by the Department of Justice gathering a multi-disciplinary group together to achieve two goals: 1) to share experiences and ideas in order to produce better strategies for addressing child sexual abuse throughout the country, and 2) to sound a loud, clear signal that child molestation is a serious criminal offense and will be treated as such.

Concurrent with these criminal justice efforts, C. Everett Koop, the Surgeon General of the U.S. Public Health Service, planned and sponsored a workshop in 1986 to study violence as a public health issue. Following this report, he encouraged mini-conferences in major cities on the subject, emphasizing that the health professions use an interdisciplinary approach to the problem of interpersonal violence.

As the problem of child sexual abuse has become more visible, research monies have become available to study child trauma. Law enforcement officials, social workers, clinicians, nurses, doctors, and researchers have amassed considerable evidence documenting both the common occurrence of child sexual abuse and serious disorders associated with its victims. While estimates of yearly rates of child sexual abuse cases in the United States range from 50,000 to over 1 million, both researchers and clinicians agree that the majority of cases remain undetected.

With child trauma cases, there is need to look not only at the child, but at the offender as well.

The Child

When abused children are not acknowledged, they fail to receive any special help or treatment. The adverse effects of child sexual abuse are numerous. Both controlled and uncontrolled retrospective studies of abused children indicate a variety of long term emotional, behavioral, social, and sexual problems. Symptoms include physical problems of headaches, stomachaches, sleeping and eating disorders; psychological reactions of fears and anxiety, depression, mood changes, guilt, and shame; social problems of school truancy and failure, and of quarreling and fighting with family members and peers; and sexual problems, such as heightened sexual activity, compulsive masturbation, exhibiting oneself, and preoccupation with sex and nudity. Running away from home, adolescent prostitution, suicide attempts, substance abuse, gender identity confusion and sexual dysfunction, and socially deviant behaviors also have been identified as possible aftermaths of untreated childhood sexual abuse.

The Offender

A parallel problem is that undetected child abusers continue to molest children. In a study of 200 non-incarcerated child molesters, it was found that child molesters involve themselves not only in child molestations, but also in various deviant sexual behaviors. Gene Abel and colleagues noted that molesters with the greatest incidence of molestation are those who molest boys. Offenders who commit incest and have never been involved with other sex crimes are rare; most are involved with children outside their homes. Both men and women can be offenders.

Research on the problem of child sexual abuse has been to assess the abuse and its effects on the child and then to offer solutions oriented toward legal considerations and interventions within the physical health, mental health, and social service systems. This approach offers only a partial solution to the problems of safety and protection of the child. A comprehensive solution to the problem involves learning ways to stop their behaviors. Controlling offenders involves the community and their families, as well as the health professions, social service agencies, law enforcement, and the criminal justice system.

This first volume in CHILD TRAUMA examines contemporary issues and research in the field.

Part I, Current Issues in Child Trauma, identifies five current issues: children's rights, newborn abductions from hospitals, memory, cognition and childhood trauma, a diagnostic category for child sexual victimization, and juvenile prostitution. In Chapter I, Essay on the Status of the American Child, 2000 A.D.: Chattel or Constitutionally Protected Child-Citizen?, the Honorable Charles D. Gill observes that children have no constitutional rights. He argues that while children are a vulnerable population who are dependent upon adults to protect and care for them during their development, statistics and literature are replete with accounts of the difficulties children have growing up in our American society. He suggests that the time has come for amending the Constitution to afford children certain inalienable rights, as adults enjoy.

The 1980s have witnessed the visibility of a crime committed against infants. In Chapter 2, Newborn Infant Abductions from Hospitals, Elizabeth B. Dowdell and John B. Rabun, Jr., write on a highly charged emotional issue. Although baby kidnapping is considered a low-incidence crime, there has been an increase in cases since 1983. As a prelude to a study that will interview the hospital staff, parents of kidnapped babies, as well as the convicted abductors, this chapter examines various aspects of the problem and discusses pre-abduction and post-abduction health policy issues.

In psychiatric and mental health circles, the 1990s are publicized as the decade of the brain. Many neurobiological contributions are being applied to childhood disorders. In Chapter 3, Memory, Cognition, and Childhood Trauma, Ann W. Burgess and Carol R. Hartman present the neurobiological findings related to the information processing of trauma. In childhood trauma, the basic assumption is that traumatic sexual abuse impacts upon basic brain functions and structures, causing disruption in primary and secondary processes of consciousness. This disruption influences development and individuals' view of themselves. The social context of the sexual abuse and the response of others interact with ongoing biological shifts adding to and shaping the response patterns and attributional cognitions of sexual abuse victims. This theoretical framework is present in the context of an adolescent case example.

Clinicians have been working on the development of a diagnostic category for childhood sexual victimization. In Chapter 4, Sexually Abused Children's Symptoms and Disorders of Extreme Stress Not Otherwise Specified: Does This Proposed Psychiatric Diagnosis Fit?, David L. Corwin reviews the literature on the emotional and behavioral effects of sexual abuse on children and adolescents. This literature clearly notes that sexual victimization is associated with significant detrimental effects. Corwin argues that the proposed diagnosis provides a suitable category for symptomatic victims of such abuse.

A neglected aftermath of child trauma is juvenile prostitution. In Chapter 5, Juvenile Prostitution: Profile of Recruitment, Evelina Giobbe describes some of the methods pimps use to procure juveniles and turn them into prostitutes. As part of the Oral History Project conducted by Women Hurt In Systems of Prostitution Engaged in Revolt (WHISPER), Giobbe notes the recruitment process used by pimps. Using examples from an interview with a 31-year-old woman who had been a prostitute for 13 years, this chapter provides insights into the complex relationship between pimp and juvenile prostitute and the difficulty endured in trying to leave the life.

As more cases of child sexual abuse are reported, there is a need for young children to testify in court. In Chapter 6, Children as Witnesses in Court: The Influence of Expert Psychological Testimony, by Eugene Borgida, April W. Gresham, Margaret Bull Kovera, and Pamela C. Regan, attention focuses on research that deals with children in court as witnesses. The authors present the results of their program of research that examines how expert psychological testimony influences perceptions of the credibility of children in child sexual abuse trials. Building upon previous research by Borgida in the area of adult sexual assault, expert psychological testimony in this context can have an influence on perceptions and judgements about child witnesses. Using a hypothetical technique and testing for where the child is perceived as unprepared or with a demeanor leads to inferences of being unprepared, the child is seen as less credible. Expert psychological testimony can inform jurors about the demeanor of the child and serves as a way to counteract these perceptions.

With the increasing numbers of child exploitation and sexual abuse cases entering the justice system, the subject of the child as a legal witness is of pressing concern. In Chapter 7, The Child Witness in Florida, Garrett J. McAvoy reports on his legal analysis of the state of Florida's procedural measures for child witnesses designed to reduce trauma to the testifying child. The implications of this study are to provide suggestions for other jurisdictions to consider adopting for trauma-reducing laws.

In Part II, Research in Child Sexual Abuse, some of the current research is reviewed. The number of reported HIV-infected individuals is increasing. In Chapter 8, HIV Transmission by Child Sexual Abuse, Laura T. Gutman and colleagues report on their study of HIV-positive children. During 1987–1989, 14 of the 96 HIV–positive children (14.6%) who were followed by the Duke Pediatric AIDS team were confirmed to have been sexually abused. Every sexually abused child was evaluated for each of the five modes of HIV transmission, and for nine of the children the pathway was found. Four of the study children had acquired HIV from sexual abuse, and for six of the children sexual abuse was a possible source. Transmission of HIV by child sexual abuse was the most frequent of the proven modes of acquiring HIV in this population. The other proven modes of acquisition were vertical transmission (3) and HIV-contaminated blood transfusion (2). None of the children acquired HIV from clotting factor cryoprecipitate or intravenous substance abuse.

Twelve males who were related to an abused child were identified (8) or suspected (4) of being perpetrators. Three knew themselves to be HIV positive at the time of an assault, and eight were aware that the child was HIV positive at the time of the assault. There was no indication from any child that "safe sex" precautions had been observed. Children with HIV infection had multiple risk factors for abuse/neglect. The sociological descriptors of the lives of the 14 abused children showed multiple known risk factors for sexual abuse, which also overlapped with known risk factors for or sequelae of the acquisition of HIV infection. These included drug abuse and alcoholism in the home, prostitution of a parent, lack of parenting, and chronic illness of the child. Preventive efforts should recognize that children as well as adults are at risk for sexually transmitted HIV infection.

One of the tasks in court is evaluating the competency of a child witness. Chapter 9, Sexually Exploited Children: Assessing Competency to Testify, by Christine A. Grant, presents a child competency tool for clinicians who interview children suspected of sexual abuse. Fifty videotaped interviews were analyzed by the process of content analysis. Through the use of coding instructions, the content of each videotaped interview was coded according to four competency categories: personal, interpersonal, academic, and truthfulness competency. Content that indicated sexual exploitation was coded according to a separate category for abuse. The content was analyzed using predetermined categories developed from the competency requirements of the Federal Rules of Evidence. The tool proved reliable among trained coders and experts in the area of child sexual exploitation.

The emotional aftermath of child victims and their parents is a new area of inquiry. In Chapter 10, Stress Responses of Children and Parents to Sexual Abuse and Ritualistic Abuse in Day Care Centers, Susan J. Kelley reports on the highly symptomatic nature of abused children and their parents years following disclosure of sexual abuse in a day care setting. The extreme forms of physical, sexual, and psychological abuse experienced by the majority of children in this study is alarming, and may, in part, explain the children's persistent symptomology. The increased psychological distress found in parents suggests that sexual victimization of a child is a major stressor for non-offending parents.

Parents have emotional reactions to their child having to testify in court. In Chapter 11, Parental Response to Child Sexual Abuse Trials Involving Day Care Settings, Ann W. Burgess, Carol R. Hartman, Susan J. Kelley, Christine A. Grant, and Ellen B. Gray, examined the stress responses of parents to whether or not their child testified in a sexual abuse trial against defendants from a day care center. Parents completed a questionnaire and the SCL-90-R, Impact of Events scale, and Life Events Survey. Parents of 17 testifying children presented higher symptoms of psychological distress than parents of 50 nontestifying children sexually abused in day care centers. In addition, the reported stress was higher in fathers than in mothers. Following disclosure of their child's sexual abuse, stressful life events of death in family, loss of income, and separation were associated with parents of testifying children.

In Part III, Treatment Interventions and Prevention Programs are discussed. As a new treatment technology, the abused child's resilient peer is proposed to assist in a structured play setting. In Chapter 12, Resilient Peer Training: Systematic Investigation of a Treatment to Improve the Social Effectiveness of Child Victims of Maltreatment, John W. Fantuzzo and Anne Holland outline the major components of their research strategy. They report the results from a series of three studies investigating a proposed intervention, Resilient Peer Training (RPT) and discuss possible next steps in this line of research. RPT basically involves using peers as treatment agents and utilizing play as a context for enhancing preschoolers' social effectiveness. Resilient peers are children who function exceptionally well even though they face the same set of environmental stressors as the target children.

Treatment perspectives are needed for working with the incest family. In Chapter 13, Intergenerational Family Processes in the Treatment of Incest, Margaret Cotroneo and Helene Moriarty note that a number of theories have been proposed to explain intrafamilial child sexual abuse and these include some understanding of problematic family systems. What is lacking, the authors argue, are well-developed family systems conceptualizations that describe intergenerational family processes that can develop into a maladaptive functioning that focuses on children. Family loyalty conflict is one relational process that increases the risk that children can become the foci of maladaptive interactions among members of a family unit. This chapter draws on clinical findings from Contextual Family Therapy to describe assessment and intervention in family loyalty conflicts.

In nonincest cases, treatment interventions need to include the child as well as the parents. In Chapter 14, Extrafamilial Child Sexual Abuse: Family-Focused Intervention, Carol R. Hartman, Allen G. Burgess, Ann W. Burgess and Susan J. Kelley conduct a secondary analysis on data reported in Chapter 11. The authors note the strong interaction of child and parent symptoms and suggest, using descriptive comments from study parents, a tri-level family focused treatment plan: crisis intervention, individual trauma therapy, and group therapies.

Many child sexual abuse prevention programs were implemented during the 1980s. In Chapter 15, Sexual Abuse Prevention Programs for Children, Jon R. Conte and Linda Fogarty note how public and professional awareness of the extent and effects of childhood sexual victimization has increased over the last decade. Concurrently, there has been a concerted interest in how sexual abuse can be prevented. The aim of this chapter is to review current efforts to prevent sexual abuse of children. In doing so, the authors discuss the nature of sexual abuse and what an understanding of that nature implies for programs to prevent sexual abuse of children, summarize the effects of sexual abuse prevention programs, and outline some of the major policy implications of this material.

Planning and implementing a curriculum on child sexual abuse requires structure and content. In Chapter 16, Developing a Child Sexual Abuse Curriculum, Thomas F. Curran presents the need for a child sexual abuse curriculum and principles and concepts on how adults learn. Considerations when planning to introduce a new curriculum into an existing academic program include: the problem approach, the emerging field approach, the discovery approach, the target population, analysis of the job to be performed, job tasks, identify individual characteristics, behavioral objectives, the learning environment and the evaluation. Student motivation, curriculum goals and objectives, prerequisites, criterion test measures, implementation plan, class size, instructional method, curriculum content, and instructor qualifications complete the discussion.

Part IV, The Aggressors, includes chapters on adolescent sex offenders, incest histories in serial rapists, rehabilitation of child molesters, serial child molesters and abductors, and juveniles who murder. In Chapter 17, Research on Adolescent Sex Offenders, Judith V. Becker and Meg S. Kaplan report on their research study of 67 adolescent males between the ages of 13 and 19, the majority of whom had been charged with or convicted of a sexual crime. Rather than a unitary profile of an adolescent sexual perpetrator, the subjects in this study could be placed into four distinct categories: (1) adolescents who engage in consensual sexual behavior with a peer-age relative; (2) adolescents who initially engage in consensual sexual behavior with a peer-age relative, but then turned to coercive sex when the relative no longer consented; (3) adolescents who have developed a deviant sexual interest pattern and meet DSM-III diagnosis for paraphilia; and (4) adolescents who engage in nondeviant sexual behavior and have incidental occurrence of deviant sexual behavior.

Childhood sexual trauma in the life histories of rapists was studied by Arlene McCormack, Frances E. Rokous, Robert R. Hazelwood, and Ann W. Burgess. Chapter 18, An Exploration of Incest in the Childhood Development of Serial Rapists, reports on the phenomenon of male incest in a sample of 41 incarcerated serial rapists. Of 31 men who reported childhood sexual abuse (penetration, exploitation, and/or witnessing), just over half were victims of incest. All incestuous experiences occurred before puberty, and the majority of the experiences were protracted in nature. When compared to non-incest victims of sexual abuse, incest victims were more likely to report parental physical abuse and to describe their childhood family structure at sixteen years of age as reconstituted (step-parent present). In all cases in which the step-father was implicated in the abuse, the abuse was of the witnessing variety; i.e., the boy witnessed sexual activity that he found disturbing. Incest victims were significantly more likely than were non-incest victims to re-enact sexually abusive behavior within the family. This finding suggests that clinical discoveries of sibling sexual activity should alert clinicians that other incestuous activities may be occurring or have occurred.

Does treatment of child molesters prevent sexual abuse? In Chapter 19, Rehabilitation of Child Molesters: A Cost-Benefit Analysis, Robert Prentky and Ann W. Burgess report on a study that examined the cost effectiveness of the rehabilitation of child molesters by designing and testing a cost-benefit model. The model uses program and reoffense data from a treatment center for offenders and costs derived from averaged figures obtained from state agencies. Results of the analysis, as well as related policy issues, are discussed.

In Chapter 20, Serial Child Molesters and Abductors, Ann W. Burgess, John Campbell, Theresa A. Delaney, Robert O. Heck, Raymond Knight, Kenneth V. Lanning, Robert A. Prentky, John B. Rabun, Jr., and Robert K. Ressler report on a study comparing demographics and crime-related variables of 97 abducting child molesters and 60 non-abducting child molesters. Three case examples are provided.

The 1980s witnessed an increase in adolescent murderers. In Chapter 21, Juveniles Who Murder, Christine A. Grant, Ann W. Burgess, Carol R. Hartman, Allen G. Burgess, Edward Shaw and Gloria MacFarland report on their study of 85 juveniles who were convicted of murder. These juveniles are male and tend to come from a household of two or more siblings where the dominant caretaker is the mother who is alone in the process of child rearing. There is a high incidence of truancy and delinquency and a relationship between alcohol and drug use. The murder classification suggests a split between young males who carry out the violent act independently as opposed to being involved with a co-defendant. Those involved in co-defendant murder most often are armed with guns and knives and assault male victims. The motive differs if the victim is known to the offender.

PART I

CURRENT ISSUES IN CHILD TRAUMA

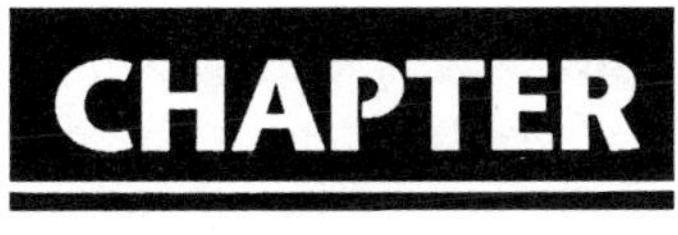

1

Essay on the Status of the American Child, 2000 A.D.: Chattel or Constitutionally Protected Child-Citizen?

The Honorable Charles D. Gill

Reprinted by permission from the *Ohio Northern University Law Review* 17 (3): 543–579.

I

We hold these truths to be self-evident, that all men are created equal, that they are endowed by their Creator with certain unalienable Rights . . . .[1]

These magnificent words, largely the inspiration of Thomas Jefferson, a slave owner, and signed by 56 white males, are the philosophical cornerstone of our democracy. This compelling phrase is permanently enshrined in each of us as school children and is frequently recited in emotional tones to hushed audiences at anniversaries and events of national significance. This belief in certain "rights" is also the foundation for the Constitution of the United States and is reflected in its preamble.

During Constitution Week of 1990, a day was set aside for each town to ring its steeple bells to celebrate the existence of our Constitution. And the bells rang. But while they were pealing for adults; the children of this country had few rights to celebrate.

The truths, the rights, justice and the blessings of liberty were not extended to all people by our fundamental documents. Slaves, children, and, to a large degree, women were excluded. They were property, mere chattel, in varying degrees. Slaves had no rights, since they were property, and the child-citizens, similarly, had no rights except to someday succeed to the rights of their fathers.[2]

The Thirteenth, Fourteenth, and Fifteenth amendments elevated the status of black citizens in the United States. One constitutional amendment, the nineteenth, improved the status of women by granting them voting rights. However, the American child remains essentially property, and its constitutionally unprotected status is more and more likely to produce disastrous consequences that threaten the viability of our democracy. This essay will examine the history of child-citizenship through present-day America and present reasons to change the status of the child via an amendment to the United States Constitution.

II

The history of childhood is a nightmare from which we have only recently begun to awaken. The further back in history one goes, the lower the level of child care, and the more likely children are to be killed, abandoned, beaten, terrorized, and sexually abused.[3]

The history of childhood is replete with suffering, well documented from biblical times to the present. One scholar notes that "from Roman times to the mid-nineteenth century [children] were treated as something akin to property and had rights which might be characterized as falling somewhere between those of slaves and those of animals."[4]

Prior to the sixteenth century, our current concept that childhood is a time for protected growth and development, free from major responsibilities, did not exist. Children were maltreated, murdered, left to die, sold into slavery, or brutally maimed so that they might become more successful beggars.[5]

Children's status began to change during the sixteenth, seventeenth, and eighteenth centuries. Although in some ways no longer considered merely "chattel," children continued to be ignored and impersonalized; they were most probably considered "replaceable" and "interchangeable." Their major value to the family was in their contributions to family work and income and supporting aging parents. The harsh upbringing they received generally produced adults who were hostile and untrusting and "incapable of developing close relationships."[6]

By the eighteenth century, most parents were "beginning to consider their children as of the same flesh and blood as themselves."[7] Parents began to accept their responsibility of maintenance, education, and protection. However, American attitudes toward the treatment of children did not begin to change until near the end of the nineteenth century.[8]

Every student of social work knows the landmark case that opened America's eyes to the children's plight.[9] The Wilson case, which arose in 1874, pricked the American social conscience as well.[10] Mary Ellen Wilson was an 8-year-old who lived in her adoptive parents' apartment in New York City. She was held there in chains, starved, and beaten. Her piercing screams brought numerous complaints to the local police. The police responded but could do nothing. After all, this was a "family matter," and families, that is, "adults," have rights.

Finally, an enterprising social worker contacted Henry Berg. Berg was only able to extricate Mary Ellen from her family torture chamber through skill and guile. Who was Henry Berg and why was he called? Henry Berg had founded a protective group the preceding year: The Society for the Protection of Cruelty to Animals.[11] Children in nineteenth-century America were eventually seen to be victimized by conditions of immigration, industrialization, and urbanization.[12] This awareness marked the beginning of a "child-saving" era, including the establishment of societies to protect children. With much trepidation, and in relatively few instances, governmental, private, and religious agencies began to intervene in family life to protect children.[13]

At the beginning of the twentieth century, child-saving took on a new meaning through the development of the "widely spread belief that children were the essential human resources whose mature form would determine the future of society."[14] However, lest the reader envision a child-perfect world based upon the foregoing statement, a step back to reality is in order. Remember that these were the days of child labor, orphanages, and the infamous "orphan trains." The orphan trains were the creation of the Children's Aid Society of New York. This nineteenth-century effort, as oblivious of past abuses as are many present efforts in the twentieth century, organized a program akin to slave distribution.[15] More than 100,000 orphaned or abandoned children were periodically removed from orphanages and herded onto railroad cars between 1853–1929.[16] In scenes reminiscent of the Holocaust, they were shipped to the western United States. The orphan trains would stop at each town, and the children would be put on display in the town hall or church. Those interested in acquiring these pieces of human property would step up and feel the children to see how strong, healthy, or otherwise attractive they were. One child survivor of the orphan trains recalled being lined up and stared at "like cows."[17]

The history of childhood in America reached its launching pad, for the predictable full protective freedoms of the twenty-first century, during the last half of the twentieth century. The last five decades have produced a number of influencing factors for change. Stuart N. Hart tells us that these factors are: Changing views of the family, economics, and education, as well as the development of knowledge from sciences and allied professions, including the legal profession.[18]

American children now stand in a transitional state between chattel and constitutionally protected child-citizen. Although there are a number of national and international forces at work to complete that transition, lawyers have yet to take a leading role in this metamorphosis.

We lawyers can be justifiably proud of our many contributions to social justice through the skillful use of the knowledge and laws that are the tools of our profession. However, when it comes to social justice for children, it seems that our profession is merely lumbering slowly along in the wake of the social and scientific professions. To some extent we are in a "Catch-22" situation as advocates. Because our profession rightly demands nearly complete loyalty to our clients, we are neutralized when client loyalty creates situations that are inherently harmful to children. The result is what other professions often term "judicially sanctioned child abuse."

The family law attorney represents his adult client's interests, with the children's interests assuming a relatively low priority. The family law attorney may wish to "win" the children for the client, which is seldom a "win" for the children. Involvement of children in this arena for any purpose may well be a loss for children, regardless of the adult outcome. There are those, including this writer, who believe that the "best interests of the child" standard is an adult conscience salve that is at best a tortured choice between the lesser of two evils. When certain people have no rights, it is a leap of great faith to believe that those who have rights will endeavor, in a legal combat situation, to protect the best interests of the rightless people, the children. The criminal defense lawyer, the corporate lawyer, the presiding judge, and even the prosecutor unwittingly contribute to this "judicially sanctioned child abuse."

The only way to provide comparable justice for a child in an adult world, or an adult courtroom, is to provide comparable protective rights for the child-citizen. This is especially true in the courtroom, where knowledge of the developmental levels and needs of children is abysmally low.

III

> *If his parents default in effectively performing their custodial function—that is, if the child is "delin-quent"—the State may intervene. In doing so, it does not deprive the child of any rights, because he has none.*[19]

Members of the general public are astonished when they learn that the Constitution does not really provide any protective rights for our children. However, even the notion that adults have certain protective rights required centuries to evolve from discourses by moral and legal philosophers to codifications in documents such as our Bill of Rights. The same cannot be said for the rights of the child, which for long periods of history were submerged within the rights of the family. The period of transition from the first assertion that children, too, have rights, to the recognition of their individual human rights by binding international law has taken barely over 100 years, and has taken place largely without the aid of social scientists and philosophers.

Although numerous other nations have recognized that children have assertible rights in their constitutions, America has made no significant move in that direction. Constitutional rights possessed by other children of the world include protective rights that shield them from parents and family. Those in the front-line trenches of child abuse know full well that the latter are the very people from whom children most often need protection. An adage of the highly reputed adolescent treatment program at the Connecticut Junior Republic reflects such beliefs: "Many abandoned children are still living at home with their families."

The early twentieth century produced the juvenile courts, where the goal shifted from punishment to rehabilitation.[20] This era also spawned child labor laws which, in hindsight, seem to be mere expressions of common sense and basic human compassion. That was not so at the time however. Some religious leaders and conservative political forces opposed such laws as being unwarranted governmental interference in the economic and privacy rights of the family.[21] It is interesting to note that these same forces are today's opposition to national and international protective rights for children.

Cynthia Price-Cohen presents an excellent review of Supreme Court decisions that many of us have falsely trusted to be statements of individual constitutional rights for children. Early child education cases decided by the Supreme Court made it clear that they were decided without regard to the interests of the children involved. Rather, they were based, as was noted by Chief Justice Earl Warren in *Brown v. Board of Education*,[22] entirely upon a doctrine of parental rights and the issue of whether the parent may not be loyal in relation to the interests of his or her child is not addressed.[23] It is ironic that, although corporations in the United States have long been held to be "persons," and thus are eligible for constitutional protection, the extent to which children, as individuals, have comparable constitutional rights is still not entirely clear. Even in the 1967 case of *In re Gault*,[24] which apparently awarded extensive due process protection to juvenile delinquents, the Court declined to settle the issue. In other words, the Court saw the child only in relation to his family and not as an individual having separate constitutional rights.[25]

More recently, in the 1972 case of *Wisconsin v. Yoder*,[26] which gave the Amish the right to keep their children out of high school, Justice Douglas, dissenting, complained bitterly of the lack of consideration given to the child's interests: "[I]t is the student's judgment, not his parent's, that is essential if we are to give full meaning to what is said about the Bill of Rights and of the right of the students to be masters of their own destiny."[27]

The past two decades have seen a growing interest in the need for protections for children in at least three settings: child abuse, custody proceedings, and children as courtroom witnesses.[28] The eighties saw the shift to a stated national policy of "family preservation" and "family reunification." These lofty goals are admirable and in some cases workable. Unfortunately, social workers and social institutions have been so firmly inculcated with these goals that they have been making varsity efforts to rehabilitate wayward parents, but few efforts for their suffering children. The individual and statistical results for children, as will be shown, are nothing short of disaster.

IV

If the emotional damage that has been done to some children could be seen on the exteriors of their bodies, we would cringe and look away at such a hideous sight.[29]

It has been said that Mother Theresa stopped the flow of adoptions from Indian orphanages to American families because of her concern for the well-being of the orphan. More recently it has been reported to this writer that Mother Theresa had to modify that position based upon the extreme poverty of India and the scarcity of Indian adoptive parents. Her most recent policy is that Americans could adopt Indian children only after the third attempt to have the child adopted by others had failed.

So much for the perceived treatment of children by the wealthiest nation in the history of the world—the United States of America. This nation is in grave danger because of its benign neglect of its only real national treasure—its children. As stated by a representative of the Children's Defense Fund, "[w]e do not have a kinder and gentler nation. As far as children are concerned, America is 'leaner and meaner.'"[30]

The Committee for Economic Development,[31] reflecting the views of corporate America, worries publicly whether our children will have sufficient education, motivation, and undamaged brains to provide the high-tech labor force necessary to lead this nation into the twenty-first century as a free and viable democracy. The National Commission on Children voiced similar warnings in its report to President Bush and the Congress in 1990. The chairman of the National Commission, Senator Jay Rockefeller of West Virginia, promises "bold proposals" in the commission's final report in March of 1991. Children's advocates, including this writer, do not expect bold proposals concerning the status of the American child to emanate from that commission. There will be no proposals for rights for children or for a change in the status of children forthcoming from this commission. It will merely propose more remedial treatment programs for child casualties rather than prevention.

President Bush's Domestic Policy Council joined the chorus and proposed directing new efforts to children's needs. The council even spoke the magic words, "It is cost effective." The drawback was that the results would be long range and not statistically visible during the tenure of President Bush. The White House decided to put the recommendation of its own council on the shelf. In the words of Press Secretary Marlin Fitzwater, when it comes to children, "There will be no new toys, we will just polish up the old ones."[32]

The White House opposition to unpaid parental leave for the care of sick, newborn, or newly adopted children is a further indication of their "back shelf for children" policy. Of the 77 so-called industrialized nations of the world, until recently, only America and South Africa denied such leave to care for children. More recently, South Africa has apparently changed its policy, leaving America standing alone, not even with her head bent in shame.

Social indicators tell us American children are in crisis:[33]

1. 500,000 American children are runaways (they are usually running away from abuse).

2. 360,000 American children are in foster care (this is a 30% increase since 1986, and some now claim the real number is 500,000 and climbing).

3. There were only 51,000 adoptions in America in 1989 (10,000 were of Korean children).

4. 14,500,000 American children suffer emotional illness or developmental deviations (75% are untreated or undertreated).

5. Apparently, over 6 million American children suffer depression.

6. Suicide is the second leading cause of death of American children.

7. There are 1,000 cocaine babies born daily.

8. Each day 3,000 children become pregnant.

9. Each year 500,000 American children give birth to children (five years later these children of children could comprise over 30,000 kindergarten classes).

10. Over 3,000,000 grandparents are raising their grandchildren in America because their own children are incompetent or unwilling to do so.

11. American children have a higher infant mortality rate than a score of other countries (the infant mortality rate in America is currently higher than that of Spain, Singapore, Hong Kong, Panama, Chile, Trinidad, and Tobago).

12. In 1989 there were 1 million American children born to unwed mothers (this is 50% higher than in 1980 and 500% higher than in 1960).

13. In 1990, 1 million children saw their parents separate in divorce.

14. Rural American children have even more difficult circumstances than urban children in 34 of 39 categories.[34]

American children lead dangerous lives even in the wealthiest of states. For example, Connecticut has the highest per capita earnings in America. Hartford, its capital, is also the insurance and health insurance capital of the world. Nevertheless, children lead dangerous lives there as well. In some Hartford neighborhoods 18% of children suffer from chronic hunger. Forty-one percent of parents report they often send their children to bed hungry in these neighborhoods. The average birth weight of a child in Hartford is 4 pounds 14 ounces, well under the expected weight of a healthy newborn.[35]

Connecticut is a small state geographically, and most of its citizens have access to a number of excellent teaching hospitals affiliated with

Yale University and the University of Connecticut schools of medicine. Those facilities and others face some astonishing health problems for children in Connecticut.

Connecticut has the highest percentage of HIV-positive babies in the nation. It has the fifth highest percentage of unwed mothers. About 21% of urban children in Connecticut have little or no prenatal care. In 1989, there were 1,200 babies born in the Yale-New Haven clinic. Ninety percent of those mothers had used illegal drugs during their pregnancies. Fifty percent had used cocaine within 48 hours of delivery.[36] Child abuse cases are up 85% in the last decade. Sexual abuse cases are up 250% in the same period.[37]

Like most states, Connecticut has a child protective agency. The Connecticut Department of Children and Youth Services (DCYS) has a child abuse hotline number. It is conceded that 60% of such calls are not afforded any response. Indeed, children and advocates for children recently sued that agency in federal court. DCYS is presently in "receivership" and is being run by a federal court mediation panel which is chaired by Judge Robert C. Zampano of the United States District Court, District of Connecticut. Other states may follow.

In the final analysis, Connecticut is probably not unlike many other states. It is true in Connecticut, as it is perhaps true in your state, that society spends more money per day to board a dog than it does to support a foster baby.

What is happening in this country? How is it that this society, which claims to be so child-centered, can be guilty of such inconceivable neglect? Ann Hartman suggests an answer:

> *[T]he plight of millions of children[] in this country*
> *is so desperate and overwhelming that the American*
> *public may be using psychic numbing to protect itself*
> *from the pain and terror, in the same way that we have*
> *defended against knowing and believing in the*
> *possibility of a nuclear holocaust.[38]*

However, Hartman is only partially correct. It is suggested that there is more than a psychic numbing. There is a numbing caused by a certain selfishness that pervades us all. Sometimes the conscience-deadening anesthesia is our own guilt and denial. In any event, the purpose of this essay is not to beg adults to sensitize their numbness, assuage their guilt, or correct their indifference. Rather, the purpose of this essay is to ask some adults to consider granting children constitutional rights commensurate with their needs, so that their success in our society is not totally dependent upon the whims of adults. We must seek a balance, a balance that can only be achieved by the granting of assertible rights to the child-citizen. The balance between the integrity of the family and state intervention is a delicate one, but one that must be made.[39]

Virtually every person receiving this message is familiar in some way with the gravity of the problem. This is most certainly true of the professionals that encounter it daily—the therapist, the educator, the police officer, the court official, the lawyer, the social worker, the nurse, the pastor, and the medical doctor. The problem is known firsthand by the many millions of Americans who are victims.

While there is indeed no magic wand, special prayer, or panacea that will make the problem disappear, we must make a dramatic national attempt to solve the problem. Although any solution obviously includes a multidisciplinary approach, the key to unlocking the correct door is the legal system. However, the legal system does not have the capacity, the understanding, the knowledge, or the desire to make any wide-ranging changes. The inherent inhibition in the legal system is its obligation to utilize existing law to follow precedent.

Present laws, however benevolently, paternalistically, or sociologically created, have failed miserably. The juvenile court system has collapsed under the weight of its charge. The legislatures do not fund buildings, programs, or personnel sufficient to salvage our children. (They do find dollars, however, to fund buildings when children mature. They are called prisons.) Court rules are adult rules which protect adults, not children.

It is time for us to view our society realistically. For better or worse, the family days of Ozzie and Harriet and Beaver Cleaver are remote history to the vast majority of American children; perhaps even unheard of to the law students of 1991.

The United States Census Bureau reports the following statistics concerning the traditional family:

1. Only 26% of the nation's 93.3 million households were composed of a married couple and children under 18 in 1990. This is a decline from 31% of the households in the 1980's and from 40% of the households in the 1970's.

2. There were 9.7 million single parents in the nation in 1989. This is 41% more than in 1980.

3. Nearly all the single parents are women. There were 8.4 million families maintained by the mother in 1990. This is up 35% from 1980. The number of single mothers grew by 82% in the 1970's. "`You could say . . . that all the increase (in households) has taken place outside of traditional families,'" said Linda Waite, a sociologist with the Rand Corporation, commenting on these statistics.[40]

The real world of America has been accurately described recently by the United States Advisory Board on Child Abuse and Neglect.[41] The board's report is really the final warning before the catastrophe:

> *For 25 years the nation has become more aware of the magnitude of child abuse and neglect. The Board has concluded that child abuse and neglect in the United States now represents a* national emergency.[42]

There are a number of social ostriches in this country who attempt to minimize the emergency as it really is. Even the media fall prey and give equal billing to the handful of adults who *may* have been unjustly accused of child abuse. The innocent reader is led to believe that the problem is exaggerated, that children fabricate these stories, that we really cannot quantify child abuse. Slick courtroom psychologists, with packaged presentations, make the circuit of family law and criminal defense seminars to peddle their contribution to the confusion of English-majors-turned-judges in the family courts and the reasonable doubt arguments to the jurors in criminal court.

> *The increase in the number of reports of child maltreatment in recent years has been astronomical. In 1974, there were about 60,000 cases reported, a number that rose to 1.1 million in 1980 and more than doubled during the 1980's to 2.4 million.*

> *Whether the increase in reports is primarily the result*
> *of a change in public awareness or whether it largely*
> *reflects actual increases in the incidence of some*
> *forms of child maltreatment, the absolute number of*
> *substantiated cases has increased at a rate as*
> *shocking as the increase in the number of reported*
> *cases. Further, there are reasons to believe that even*
> *that number is just a fraction of the actual incidence*
> *of child abuse and neglect. Surveys consistently show*
> *that large proportions of cases of suspected child*
> *maltreatment remain unreported.*[43]

The American child national emergency led the Advisory Board to make the following observations:

1. Not only are child abuse and neglect wrong, but the nation's lack of an effective response to them is also wrong. Neither can be tolerated. Together they constitute *a moral disaster.*

2. All Americans share an ethical duty to ensure the safety of children. Protection of children from harm is not just an ethical duty: it is a matter of *national survival.*

3. All Americans should be *outraged* by child maltreatment.[44]

The sad truth is that not enough Americans are even momentarily concerned, no less outraged.

The Advisory Board made three findings:

1. Each year hundreds of thousands of children are being starved and abandoned, burned and severely beaten, raped and sodomized, berated and belittled;

2. The system the nation had devised to respond to child abuse and neglect is failing; and

3. The United States spends billions of dollars on programs that deal with the result of the nation's failure to prevent and treat child abuse and neglect.[45]

These findings are an indictment of the American approach to "curing" child abuse. We know we have a problem. We know the present system has failed. We know we spend billions of dollars on programs to fix what we allowed to break. In other words, we provide programs that treat the casualties but provide nothing to prevent them from being casualties in the first place!

If America had solved the problem of polio using the same strategies it utilizes to "solve" the child abuse problem, we would have an interesting country. It would be a country with countless people sporting high-tech leg braces, scientifically advanced crutches and state-of-the-art, computer-age iron lungs. And, naturally, we would have programs and telethons to make sure that each new victim had the appropriate apparatus.

Dr. Jerry Weiner, the past president of the American Academy of Child and Adolescent Psychiatry (the Academy has endorsed this constitutional amendment) tells the following story which makes the point beautifully: A group of people were standing by the side of a fast moving stream when one of them saw a baby floating in the rapids. The people quickly formed a human chain, entered the stream, and brought the baby to shore to a zone of safety. They looked back and saw three more babies and again locked arms, formed a human chain, and brought the three babies to shore, a zone of safety. They looked again and saw twelve babies floating to disaster, and, as they formed the chain again, one of them walked away. The group was agitated and shouted at the departing person to return and help them save the imperiled babies. "No," the person replied. "You save these babies, I am going upstream to find out who is throwing them in."[46] Upon hearing this story, a regional director of the Connecticut DCYS remarked to a group of children's advocates that "even the babies we are able to locate in the stream slip by us. God knows how many we do not even see." The policies, programs, and dollars of today are all at the side of America's stream of life. No one is going upstream to prevent the trip in the first place.

It is probably difficult for you, the reader, to feel the impact of this national emergency on children and our society by merely reading these printed words. You are probably relaxed in a law library, a comfortable office, or a tranquil home. You are warm, well fed, adequately clothed, and on the road to success because of an adequate family rearing effort. (Or, absent the latter, much good luck.)

Lawyers are trained to be analytical and objective. We shunt aside the irrelevant and guard against the emotional. These are desirable attributes, most of the time.[47]

You, the readers, are asked to forget who you are for a moment. Forget about your legal training. Instead, let us engage in a little role playing. Let us pretend that you are the chairperson of a commission for the city of Cleveland. Presume also that the stork delivers babies. Today the stork has delivered three babies, and it is your task to distribute them to families. Being a conscientious and diligent person, you are about to interview applicants for the positions as parents.

Couple number one is married. Husband and wife are in their mid-thirties. Dad is a raging alcoholic who is abusive of Mom and the other children. Mom is an alcohol abuser herself and is unable to defend the children from Dad's physical and verbal abuses. Dad has been arrested several times and has been hospitalized twice with alcohol-related illnesses. He does not perform well at work and relates poorly to fellow workers. His continued employment is always tenuous. There are three children in the family already. The oldest is in sixth grade and is in special education. He has brain damage of unknown etiology. The middle child is in second grade and receives medication for his hyperactivity and lack of concentration. The youngest child is a preschooler, and little is known about her at this time.

The second applicant is an unmarried couple. The man and woman are both in their twenties. They have been living together, off and on, for two years. They are both cocaine abusers. The female has had three medical interventions and is willing to enter another program if she can get this "kid." The male works sporadically as a house painter. They have resided at three locations in the past year and have done some traveling with friends.

The third applicant is a single female. She is 15 years old. She lives at home with her mother, who is 32 years old, and her mother's current boyfriend. The applicant is madly in love with 19-year-old Lenny. She and Lenny do not "do" heavy drugs. They only do alcohol and marijuana on weekends, recreationally. At present, Lenny is in jail for some minor larcenies. But, when he gets out, he is going to get two good jobs, a super apartment, a new car, and great toys for the kid.

Well dear chairperson, let us start the distribution of these three babies. What is this? You hesitate? Stop looking through the eyes of these babies. This is only pretend. In the real word distribution is automatic. Whoever begets them, gets them.

One baby, perhaps with fetal alcohol syndrome, goes to couple number one. Now we have four children in that family in the stream. The second baby, perhaps with the relentless wailing characteristic of cocaine withdrawal, goes to couple number two. The third baby, perhaps with low birth weight and the problems associated therewith, goes to the 15-year-old and Lenny.

If there is anything predictable in life it is the nonexistence of safe and fulfilling lives for these children—these victims. Ann Hartman reports that "Americans believe that a person's destiny is appropriately determined by the 'accident of birth'—by the parents he or she is born to."[48]

What if one of these children was enormously gifted? What if that child had an I.Q. over 150? Or, had the potential to be the finest pianist the world had ever heard? Or to be a scientist with the genius to solve the riddles of cancer and AIDS? What if the child was you?

These three examples are just a sample of the myriad of situations that threaten American children at birth and thereafter. They are by no means the most graphic. This is a new glimpse of what is happening "upstream" in America everyday. We see it in the hospitals, the courts, the schools, the prisons, and the television programming. We wonder why. The complete answer will be found in the correction of a myriad of societal deficiencies. The first answer is to change the status of children from quasi-chattel to full child-citizens. This change, if accomplished by constitutional mandate, will be the catalyst, the driving force, to correct these deficiencies.

It may be difficult for some lawyers to view the day-to-day national emergency even in the three pretend examples. It is perhaps better to approach the problem in the more familiar setting of case law.

As prologue to these cases one must be aware of our national policy, i.e., our national "adult" policy, as it effects children. The previously mentioned national adult policy is called "family preservation" or "family reunification." On the surface, these are rational goals. And, in some situations, they are even workable for adults and children alike.

Unfortunately, this national policy plays out quite differently in actual practice for hundreds of thousands of children. The national policy pendulum has swung so far to the adult side that we are leaving children in emotional limbo, or zones of danger, for often fatal periods of time. There are two practical reasons why the pendulum favors the adults. The first is money. It is cheaper for government to continue to keep children at "home" with their biological parent or parents. Second, it sounds good to the underinformed public, religious theorists, and ultra conservatives that we are making "reasonable efforts" to preserve families. The truth is we are disregarding the security, love, and bonding needs of our most helpless children. Their universally recognized needs as developing persons from birth to three years are largely ignored in order to attempt unreasonable efforts at salvaging their harmful biologic caretakers. There is, as one influential medical journal recently pointed out, a "bias in favor of the biologic family . . . . "[49] The end results of that bias, according to one journal, are that (1) 39% of children in foster care spend more than two years in "temporary placements," and that (2) the average wait for a permanent home for a child in 1984 in New York City was six years; in 1989, in Maryland it was five years; and most of the children who entered the court process in Boston in 1985 and 1986 remain in temporary placements.[50] The study also showed that as the children became older, they had more emotional, behavioral, and academic problems and were less likely to be adopted. Many of them are next seen in the delinquency courts.[51]

This essay is not intended to be a criticism of the variety of parenting practices and cultural beliefs that are present in America. Rather, it seeks to expose the desperate situations children find themselves in because of the biologic bias.

Studies of families brought before the Boston Juvenile Court indicate that more than half included a parent with a serious psychiatric disorder. Eighty-one percent had an average of four reports of abuse and neglect in the preceding three-year period![52] Parental substance abuse and alcoholism are major factors in the lives of the children presented to the Boston Juvenile Court, especially in cases of severe neglect.[53]

The study warns physicians who treat these children not to assume that "the child will be rescued" and "will be safe from further harm and that child's long-term development will become the highest priority"[54] after referral to a child protective agency, the police, or the courts. Nothing could be farther from the truth in America. As an example of how these policies and biases actualize in the courtroom, the court in *DeShaney v. Winnebago County Department of Social Services*[55] stated: "[T]he State does not become the permanent guarantor of an individual's safety by having once offered him shelter. Under these circumstances, the State had no constitutional duty to protect Joshua."[56]

Joshua was born in 1979. In 1980, his father, Randy DeShaney, was awarded custody of the child in a divorce proceeding. In 1982, Randy's second wife complained to the police that Randy was physically abusing Joshua. The Wisconsin Department of Social Services (DSS) investigated. The father denied the accusations and the investigation stopped. In 1983, Joshua was admitted to the hospital with multiple bruises and abrasions. The doctor suspected child abuse and notified the DSS. The Juvenile Court ordered him held in the hospital for three days. Three days later an ad hoc child protection team met and found there was insufficient evidence of abuse to retain custody in the court. Joshua's dad did agree to enroll him in a preschool program. A month later emergency room personnel called the DSS to report that Joshua was again being treated for suspicious injuries. The DSS worker concluded that there was no basis for action. For the next six months the caseworker made monthly visits to Joshua's home, during which she observed a number of suspicious injuries on Joshua's head. She also noticed that he had not been enrolled in school and that Randy's girlfriend, previously ordered to move out, was still in the home. The caseworker dutifully recorded these incidents in her files, along with her continuing suspicions that someone was abusing Joshua. Still the agency took no action.

In November of 1983, the emergency room again notified the DSS that Joshua was being treated for injuries that they believed to be caused by child abuse. On the caseworker's next two visits to Joshua's home, she was told that Joshua was too ill to see her. Still the DSS took no action.

In March of 1984, Randy beat 4-year-old Joshua so severely that he fell into a life-threatening coma. Emergency brain surgery revealed a series of hemorrhages caused by traumatic injuries to the head inflicted over a long period of time. Joshua did not die, but he suffered brain damage so severe that he will spend the rest of his life confined to an institution for the profoundly retarded. Randy was convicted of child abuse.

Joshua and his mother sued the state, claiming that the state's failure to intervene to protect him against a risk of violence at his father's hands, of which they knew or should have known, was a violation of his liberty without due process.[57] Joshua and his mother relied on a third circuit case, *Estate of Bailey by Oare v. County of York.*[58]

The *Bailey* case held that, once the state learns that a particular child is in danger of abuse from third parties and actually undertakes to protect him from that danger, a "special relationship" arises between it and the child. This special relationship imposes an affirmative constitutional duty on the state to provide protection.[59] The United States Supreme Court flatly rejected these holdings.

The Court agreed that the due process clause protects *adults* who have been made *helpless* by their circumstances.[60] But a child, according to the Supreme Court, finds no constitutional protection:

> *The Estelle-Youngberg analysis simply has no*
> *applicability in the present case. Petitioners concede*
> *that the harms Joshua suffered did not occur while he*
> *was in the State's custody, but while he was in the*
> *custody of his natural father, who was in no sense a*
> *state actor. While the State may have been aware of*
> *the dangers that Joshua faced in the free world, it*
> *played no part in their creation, nor did it do anything*
> *to render him any more vulnerable to them. That the*
> *State once took temporary custody of Joshua does not*
> *alter the analysis, for when it returned him to his*
> *father' custody, it placed him in no worse position*
> *than that in which he would have been had it not*
> *acted at all; the State does not become the permanent*
> *guarantor of an individual's safety by having once*
> *offered him shelter. Under these circumstances, the*
> *State had no constitutional duty to protect Joshua.*[61]

The Court was admittedly sympathetic, but visualized a scenario where the violation of the adult parent's due process rights of family privacy would be violated if they had acted otherwise:

> *Judges and lawyers, like other humans, are moved*
> *by natural sympathy in a case like this to find a way*
> *for Joshua and his mother to receive adequate*
> *compensation for the grievous harm inflicted upon*

> *them. But before yielding to that impulse, it is well to remember once again that the harm was inflicted not by the State of Wisconsin but by Joshua's father. The most that can be said of the state functionaries in this case is that they stood by and did nothing when suspicious circumstances dictated a more active role for them. In defense of them it must also be said that had they moved too soon to take custody of the son away from the father, they would likely have been met with charges of improperly intruding into the parent-child relationship, charges based on the same Due Process clause that forms the basis for the present charge of failure to provide adequate protection. The people of Wisconsin may well prefer a system of liability which would place upon the State and its officials the responsibility for failure to act in situations such as the present one.*[62]

The people of Wisconsin and the rest of the United States of America now have the opportunity to right the wrongs *DeShaney* perpetuates, by passing a new responsibility-balancing constitutional amendment. Justice Blackmun said it all in dissent:

> *Today, the Court purports to be the dispassionate oracle of the law, unmoved by "natural sympathy." But, in this pretense, the Court itself retreats into a sterile formalism which prevents it from recognizing either the facts of the case before it or the legal norms that should apply to those facts . . . .*

> *Poor Joshua! Victim of repeated attacks by an irresponsible, bullying, cowardly, and intemperate father, and abandoned by respondents who placed him in a dangerous predicament and who knew or learned what was going on, and yet did essentially nothing except, as the Court revealingly observes, . . . "dutifully recorded these incidents in [their] files." It is a sad commentary upon American life, and constitutional principles—so full of late of patriotic fervor and proud proclamations about "liberty and justice for all," that this child, Joshua DeShaney, now is assigned to live out the remainder of his life profoundly retarded.*[63]

There is an interesting case of academic debate on adult constitutional rights, while the child, whose interests were supposedly being considered, had already been thrown in the stream and is now probably dead. Jacqueline Bouknight was the birth parent of Maurice M.[64] Jacqueline Bouknight was a drug abuser with significant psychological problems. Maurice was an abused child from birth, and perhaps even before. From the first days of his life he was subjected to "severe physical abuse."[65] He had several bone fractures and other indications of that severe abuse. He was finally hospitalized at age 3 months with a fractured left femur.[66] Those readers familiar with the medical significance of that injury know the absolute force and severity of the assault that broke that large bone. While in the hospital a spica cast was applied to his body. Hospital staff observed Maurice's birth-mother shaking Maurice, dropping him in his crib (cast and all), and otherwise handling him in a manner "inconsistent with his recovery and continued health."[67] The hospital staff notified the child protection agency of "suspected child abuse."[68]

A court order removed him from his mother and placed him in shelter care. Several months later, for unstated but not unknown reasons ("family preservation," "family reunification"), Maurice was returned to birth-mother Bouknight.[69] A subsequent juvenile court hearing led to the declaring of Maurice a "child in need of assistance."[70]

The child protection agency asserted its jurisdiction over Maurice and then followed our national policy. They had birth-parent Bouknight continue as the custodian of Maurice! Of course, as a person with no parenting knowledge, a negative psychological profile, and an addiction to illegal drugs, she was told that she could only continue to be the custodian of Maurice if she followed certain extensive "conditions" set forth in the court orders. Bouknight was ordered to cooperate with the protective agency, to continue in therapy, to participate in parental aid and training programs, and to "'refrain from physically punishing [Maurice]'" who was under the age of one, in diapers, but presumably out of his body cast by now.[71] Bouknight and her lawyer signed the order and she agreed to its terms.

Eight months later, the protective agency, citing a concern for Maurice's safety, brought the case back to court. The agency stated for the record "that Bouknight would not cooperate with them and had in nearly every respect violated the terms of the protective order."[72] Surprise, surprise! A mentally ill person, addicted to illegal drugs, with a known history of severely abusing a helpless infant, did not follow such a logical program.

It would be nice to think that the return to court was prompted by the twenty observations of Maurice by the protective agency during those eight months. It is more likely that the renewed interest in Maurice's safety was prompted by the reported murder of his father in a drug-related shooting incident.

The protective agency by then concluded that Bouknight, in light of her psychological and drug history, could not provide adequate care for Maurice.[73] When Maurice would have been about a year and one half old, the court ordered him removed to foster care. Unfortunately, Maurice was nowhere to be found. Bouknight refused to produce him, saying she feared the state would "'snatch the child.'"[74] Perhaps a reasonable thought, but 18 months too late. The court was concerned that Maurice "was endangered or perhaps dead . . . ."[75] The answer to these concerns has never been provided.

The court found Bouknight in contempt for failure to produce Maurice and she was imprisoned.[76] The issue was Bouknight's Fifth Amendment right not to incriminate herself.[77] It was midway through the academic oral argument on the adult issue when Chief Justice Rehnquist interjected into the case, the children's issue: "Could not reasonable people see what was happening to Maurice here?"[78] The answer is, "Of course they could. Why are we looking at this case in hindsight?"[79] Because Maurice was still a quasi-chattel, he had no constitutional right to protection. His birth-mother has rights akin to ownership. And when danger, or even death, is visible to the naked eye of reasonable people, a national policy of family-adult rights is set in motion without balancing protective rights for children. This inequity hardly reaches the theoretical goal of our system, i.e., justice for all.

Recently, the American Bar Association Center on Children and the Law drafted a model family preservation code which is designed to further our failing national policy. Well-intentioned and competent authors Howard Davidson and Mark Hardin have, in 179 pages, revealed in writing what the nation has been doing in practice to gamble the lives of children in the adult game of chance.

This unpublished work is the penultimate vehicle for judicially approved child abuse. This proposed code creates not only unrealistic, but nearly impossible, barriers for trial judges to overcome to save a child. The only parents *not* allowed to keep their children in zones of danger under this proposal would be dead ones.

The ABA *Children and the Law* proposal utilizes in its commentary essentially this well-worn syllogism:

1. Children need a loving and protective environment to thrive.

2. Families provide such a loving and protective environment.

3. Therefore, we must expend efforts to preserve families.

The proposers cite as authority for the syllogism the works of Joseph Goldstein, Albert Solnit, and Anna Freud.[80] It is hard to quibble with the logic on its face. It is only when we realize that the efforts to be expended to preserve the adult's version of family exceed the heroic, and near the impossible, that we see the existing dangers to virtually unprotected children.

Anna Freud herself worried about how realistic this syllogism was back in 1978! The following is an excerpt from a letter she wrote to Goldstein and Solnit on the issue.

> *This brings me to a worry about our new book
> which I have had all the time, and which I can never
> express convincingly enough for you and Al Solnit. In
> your endeavor to protect the family from unwarranted
> intrusion, you and the book have built up a picture of
> family life and its benefits which many people will
> feel to be quite unrealistic nowadays, and this
> criticism may well interfere with an appreciation of
> the book.*

It is true that we make two important points:

1. That only the intact family can really fulfill all the child's developmental needs. But in extension of this, do we also make it clear enough that we realize how many families fail in this respect? And that every year, fewer and fewer come up to the ideal pattern which we describe?

2. I do not ignore the fact that we say in one paragraph that the very complexity of parental duties causes failure in many cases, but it seems to me that this paragraph is too short in comparison with all the paragraphs in praise of the family. In short, I don't know what the right balance is that we should strike, but my feeling is that we have not achieved it yet.[81]

The right balance was not struck when the letter was written nor in the tragic 13 years since.

The status of children as constitutional outsiders is not limited to the abuse situations described herein. The exclusion of children from constitutional protection is evident in other areas, such as education, health, and even the courtroom process itself. All such deficiencies are the inheritance of our legal history.

It is hardly a novel idea in the world to include protections for children in national constitutions.[82] Unlike America, the constitutions of 79 nations at least mention children. Every new idea has to start with words reduced to writing. The National Task Force for Children's Constitutional Rights has done this. This idea is not presented as a final, unchangeable, document of perfect content and draftsmanship. It is presented as a starting point only. An agenda to initiate discussion, constructive criticism, and even unconstructive criticism. The language of section one is no more than a description of the basic needs of children as generally agreed upon by reasonable people. Sections two through four are an attempt to equalize the child in the courtroom and to put a child's developmental needs in a position of understanding and respect in the adult arena.

Read this not with cynical eyes of the lawyer, but with the eyes of a child. Your eyes as a child in need, or those of your child.

This is the amendment that is proposed for discussion and dialogue on the American agenda as we approach the year 2000 A.D.:

Section 1

All citizens of the United States who are 15 years of age or younger shall enjoy the right to live in a home that is safe and healthy; the right to adequate health care; the right to an adequate education; and the right to the care of a loving family or a substitute thereof, which approximates as closely as possible such family.

Section 2

*All citizens of the United States who are 15 years
of age or younger shall be allowed to testify in any
legal proceeding without having to view any person
accused of abusing said citizen, notwithstanding any
other provision of this Constitution.*

Section 3

*All citizens of the United States who are 15 years
of age or younger shall enjoy the right in any legal
proceeding to have the trier receive evidence as to such
citizen's developmental level as it pertains to that
citizen's credibility.*

Section 4

*All citizens of the United States who are 15 years
of age or younger shall enjoy the right to counsel in
any legal proceeding that effects that citizen's
interests.*[83]

Law students, lawyers, and most law professors may find this proposal difficult to deal with. To some degree, law training is designed to be an expansion of our society's ability to have learned and creative people mold and shape the law for society's benefit. Lawyers, building primarily upon "bricks" laid by others, artfully expand and contract the law to comport with the needs of their clients. The law library provides the source of the bricks and the appellate courts the parameters of their use.

The ultimate arbitrator of any new legal architecture is the then sitting United States Supreme Court. Serious societal concerns, such as the protection of children, have been presented to that body. The Court's decisions, whether based on precedent, personal philosophy, theological belief, or political nose-counting will provide no relief for children this century. The present Court's reticence to expand individual rights is the first reason why this suggested amendment creates difficulty for the legal profession. There are no bricks! Such a decision would extend beyond accepted parameters.

Practically all of the legal people who read this suggested amendment first focus their eyes on the phrase "a loving family." Their lawyer's training sends "does not compute" messages to their legal brains. How does one enforce a right to be in a loving family? How do we define love? (It always brings a smile to this writer's face when his profession has difficulty dealing with an "abstraction" such as "love" but has no difficulty dealing with a "scintilla of evidence," "probable cause," "reasonable doubt," "fundamental fairness," and a "fair preponderance of evidence.")

It may well be that a final amendment would exclude the word "love." It is fascinating to watch law colleagues squirm at the concept of that term which other professions have no difficulty evaluating. This mysterious and indefinable term is promised by adults at the time of their marriage contract, used to describe their acts of sexual intimacy, sworn to exist for their children in custody proceedings and recited as being absent in their divorce hearings. Scientifically, we know babies die without it and adults die for it. My legal colleagues will also be disturbed by section four of the suggested amendment, which provides for legal counsel for children. Imagine! A quasi-chattel having the right to counsel in any legal proceeding that effects that "helpless" child-citizen's interests! Outlandish!

Or is it? Do we not provide counsel or representation for a "helpless" adult in any legal proceeding affecting the adult's interest? Does not modern society provide protection rights for adults who are retarded, mentally ill, or so disabled as to be helpless?

Sections two and three give rise to "adult" concerns over "adult" trials of "adults." Adults can see no farther than their Bill of Rights of 1791. Even the drafters of the Constitution knew it was imperfect and expected change. They provided for two amending processes within the Constitution itself.[84]

In 1991, some adults may feel that justice for an adult accused in a criminal case includes the right to force a 5-year-old child witness to look the adult defendant straight in the eye. All capable adults can easily avoid such a process. Some adults feel this is just. Others feel that, based upon our depth of modern knowledge of child development, it is court-sanctioned child abuse.

Some may feel that section three works an injustice to adults while providing justice to children. Would a judge or jury more likely reach an unjust result by having access to information that facilitates the fact-finding process?

Would evidence as to a child's development level help or harm a jury trying to determine credibility? Is it fair to say that the jurors' present ignorance of the child witnesses' developmental level has produced unjust verdicts? Has juror ignorance in this area helped in the search for truth that we claim is the goal of the American trial?

Ignorance of developmental and cultural norms has led many a good jurist astray. One colleague of this writer was always able to "size up" youthful offenders of a certain ethnic group who appeared before him. He noted how they were afraid to look him in the eye. One wonders how many children suffered incarceration or were not believed by this judge. He did not realize that young men of that culture were trained not to look an older man in the eyes, because it would be disrespectful.

According to Professor Phillip Alston, other countries of the world have given children the following rights in constitutional form:

> 1. *The right to health care.*
>
> 2. *The right to protection.*
>
> 3. *The right to education.*
>
> 4. *The right not to be exploited.*
>
> 5. *The right of "special consideration in judicial and administrative procedures . . . ."*[85]

The proposed amendment intentionally creates exclusions. It does not protect fetuses. The amendment's proponents certainly do not intend to confer these rights on children, only to have them delayed or defeated by the national "fetus rights" battles. Supporters of the proposed amendment have diverse positions on the fetus issue. They have chosen to shelve these positions in this effort so as not to deny protections to those who have been born and who are now suffering.

The proposed amendment defines a citizen, as does the Constitution, as a person *born* in the United States. The proposed amendment likewise excludes children ages 16 and 17. It is fully realized that children of those ages have special needs also, and are often found in dire circumstances "slipping through the cracks." ([The]

16- and 17-year-olds can be the Achilles heel of this movement.) The example of a 17-year-old drug dealer, in a BMW surrounded by money and possessions, who cries for protection under this proposed amendment in a courtroom would surely insure the defeat of the amendment for those children who clearly need it—the proposal's "Willie Horton" if you will.

Discussions of this proposed amendment invariably lead to a comparison to the Equal Rights Amendment (ERA). Some immediately rush to the conclusion that "equal rights" for children are sought here. Obviously, such is not the case. The rights here, like the needs, are special. They fulfill those basic needs of children and protect them from adults and adult courtroom procedures.

The proposal does not ask, for example, that 4-year-old children have the right not to incriminate themselves. It does ask that these children have the right to avoid people or circumstances that constitute dangers to them at home or in a courtroom.

Pessimists observed that the ERA was defeated, and, if voting adult females cannot prevail, how can voteless children? Did the ERA fail? Were the efforts toward it unsuccessful? Technically, the ERA was defeated. But it was also successful. In the wake of these ERA battles much was won and realized for the adult American female. Nearly half of our states have enacted an equal rights amendment. Nearly all state legislatures have passed legislation that alters the status of women. Nearly all courts have made efforts to become sensitized to women's issues. Private industry, the professions, and even government itself have changed policies and procedures, written and unwritten, that effect women positively. Although there is perhaps much more to be done for the status of the adult female in America, the ERA movement was by no means unsuccessful.

The success of the last great movement in America, the women's movement, should be a model for the "Next Great Movement in America,"[86] the Children's Rights Movement. The women's success occurred when they shared a single banner, a unified goal, an agreed-upon focal point. Unfortunately for children, the children's rights movement is splintered into thousands of largely ineffective shards of interests. Older established children's groups suffer "hardening of the arteries" with clear symptoms of terminal complacency. They search for crumbs from the federal table in a style some colleagues call "disjointed incrementalism." They see modest legislative achievements as "breakthroughs" and crow about tomorrow's increments at each annual meeting. Other smaller groups have set their sights on only a narrow facet of the total child-rights dilemma. Some focus on spanking, denial of health care to children whose parent's religions disdain modern medicine, or on creating support groups for the identified casualties.

All of these forces have done little to meet our "national emergency." And such will be the case until they all gather behind a single banner. Until enough bodies and groups speak with a single, powerful, and politically intimidating voice for children, the status of children will not change.

The point where all groups believe, unite, and demand action will be when they reach what Jim Lardie, Executive Director of the Association of Child Advocates, calls the "critical mass," i.e., the gathering of enough bright and angry children advocates.

This may well be happening. In January of 1991, the groundwork for the National Committee for the Rights of the Child was laid in Washington, D.C. Dozens of national groups, old and new, met to initiate "The Next Great Movement in America." If successful, it would be Jim Lardie's "critical mass," for these organizations represent literally millions of Americans.

The litmus test for all social changes in America these days seems to be based on the politics of those who propose the changes. But before we engage our adult political baggage, whether the proposal to give American children protective constitutional rights is one that must immediately give rise to a liberal versus conservative position, or pro-family—anti-family platforms, the Republicans versus Democratic concerns or right wing versus left wing . . . stop! Stop. We must not embroil American children in the unproductive morass of those wars. Let us put our adult philosophical baggage on the shelf, for the children's sake. If Americans cannot reach a consensus on the Joshua DeShaneys of the nation, then there never will be a consensus, and there will always be Joshua DeShaneys.

Looked at through the eyes of children and open-minded adults, the creation of constitutional protections for children is hardly a radical idea in 1991—certainly not in the eyes of the American

Academy of Child and Adolescent Psychiatry, church leaders, and other professionals who have endorsed it. And certainly not in the mind of the great American whose signature is affixed to the following:

> For every child a home and that love and security which a home provides: and for that child who must receive foster care, the nearest substitute for his own home. For every child a school which is safe . . . and properly equipped. For younger children nursery schools and kindergartens to supplement home care.

> For every child an education which, through the discovery and development of his individual abilities, prepares him for life; and through training and vocational guidance prepares him for a living which will yield him the maximum of satisfaction.

> For every child who is blind, deaf, or otherwise physically handicapped, and for the child who is mentally handicapped, such measures as will early discover and diagnose his handicap, provide care and treatment, and so train him that he may become an asset to society rather than a liability. *Expenses of these services should be born publicly where they cannot be privately met.*

> For every child protection from abuse, neglect, exploitation or moral hazard.

> *For every child these rights, regardless of race, or color, or situation, wherever he may live under the protection of the American flag.*[87]

The signature affixed to this work was that of President Herbert Hoover, the year, 1930. The occasion, the White House Conference of Children.

Is this really not an idea whose time has come . . . again? In President Hoover's words:

> *Let no one believe that these are questions which*
> *should not stir a nation: That they are below the*
> *dignity of statesmen or governments. If we could have*
> *but one generation of properly born, trained, educated,*

> *and healthy children, a thousand other problems of*
> *government would vanish.*[88]

It is unlikely that problems will vanish until children's rights appear. Any group that proposes a substantial change in the status quo must be ready to present concrete advantages to the change. A "No One Knows" position will not do. The proposed amendment initially entitles American children to receive that which all reasonable people believe to be their basic needs: health care, education, safety, and a nurturing environment seem beyond dispute.

Once entitled, the satisfaction of these needs is not obtained from the bended knee of the child advocate at a legislative hearing. The legislature would be no longer able to choose which bone is thrown to the child, along with the highway department, the state police, and the university basketball team. The child advocates can leave their well-worn knees and demand that government provide for these needs where parents cannot, or will not, provide.

The proposed amendment is merely to initiate dialogue. It is offered for concept rather than legislative detail. Does the reader agree that American children should be protected? Are these protections and entitlements generally palatable? If so, let the dialogue begin. Let the drafters, the word mechanics, the debaters, and the philosophers loose their weapons and skills. In doing so, let them remember that the adult protective rights are already in the repository of the United States Constitution. Let them remember that speculation and flyspecking did not prevent the passage of the adult Bill of Rights. For example, speculation as to whether yelling "fire" in a crowded theater or burning the flag constitutes free speech was not an impediment to the adoption of the First Amendment.

What might have happened to certain children had they had these constitutional protections a decade ago? The answer is that virtually every case we know by its infamy could have had a different outcome. Joshua DeShaney, instead of lying in an institution being fed, changed, and nursed 24 hours a day, would be in seventh grade. He might be studying introductory algebra, social science and reading adventure stories. He might be playing soccer after school and worrying about his first girl-boy party. If Joshua had had a constitutional right to safety and a right to a lawyer when his safety was being decided in the court and in the hospital, he might never have been the victim of the final assault from his criminal birth-parent.

The real point of protection is not the ability to maintain a tort action *after* the assault or for the perpetrator to be successfully prosecuted *thereafter*. The real protections [are] to prevent the child from being in the zone of danger to begin with, or removing him from it forthwith.

Maurice M., instead of being missing or dead, would be in a preschool program prior to entering kindergarten this fall. He would be learning colors and letters. He would be making treasures for his new mom and dad out of string, cardboard, and glue. He would be tucked in a clean, warm bed at night and be whispered a "good night, I love you" before sleeping.

Maurice with protective constitutional rights would face no more than a broken femur and a spica cast before his rights to safety would be triggered. He would not have to wait for a birth parent to detox, medicate, or be educated. Children do not have a lot of time to be children. In Maurice's case, he had none at all.

Hillary Morgan, instead of spending nearly two years in a foreign country with relatives who were virtual strangers, may have been at home with a loving and protective birth-parent during those crucial developmental years of her life.

The judge, entitled, of course, to vindicate the authority of his court by finding contempt on the part of Hillary's mother, would have been forced to factor Hillary's right to live in a loving environment with her family in the equation. She might not have lost those crucial years.

Robyn Twitchell, the 2-year-old Massachusetts boy who died of a bowel obstruction, would be alive if he had had the right to live in safety and the right to health care. The religious rights of his parents to follow their Christian Science beliefs and pray for Robyn's healing would remain intact. But Robyn would not have had to die or endure five days of excruciating abdominal pain and the vomiting of his own fecal matter if he had a constitutional right equal to that of his parents. Instead of his death and his parents' conviction for manslaughter, we would have a healthy, happy, and free family. The list goes on: Lisa Steinberg, Baby M., Bradley McGee.

Modern science amplifies the need for protective rights. The case of Baby Calvert in California makes the point. There the fertilized egg of one woman was implanted in the womb of another woman. When the baby was born, the birth-parent did not wish to surrender the child to the genetic-parents as agreed (the "natural" parents?). The question for the court was, "Who owns the chattel, the baby?"

The judge was on the horns of a dilemma. He had an onerous decision to make as to the temporary custody of the infant while the "ownership" issue was decided. The birth-mother, capable of breast feeding the infant, pleaded for the child of her womb. The genetic-mother, treating the birth-mother as a human warehouse-bailee, demanded possession of the chattel originated by her genes and those of her husband.

In a scene from the Old Testament, the judge attempted to act like Solomon. He did not threaten to slice the baby in half to learn who the real mother was. Instead, he used the modern equivalent. He ordered the child separated from both parties and placed in foster care. The birth-mother then relented and allowed the genetic mother to take temporary custody.

The judge was alleged to have said that the foster care option was to insure that neither mother "had a bonding advantage." The adults were ready to sacrifice that baby's bonding needs while their owner-ship rights were litigated! The foster care option would not have been such a ready alternative if the child had had constitutional rights to be considered. A final legal decision on "ownership" could not be postponed for the first two years of the baby's life if it had certain constitutional rights. Recently, the federal administration has considered two constitutional amendments. The first would give a fetus the right to be born. The second would give the symbol of America's promise to provide justice for all, the American flag, constitutional protection. Is it not logical to ask protection for these American children who have been born under the American flag?

Protections have recently been extended to children internation-ally. On November 20, 1989, the United Nations (UN) unanimously adopted the UN Convention on the Rights of the Child:

> *Whatever the reason for the final form of the convention on the rights of the child, it is, indeed, a Magna Charta for children. It does not matter that it was drafted without reference to a comprehensive theory of children's rights. Now that it exists, it creates a theory of its own, a theory which upholds the right of the individual child to dignity and respect.*[89]

This Magna Charta provides for a number of rights, some of which mirror the proposed amendment. Some relevant provisions are presented here:

Article 2

1. States Parties shall respect and ensure the rights set forth in the present Convention to each child within their jurisdiction *without discrimination of any kind, irrespective of the child's or his or her parent's or legal guardian's race, sex, language, religion, political or other opinion, national, ethnic or social origin, property, disability, birth or other status.*

Article 3

1. In all actions concerning children, *whether undertaken by public or private social welfare institutions, courts of law, administrative authorities or legislative bodies,* the best interests of the child shall be a primary consideration.

2. States Parties undertake to ensure the child such protection and care as is necessary for his or her well-being, *taking into account the rights and duties of his or her parents, legal guardians or other individuals legally responsible for him or her, and, to this end, shall take all appropriate legislative and administrative measures.*

3. States Parties shall ensure that the institutions, services and facilities responsible for the care or protection of children shall conform with the standards established by competent authorities, particularly in the area of safety, health, in the number and suitability of their staff as well as competent supervision.

Article 4

States Parties shall undertake all appropriate legislative, *administrative, and other* measures for the implementation of the rights recognized in this Convention. *In regard to economic, social and cultural rights, States Parties shall undertake such measures to the maximum extent of their available resources and, where needed, within the framework of international cooperation.*

Article 12

1. States Parties shall assure to the child who is capable of forming his or her own views the right to express those views freely in all matters affecting the child, the views of the child being given due weight in accordance with the age and maturity of the child.

2. For this purpose, the child shall in particular be provided the opportunity to be heard in any judicial and administrative proceedings affecting the child, either directly, or through a representative *or an appropriate body,* in a manner consistent with the procedural rule of national law.

Article 19

1. States Parties shall take all appropriate legislative, *administrative, social and educational* measures to protect the child from all forms of physical or mental violence, injury or abuse, neglect or negligent treatment, maltreatment or exploitation including sexual abuse, while in the care of parent(s), legal guardian(s) or any other person who has the care of the child.

2. Such protective measures should, as appropriate, include effective procedures for the establishment of social programmes to provide necessary support for the child as well as for other forms of prevention and for identification, reporting, referral, investigation, treatment and follow-up of instances of child maltreat-

ment described heretofore, and, as appropriate, for judicial involvement.

Article 20

1. A child temporarily or permanently deprived of his or her family environment, or in whose own best interests cannot be allowed to remain in that environment, shall be entitled to special protection and assistance provided by the State.

Article 23

1. States Parties recognize that a mentally or physically disabled child should enjoy a full and decent life, in conditions which ensure dignity, promote self-reliance and facilitate the child's active participation in the community.

2. States Parties recognize the right of the disabled child to special care and shall encourage and ensure the extension, subject to available resources, to the eligible child and those responsible for his or her care, of assistance for which application is made and which is appropriate to the child's condition and to the circumstances of the parents or others caring for the child.

3. Recognizing the special needs of a disabled child, assistance extended in accordance with paragraph 2 shall be provided free of charge, whenever possible, taking into account the financial resources of the parents or others caring for the child, and shall be designed to ensure that the disabled child has effective access to and receives education, training, health care services, rehabilitation services, preparation for employment and recreation opportunities in a manner conducive to the child's achieving the fullest possible social integration and individual development, including his or her cultural and spiritual development.

Article 24

1. States Parties recognize the right of the child to the enjoyment of the highest attainable standard of health and to facilities for the treat-

ment of illness and rehabilitation of health. The States Parties shall strive to ensure that no child is deprived of his or her right of access to such health care services.

Article 27

1. States Parties recognize the right of every child to a standard of living adequate for the child's physical, mental, spiritual, moral and social development.

2. The parent(s) or others responsible for the child have the primary responsibility to secure, within their abilities and financial capacities, the conditions of living necessary for the child's development.

3. States Parties in accordance with national conditions and within their means shall take appropriate measures to assist parents and others responsible for the child to implement this right and shall in case of need provide material assistance and support programmes, particularly with regard to nutrition, clothing and housing.

Article 28

1. States Parties recognize the right of the child to education, *and with a view to achieving this right progressively and on the basis of equal opportunity, they shall, in particular:*

(a) Make primary education compulsory and available free to all;

(b) Encourage the development of different forms of secondary education, including general and vocational education, make them available and accessible to every child, and take appropriate measures such as the introduction of free education and offering financial assistance in case of need;

(c) Make higher education accessible to all on basis of capacity by every appropriate means;

(d) Make educational and vocational information and guidance available and accessible to all children;

(e) Take measures to encourage regular attendance at schools and the reduction of drop-out rates.

Article 32

1. States Parties recognize the right of the child to be protected from economic exploitation and from performing any work that is likely to be hazardous or to interfere with the child's education, or to be harmful to the child's health or physical, mental, spiritual, moral or social development.

Article 33

States Parties shall take all appropriate measures, *including legislative, administrative, social and educational measures,* to protect children from the illicit use of narcotic drugs and psychotropic substances *as defined in the relevant international treaties,* and to prevent the use of children in the illicit production and trafficking of such substances.

Article 34

States Parties undertake to protect the child from all forms of sexual exploitation and sexual abuse. *For these purposes,* States Parties shall in particular take all appropriate national, *bilateral and multilateral* measures to prevent:

(a) The inducement or coercion of a child to engage in any unlawful sexual activity;

(b) The exploitative use of children in prostitution or other unlawful sexual practices;

(c) The exploitative use of children in pornographic performances and materials.

Article 40

1. States Parties recognize the right of every child alleged as, accused of, *or recognized as* having

> infringed the penal law to be treated *in a manner*
> *consistent with the promotion of the child's sense of*
> *dignity and worth, which reinforces the child's respect*
> *for the human rights and fundamental freedoms of*
> *others* and which takes into account the child's age
> and the *desirability of promoting the child's re-*
> *integration and the child's assuming a constructive role*
> *in society.*[90]

This Convention went into force as international law on September 2, 1990, when it was ratified by the twentieth nation.[91] Approximately 70 nations have now ratified the Convention thus becoming legally bound by its standards. Another 70 nations have indicated their intent to ratify it.

The notable holdouts are Iran, Iraq, Libya, South Africa, and the United States of America. Since we are "known by the company we keep," our administration has raised several strawmen as impediments. All of these impediments can be resolved by merely taking reservations and thus allowing American children to be brought into the twenty-first century in the safety of the majority of the Convention provisions.[92]

It is supremely ironic that American children now, theoretically, have more protective rights under international law than they have here in the land of the free, home of the brave.

The Convention is a remarkable document. It tells us that a "worldwide consensus has emerged that children are indeed persons, that they are entitled a fortiori to respect and protection, and that nation-states should ensure the fulfillment of such rights with the force of law."[93]

There are those who believe that the United States Supreme Court has fully declared children to be persons. These beliefs were shaken when that Court allowed unadjudicated juveniles to be detained in a locked facility because "[j]uveniles, unlike adults, are always in some form of custody."[94]

The Convention makes a total break from previous approaches to children's rights. Previous "rights" were paternalistic, whereas the Convention makes the state directly responsible to the child. The pervading themes of the Convention are the dignity of the child and the individual child's best interests.

> *This is true even when the child's interest may come into conflict with the rights of parents. The child has a right to be brought up by his or her parents, but he or she also has the right to be placed in an alternative family setting should this be necessary. The child has a right to be protected from all types of abuse, including that which occurs within the family unit. Under the Convention, the rights of the individual child are paramount.[95]*

The Convention also requires that nations ratifying it shall have 2 years and 30 days from ratification to submit the extent of their acts of compliance. Presuming eventual ratification, ways must be sought in which to implement its proposals.

Do we need state by state legislation? Do we need federal legislation? Or shall children's rights be placed alongside the adult's rights in the Constitution? Professor Alston suggests that in lieu of a specific, constitutional amendment as is suggested here, a simple constitutional amendment such as the following may be sufficient: "Children shall enjoy the protection provided in international agreements which safeguard their rights."[96]

> *Children's rights are now the central issue in the human rights movement. Child rearing at home, in school, and in the community will determine both the course of society, nationally and internationally, and the dignity accorded all persons. During the last few hundred years, children have progressed through property and potential person status, with protection and nurturance rights, to partial personal status, with some self-determination rights. Public opinion, policies, and laws are converging in support of assuring self-determination rights for children to validate their person status.[97]*

This essay began with the Declaration of Independence. Perhaps it should conclude with a contemporary reference to it.

> *The Constitution was indeed a fulfillment of the promises of the Declaration of 1776. But that it did not go as far as the Declaration of Independence was shown when, in 1857, the Supreme Court decided that Dred Scott could not be a citizen because he was black and when, in 1896, it held that a state could require blacks to ride in separate railways cars so long as the cars were equal to those for white passengers. In 1954, the court struck down the idea that "separate" could be equal. Even today, we must change many attitudes and practices before we can say the promises of 1776 have really been fulfilled.*[98]

NOTES

1. Declaration of Independence (U.S. 1776).

2. *See* Dred Scott v. Sandford, 60 U.S. (19 How.) 393, 476 (1856).

3. De Mause, *The Evolution of Childhood*, in *The History of Childhood* 1 (L. de Mause ed. 1974).

4. Cohen, *Relationships Between the Child, the Family, and the State*, in *Perspectives on the Family* 293 (M. Bayles, R. Moffat, & J. Greie eds. 1990).

5. For a historical analysis of the maltreatment of children, see Pappas, *Law and the Status of the Child*, 13 *Colum. Hum. Rts. L. Rev.* XXV, XXVII-XXVIII (1981–82).

6. L. Stone, *The Family, Sex and Marriage in England 1500–1800* 409–11 (1977).

7. R. Bayne-Powell, *The English Child in the Eighteenth Century* 1 (1939).

8. Hart, *From Property to Person Status: Historical Perspective on Children's Rights*, 46 *Am. Psychologist* 53, 53 (Jan. 1991) [hereinafter *Historical Perspective*].

9. The case of Mary Ellen Wilson was not a case which reached the courts. This case, however, has been reported and discussed extensively throughout literature pertaining to children's rights. *See generally* Zigler & Hall, *Physical Child Abuse in America: Past, Present and Future* in *America: Past, Present and Future* 38–75 (D. Cicchetti & Z. Carlson eds. 1989).

10. *Id.*

11. Even to this day, American activism seems more directed to animal rights rather than children's. America is more likely to have dolphin-free tuna than drug-free children.

12. *Historical Perspective, supra* note 8, at 53.

13. *Id.*

14. The only known group in America which advocates for constitutional protection for children is the National Task Force for Children's Constitutional Rights, Inc. This is a multidisciplinary organization founded at the University of Pennsylvania in 1988.

15. *See generally Historical Perspective, supra* note 8, at 53–58.

16. *Id.*

17. *Id.*

18. *Id.* at 54.

19. *In re* Gault, 387 U.S. 1, 17 (1967).

20. A. Platt, *The Child Savers: The Invention of Delinquency* 9–14 (1969).

21. *See* Hammer v. Dagenhart, 247 U.S. 251 (1918), which provides an example of the tensions surrounding the move to stop child labor. *See also* R. Mnookin, *Child, Family and State* 646–68 (1978).

22. 347 U.S. 483 (1954).

23. *Id.*

24. 387 U.S. 1 (1967). 25. *Id.* at 12–16. Some scholars, such as Professor Joseph Goldstein of the Yale Law School, suggest in conversation that even these due process protections were urged by and possessed by the parents and not necessarily the children.

26. 406 U.S. 205 (1972).

27. *Id.* at 245. (Douglas, J., dissenting in part). One slight break from the mold is the apparent retreat from the old doctrine of interfamily tort immunity which prevented a child from suing a parent for tortious conduct. *See, e.g.,* Colter v. White, 20 Wis. 2d 402, 122 N.W.2d 193 (1963).

28. *See* J. Goldstein, A. Freud, & A. Solnit, *Beyond the Best Interest of the Child* (1979); Kempe, Silverman, Steele, Droegemuller, & Silver, *The Battered-Child Syndrome*, 17 *J. Am. Med. Ass'n* 181 (1962).

29. Testimony by John Fitzgerald, Ph.D., in Waterbury Superior Court (1984) appearing before Judge Gill.

30. Marian Wright Edelman, Children's Defense Fund (television interview, Sept. 1990).

31. The Committee for Economic Development is composed of 250 of the nation's top corporate executives and university presidents.

32. Statement of Marlin Fitzwater, Presidential Press Secretary.

33. These statistics were prepared by federal and state agencies and reported in the media. A specific source is available by writing the National Task Force for Children's Constitutional Rights, Suite 602, 952 Main Street, Hartford, CT 06103.

34. *Id.*

35. These statistics were obtained in 1989 from Saint Francis Hospital and Medical Center, Hartford, Connecticut.

36. *Id.*

37. A decade ago, in the Litchfield, Connecticut Superior Court, it was rare for a prospective juror to request excusal in a sexual abuse case because of a similar experience. Presently, one-third of prospective jurors reveal that they, or someone close to them, has been the victim of sexual abuse.

38. Hartman, *Children in a Careless Society*, 35 *Social Work* 483, 483 (1990).

39. J. Goldstein, realizing the delicacy between state intervention into family matters has stated:

> *We had to remind ourselves that neither law, nor medicine, nor science has magical powers and that there is no societal consensus about what is "best" or even "good" for all children. More than that, we had to address the tension between the fear of encouraging the state to violate a family's integrity before intervention is justified and the fear of inhibiting the state until it may be too late to protect the child whose well-being is threatened.*

Goldstein, *Anna Freud*, 92 *Yale L.J.* 219, 226 (1982).

40. *The Hartford Courant*, Jan. 30, 1991 at A3.

41. *Child Abuse and Neglect: Critical First Steps in Response to a National Emergency* VII (Aug. 1990) (for copies contact: U.S. Government Printing Office, Superintendent of Documents, Washington, D.C. 20401 No: 017-092-00104-5 $7.50). This board was established under the provisions of the 1988 Amendments to the Child Abuse Prevention and Treatment Act and operates under the aegis of the United States Department of Health and Human Services.

42. *Id.* (emphasis added).

43. *Id.* at X.

44. *Id.* at VIII.

45. *Id.* at VII.

46. The story was told at a speech given by Dr. Weiner upon the installation of the American Academy of Child and Adolescent Psychiatry (1987).

47. It has been this writer's experience that, when lawyers become parties to litigation, objectivity is quickly replaced by the highest degree of unleashed emotions.

48. Hartman, *supra* note 38, at 484.

49. Jellinek, Murphy, Bishop, Poitrast, & Quinn, *Protecting Severely Abused and Neglected Children—An Unkept Promise*, 323 New Eng. J. Med. 1629 (1980) [hereinafter *An Unkept Promise*].

50. *Id.*

51. *Id.*

52. Murphy, Jellinek, Quinn, Smith, Poitrast, & Goshko, *Substance Abuse and Serious Child Mistreatment: Prevalence, Risk and Outcome in a Court Sample, J. Child Abuse Negl.* (in press); Taylor, Norman, & Murphy, *Diagnosed Mutual and Emotional Impairment Among Parents Who Seriously Mistreat Their Children: Incidence, Type, and Outcome in the Court Sample, J. Child Abuse Negl.* (in press).

53. According to the study, prevalence rates of 33, 50, and 80% have been reported in Florida, Massachusetts, and Washington D.C., respectively. *United States House of Representatives Select Committee on Children, Youth, and Families, 101st Cong. 1st Sess., No Place To Call Home: Discarded Children in America* (Gov't Print. Office 1989).

54. *Id.*

55. 489 U.S. 189 (1979).

56. *Id.* at 201.

57. *Id.* at 191.

58. 768 F.2d 503, 510–11 (3d Cir. 1985).

59. *Id. See* Jenson v. Conrad, 747 F.2d 185, 190–94 (4th Cir. 1984), *cert. denied* 470 U.S. 1052 (1985).

60. *See* Estelle v. Gamble, 429 U.S. 97 (1976) (holding that an *adult* prisoner is entitled to adequate medical care); *See also* Youngberg v. Romeo, 457 U.S. 307 (1982) (holding *adult* mental patients have a right to such services as are necessary to ensure their reasonable safety, as well as shelter and medical care).

61. *DeShaney*, 489 U.S. at 201 (Rehnquist, C.J.).

62. *Id.* at 202–03.

63. *Id.* at 212–13 (Blackmun, J., dissenting).

64. Baltimore Soc. Serv. v. Bouknight, 110 S. Ct. 900 (1990). States have a custom of concealing the last name of a child in judicial proceedings. The rationale is ostensibly that it protects the child's identity and privacy. In this case, the state protected his last name but not his life. *See id.*

65. *Id.* at 903.

66. *Id.*

67. *Id.*

68. *Id.*

69. *Id.*

70. *Id.* The record does not disclose whether he was still wearing his spica cast at the time.

71. *Id.*

72. *Id.*

73. *Id.*

74. *Id.* at 904.

75. *Id.*

76. *Id.*

77. *Id.*

78. *Id.* (statement by Chief Justice Rehnquist during oral argument).

79. *Id.*

80. *See* J. Goldstein, A. Freud, & A. Solnit, *supra* note 28.

81. Goldstein, *Anna Freud,* 92 *Yale L.J.* 219, 225–26 (1982) (quoting letter from Anna Freud to Joseph Goldstein (Nov. 13, 1978).

82. P. Alston, *Background Note on Children's Rights and National Constitutions* (Dec. 1990) (unpublished manuscript) (the author is professor and director for the Center for Advanced Legal Studies at the Australian National University, Canberra, Australia). Alston states:

> *At present, there are at least 79 national constitutions containing provisions dealing explicitly with the rights of children. These range from comprehensive and detailed provisions, such as those found in the Brazilian Constitution of 1988, to the very brief and narrowly focused provisions such as that contained in*

> *the 1946 Constitution of Japan which provides that*
> *"children shall not be exploited." [sic] To some*
> *extent, these differences might reflect factors such as*
> *the age of the constitution (the more recent the*
> *constitution, the more detailed the provisions), and*
> *the assumption that children are adequately covered*
> *by provisions applicable to all citizens.*

Id. at 6. 83. These sections were proposed by the National Task Force for Children's Constitutional Rights.

84. *See U.S. Const.* art. V.

85. P. Alston, *supra* note 82, at 8.

86. This was the slogan of the annual meeting of the Child Advocate Association held in San Francisco in October 1990.

87. W. Myers & W. Newton, *The Hoover Administration, A Documented Narrative*, 458–61 (1936) (emphasis added).

88. *Id.* at 456–57.

89. Cohen, *supra* note 4, at 308.

90. *Id.* at 319–35.

91. *Id.*

92. The American concerns are fetal rights and the desire to have teenagers subject to the death penalty. The latter concern is exclusively American. Through technical arguments, America had the convention allow the conscription of children age fifteen in the armed forces and to participate in combat.

93. Melton, *Socialization in the Global Community, "Respect for the Dignity of Children, "* 46 *Am. Psychologist* at 66–71 (Jan. 1991).

94. Schall v. Martin, 467 U.S. 253, 265 (1984) (quoting Lehman v. Lycoming County Children's Servs., 458 U.S. 502, 510–11 (1982)).

95. Cohen & Naimark, *United Nations Convention on the Rights of the Child: Individual Rights Concepts and Their Significance for Social Scientists*, 46 *Am. Psychologist* 60, 60 (Jan. 1991).

96. Constitucion [Constitution] art. 39 (Spain).

97. *Historical Perspective, supra* note 8, at 57.

98. Buger, *What It Means to Us, Parade*, Jan. 27, 1991 [magazine], at 6.

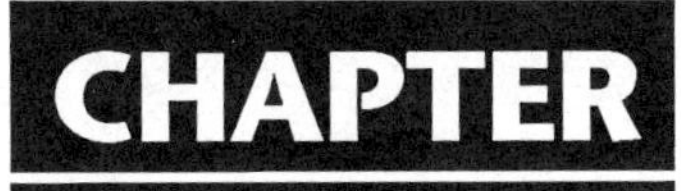

2

Newborn Infant Abductions from Hospitals

Elizabeth Burgess Dowdell
John B. Rabun, Jr.

It is Tuesday morning. A young mother sits with her newborn baby in her room in a secure and well-managed private hospital. A woman dressed as a nurse comes in the room and tells the mother that she is taking the baby to weigh him. The mother hands her baby over, and within minutes, the baby is out of the hospital, abducted by a woman impersonating a nurse.

The abduction of newborn infants from hospitals poses a serious threat to the abducted children, the parents, and the medical facilities involved. There has been a curious rise in the number of newborn infant abductions since 1985, and this problem has had an impact upon the health-care delivery system. Indeed, the abduction of an infant from a facility is a traumatic and stressful event for everyone involved. A multidisciplinary approach in the development of specific health policies is needed to combat effectively this infrequent and highly visible crime. The purpose of this article is to (1) examine various aspects of the problem of infant abduction and (2) discuss preabduction and postabduction health policy issues.

THE PROBLEM OF NEWBORN INFANT ABDUCTION

Scope of the Problem

The National Center for Missing and Exploited Children (NCMEC) (1990) has on record 109 abductions by nonfamily members of newborns and infants since January 1983. Of these 109 babies, 69 were reported as being abducted from hospitals. Of these 69, 65 have been recovered in good health, while 4 remain missing. There were 6 attempted abductions from hospitals also reported during this time period.

Based on a study of NCMEC cases (1989) from 1983 through 1988, the best estimate for the incidence of hospital abductions is between 12 and 18 newborn infants yearly nationwide. Because a number of cases may not be reported to the NCMEC or other organizations, it is believed that this estimate is conservative. Of all the newborn infants abducted from the hospital, 90 % were located and safely returned, usually within a few days to two weeks.

Abductor Profile

Abductions are as unique as the infants being abducted. However, there is a familiar pattern and type of individual who undertakes such abductions. The typical hospital abduction case involves an abductor impersonating a nurse, hospital employee, volunteer, or relative in order to gain access to an infant. The obstetrics ward is, for the most part, an open and inviting one. It can be filled with medical and nursing staff, visitors, students, volunteers, delivery persons, and participants in parenting and newborn care classes. The number of new and changing faces on the floor is high, thus making the ward an area where a stranger is unlikely to be noticed.

In cases of newborn infant abduction, the abductor is almost always a female, generally with no prior criminal record. The motivation in the majority of these cases is the woman's wish to obtain or replace a baby she has lost or desiring a vicarious birthing of a child she is, for some reason, unable to conceive. While the crime is often precipitated by impulse and opportunity, these women demonstrate a capability to care adequately for the abducted baby.

The crimes are not always committed by our stereotypical view of a stranger. In most cases the abductors make themselves known and achieve some degree of familiarity with hospital personnel and even with the victim parents. The abductor may visit the nursery unit for several days in a row before the abduction, repeatedly asking detailed questions about hospital procedures and the layout of the maternity floor. She usually appears pregnant and is thought to be a expectant mother visiting the ward prior to giving birth. Looking pregnant aids the abductor in deflecting suspicion when she brings the abducted infant home. Most abductors have a recent history of miscarriage; however, few disclose this information to a spouse or to family members.

An abductor does not necessarily target a specific baby for abduction. When the opportunity arises, she may immediately snatch an available victim and run. For example, one abductor told police that she went to the hospital seeking employment, not to abduct a baby. But when she saw the baby in a room and he smiled at her, she decided to take him. She went into the room, cut his IV line, placed him in a gym bag that contained some of his clothing, and left the scene (Presseley & Churchville, 1987).

An important difference is evident in the abduction style and technique used in hospital versus nonhospital abductions. Hospital abductors use little or no violence when kidnapping the infant. In contrast, in cases of infants taken by nonhospital abductors, primarily from the infant's home, a high rate of violence is present. Of the 40 nonhospital abduction cases reported to NCMEC from 1983 to 1991, 6 involved killing the mother and 1 involved killing both mother and father (National Center for Missing & Exploited Children, 1991).

Liability Issues

The changing world of health care involves an intricate system in which the influence of the legal discipline has been felt. When an infant is abducted, a number of liability issues immediately are raised by the involved parties. The major issue concerns who is responsible and what legal ramifications are associated with negligence and compensation.

In cases of newborn infant abduction, the hospital is potentially liable on two grounds. The first is based on its general duty to take reasonable care to prevent the occurrence of foreseeable harm to its patients. The hospital would be liable for any physical or psychological harm suffered by the abducted infant.

The second area of liability is based on the hospital's contractual duty to use reasonable care to prevent the occurrence of foreseeable injury to third parties. Thus, the hospital would be liable to the parents for the costs of any searches and for psychological harm. Parental recovery for emotional injury if the child has not been physically harmed depends on state law. Some states find liability if gross negligence exists, regardless of whether physical harm occurred; others require physical harm to have occurred. Some states would find liability only if the parents are direct victims rather than bystanders.

An example of the latter is the case of *Johnson v. Jamaica Hospital* (467 N.Y.S. 2d 634, NY 1983). In this case the parents sued the hospital when their baby was abducted from the newborn nursery and not recovered for over four months. The appellate division of the New York Supreme Court affirmed the trial court's denial of the hospital's motion to dismiss. The appellate court viewed the parents as the direct victims. Therefore, under New York law they were able to recover damages for emotional injury that did not involve physical harm.

In response to two 1987 incidents of newborn infant abduction within weeks of each other at two separate hospitals, the Maryland General Assembly enacted Sections 20-401 and 20-402 of the state health code requiring hospitals to perform identification procedures on newborns (obtaining and retaining umbilical cord blood samples and footprints or using other procedures designated by the secretary of health). These procedures would aid in the positive identification of infants recovered after abduction. If an abduction occurred and the police had difficulty in ascertaining whether a particular child was the abducted one, the failure of the hospital to have followed the statutory procedures might be an additional ground for liability.

Such failure also might be persuasive in showing that the hospital was negligent in allowing the abduction to occur.

The New York case and the annotated Maryland Health Code are significant in view of institutional legal liability. A common early response, after panic, by victim parents is placing blame. Once accusations are made, legal counsel is called in, and negotiations for compensation begin. Most hospitals and administrators dislike this particular interaction and have gone to great lengths to prevent such an event. As a result, they are quick to pay for the maternity stay and the physician's services; additionally, it is not unusual for them to make a cash settlement (Grant, 1990).

REACTIONS TO NEWBORN INFANT ABDUCTION

Parental Reaction

Experiencing the abduction of a newborn infant is intensely traumatic and stressful. The crime can shatter the emotional equilibrium of the parents involved as the event is one of the most devastating things that can happen to new parents.

Victimization has several key cognitive, psychological, and social consequences. These include "social network disruption, family conflicts, new symptoms of fear and phobia, diminished involvement with others, and continual preoccupation with the criminal event" (Rich & Burgess, 1985). The impact of the abduction can manifest itself in feelings of guilt, fear, anxiety, anger, and anguish. Because there is easier access to a patient's room than to the newborn nursery, almost all abductors take the infant directly from the mother's arms (Grant, 1990). Hence, the feelings of guilt experienced by these mothers can be overwhelming. As one victim mother stated, "When it sunk in that my baby had been kidnapped, I felt all at once that my life was over. Having your child stolen from you is like having someone rip your heart out."

The psychological effects on the parents, specifically mothers, are now being studied. Anecdotal reports from victim parents indicate that they maintain high levels of anxiety during the abduction period. Even after the infant is returned, the impact of the event cannot be minimized. Length of abduction also may have an influence. As one mother whose newborn infant was abducted for 36 hours stated after two years had passed, "I will never forget it. She is never out of my sight now. I won't use a babysitter, except my mother. I take her to day care so she can play with other children, but I stay with her, even there."

Infant Reaction

To date, the majority of the recovered infants have suffered no ill effects and have been found in good physical health. The abductors, in fact, have considered the babies to be their own and have treated them as such. The influence of the abduction on these newborn infants as they have grown and matured has not been studied. Given the careful physical care and treatment the infants received while abducted, one can hypothesize that the greatest effect must be the emotional/psychological one. Proceeding further, one can speculate that the influence of the abduction experience is greatest once the infant is returned to the parents. The infant can become the identified target of intense parental anxiety. This focused attention and its duration raise a number of questions: How do these children progress developmentally? Do the children have more phobias than other children? How do they develop a sense of independence and self-esteem? How do they relate to peers? How do the parents react when the children reach milestones (i.e., going to school, reaching adolescence, participating in peer group activities such as sleep-overs, leaving for college, etc.).

Hospital and Staff Reactions

When a newborn infant is abducted, the hospital reacts quickly. The first response is to search the buildings and grounds for the infant. Notification of the police and usually the FBI are the next steps. Often the hospital will use the news media to assist in finding the infant. This technique has proved very effective in locating missing children.

In the 1986 case of the one-day-old infant abducted at Grand View Hospital, in Sellersville, Pennsylvania, the news media was most helpful (Doyle, 1990). When the director of public affairs was notified of the abduction, he immediately called the local police, the county district attorney, and police detectives. His next move was to use the news media to help locate the infant. He kept the story visible primarily by supplying fresh information to the media, and he controlled the flow of information by staying close to the parents and in touch with the law enforcement agencies. Open communication and maximization of resources proved to be the key in this case.

Although the abduction of a newborn infant is unnerving for all hospital staff members, the psychological effects are not well known. The influence upon delivery of care can be hypothesized to be moderate. If the abduction occurred in the nursery, the nursing staff often feel responsible either for giving the infant to the abductor or for not somehow knowing that the abductor was an imposter. A nurse who had one of her primary newborn infants abducted stated that she is "so careful now when releasing infants out of the nursery. I check everything—the mother's ID bracelet, the baby's, what room the mother is in—and compare it to which one she came from. Sometimes I'll even follow them back to her room, just to make sure".

One interesting note is the strong reaction to nonfamily-member abductors by nursing and other medical personnel when compared with family-member abductors. When a family member takes an infant, the response is often, "Well, it could have been a stranger." Security measures are less rigidly applied, typically, in these types of cases by staff members.

HEALTH POLICY IMPLICATIONS

Reducing the risk of newborn infant abduction is the primary focus of the policy issues to be discussed in this section. When faced with the problem, institutions first generally consider security and protection issues. While these areas are key to any policy development, addressing the needs of the victim parents, infant, staff, and community are also important.

Risk Management

"In the health-care system, needs are infinite and resources are finite" says Dr. William L. Kissick, professor of health care systems at the Wharton School, the University of Pennsylvania. Although some preventive measures suggested are instructive and informative, the majority have the potential to be expensive to implement. The use of expensive monitoring devices coupled with the manpower and hours needed to utilize such devices may be difficult to justify in a budget. Being alert to a risk and using the protections available can lead to safer practice and reduction in potential hazards (Jacobson, 1990).

Preabduction Policy Implementation

Several steps to assist in the prevention of newborn infant abductions have been suggested to all hospitals nationwide by NCMEC. First, the facility should develop a specific policy regarding the security of newborn infants. The burden of providing adequate security and reasonable care lies with administrators, physicians, nurses, allied professionals, and security personnel. Since foresight is perhaps the best defense against the occurrence of a crime, the policy should identify the preventive and search measures to be taken and the administrators and staff who have responsibility for implementation and monitoring of the policy.

Second, a thorough review should be made of the physical plant to identify areas of uncontrolled access and impaired surveillance. Depending on budgetary constraints and fire code requirements, a number of modifications may be made. The facility may choose to address problems by reducing or eliminating multiple exits so that all entrances to and exits from maternity and nursery areas have security checkpoints. Nurses' stations may be positioned so that all persons who enter and leave can be informally screened. Cameras for closed-circuit TV may be positioned to increase observation of areas where infants usually are located. Access to staff locker rooms may be more rigidly secured.

Third, a variety of identification procedures may improve security. These include measures to identify each infant, such as umbilical cord blood samples or footprinting (data collected from these procedures have been instrumental in making positive identifications of infants who had been abducted for long periods of time, i.e., greater than four weeks). The facility should consider the use of log books for visitors and the issuance of duplicate badges for employees (including photos) and visitors, with one badge being left in the infant's crib if the infant is removed for medical or other reasons. Uniforms for staff working in the maternity and nursery areas should be color coded and should not be left in carts in the hallways.

Fourth, all employees must be thoroughly trained, both in the specific procedures the facility elects to use and in the steps to take once a potential incident is identified. The identification of potential trouble spots, dangerous situations, and common strategies used by abductors may help employees to recognize suspicious behaviors. Staff members must concentrate not only on danger from third persons, but also a danger of parental abduction when parents are in the process of separation or are involved in custody litigation over the infant.

Finally, security personnel must be able to intervene effectively in any crisis situation involving the abduction of a patient. Their training is an important preventive and crisis management measure and should include role playing of potential and actual abductions. This will help develop their skills in working sensitively with the parents and general public and in understanding the legal and public relations issues involved. It will also improve their working relationships with others on these issues (Phillips & Lloyd, 1989).

The group identified to implement these five suggested steps are nurse managers. The main reasons for this recommendation are the holistic philosophy of nursing, the large numbers of nurses working in the obstetrics wards, the large amount of nursing time spent with parents and infants, and the educational component of nursing care and the ability to incorporate teaching infant safety to parents. Additionally, OB and nursery nurses, given the nature of maternity services, have a close working relationship that would facilitate implementation of effective policies.

Postabduction Policy Implications

Family and friends are a normal part of the traffic pattern. However, when a newborn infant is abducted, security often is identified as weak, and new policies concerning families and friends are implemented immediately. Frequently there can be a reciprocal overreaction. For example, at Prince Georges County Hospital Center in Cheverly, Maryland, changes in security were made after an abduction. Nurses on the obstetrics ward now wear a different color of scrub suits than the rest of the hospital. Alarms have been added to all the stairwell exits leading to the maternity ward. Additionally, only fathers who can produce photo cards bearing the same last name as the infant are allowed to take the baby out of the nursery. If the father has a different last name, a nurse must deliver the infant to the mother (Gregg, 1989).

Victim Assistance

Quick reactions to abductions by securing the facility involved have influenced how a hospital views itself and the message that is given to the community. While maintaining a safe and secure environment is important, support and crisis intervention for families and staff also are of concern. Historically, the primary focus of resources after a crime has been committed is usually on the offender. In the situation of newborn infant abductions, there are few exceptions. The focus is on the safe return of the infant; once that occurs, attention shifts to the abductor in terms of providing psychological help and/or incarceration (Valentine & Jennings, 1987). There often are few supports extended to victim parents or staff. The violation of trust that victim parents feel toward the hospital, and the guilt individuals direct toward themselves make the parents emotionally vulnerable. Victims of other crimes are given support. These victims should receive the same assistance. Development of health policy in this area is crucial.

Community Relations

For most hospitals obstetrics is a money-making enterprise. Keeping patient numbers high is key in maintaining revenue. A hospital's image as providing quality health care is crucial to good public relations. When a newborn infant is abducted, the institution's reputation is blemished. In addition, many individuals today see the hospital as the enemy of the people (Sigmond, 1989). Thus, maintaining a good relationship with the community is significant. In the case of Grand View Hospital, the positive attitude that the community has maintained toward the hospital is attributed to Grand View's efforts to recover the infant (Doyle, 1990). Its role in reacting to the incident and in finding the infant was strategic in preserving an established community image.

CONCLUSION

The abductions of newborn infants from hospitals is a different investigative challenge and prevention problem than other suspicious disappearances of children. As the numbers increase in this high-profile crime, so do the implications for the health care delivery system to be proactive. Development of productive, protective, and effective health policies are key in reducing the numbers of abductions. Prevention techniques to avert infant abductions must rely on hospital staff awareness of persons and their conduct in and around the maternity ward that might signal or conform the pattern of an abductor. Assistance to the victim parents and staff members is imperative in maintaining optimum mental health and public relations. No one group of persons or discipline can do it alone. Hospital maternity wards cannot be isolation wards or armed security camps. Collaboration and communication remain critical in finding safe, effective, and realistic solutions to the traumatic event of newborn infant abduction.

REFERENCES

Doyle, E.T. (1990). Abducted infant kidnappings and the effects on three hospitals. *Health Care Communicator* 1 (February): 2–23.

Grant, R. (1990). The new babysnatchers. *Redbook* (May): 151–154.

Gregg, S.R. (1987). Incident spurs search for better ward security. *Washington Post*, A31, October 30.

Jacobson, E. (1990). Hospital hazards, part II. *American Journal of Nursing* 90 (April): 48–53.

National Center for Missing & Exploited Children (1989). For Hospital Professionals: Guidelines on Preventing Abduction of Infants from the Hospital. Arlington, Va.: The Center.

National Center for Missing & Exploited Children (1990). Memorandum of Newborn/Infant Abductions. Arlington, Va.: The Center, July.

Phillips, L., & Lloyd, D.W. (1989). Abduction of infants from hospitals: issues of risk management. Unpublished paper.

Presseley, S.A., & Churchville, V. (1987). Coincidence solved baby's kidnaping. *Washington Post*, A1, A22, October 30.

Rich, R.F., & Burgess, A.W. (1985). The aftermath of crime a mental health crisis. Final statement of the Assessment Panel from a Services Research and Evaluation Colloquium.

Sigmond, R.M. (1989). A catalyst for change. *Health Progress* (December): 40–42.

Valentine, P., & Jennings, V.T. (1987). Kidnaped Kernes baby reunited with parents. *Washington Post*, A1, A31, November 1.

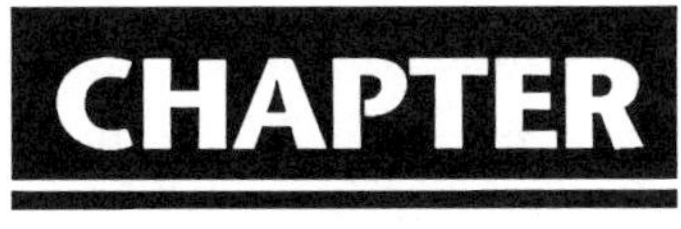

3

Memory, Cognition, and Childhood Trauma

Ann Wolbert Burgess
Carol R. Hartman

A 19-year-old male college student, pseudonym John, seeks consultation because of a "declining interest in school and inability to concentrate." The eldest of three children, he grew up in a traditional intact family in a suburban home environment. He attended private school and was an excellent student until the seventh grade. Teacher reports noted him to be conscientious, energetic, productive, warm, popular, and intelligent. He participated in school activities, had positive and substantive interpersonal relationships with parents, siblings, teachers, classmates, and friends. John described himself, prior to the fall of seventh grade, as happy, outgoing, and challenged by life and school. During the consultation John acknowledged sexual abuse by a teacher during his seventh grade but was unable to provide details of the abuse. After seventh grade there was a dramatic shift in his goal-oriented activities and a marked negative change in behavior until the present time.

What would account for the memory fade of cognitive details for the sexual abuse and presentation of negative self-defeating behaviors? Part of the answer lies in the current research on memory, cognition, and childhood trauma.

This chapter describes a neuropsychosocial model of information processing of trauma that emphasizes the limbic system as being the primary system for coding incoming information. This encoding relates to the process of memory retrieval and recall. When the limbic system is overwhelmed by incoming information, there is an initial altering response that, if unsuccessful in managing and responding to the information, becomes the survival response of numbing (dissociation). Implications for this response of hyperarousal and dissociation can lead to disruption of the interconnections of key processes operant in the construction of memory and in associative learning. The case example of John will be discussed following the presentation of research in the area of memory and childhood sexual abuse.

MODELS OF CHILD SEXUAL ABUSE

Four models describing the consequences associated with child sexual abuse help set the stage for our contrasting fifth model of information processing of trauma. First, the *psychoanalytic model* emphasizes the overstimulation in children of Oedipal fantasies and the ensuing anxiety associated with the emergence of personal concerns of control over sexual impulses (Ferenczi, 1949; Freud, 1920; Lewis & Sarrel, 1969; Sugar, 1983). Fixation, a major concept regarding premature introduction to excessive sexual stimulation, accounts for the dominance of constructs regarding oneself, others, the world, and intentionality. Sexual gratification is paired with socially inappropriate objects, such as a child, clothing, or behaviors. This model plus developmental theories has been basic to classify and develop a taxonomy of sex offenders, both rapists and child molesters (Knight, 1988; Prentky, Knight, & Rosenberg, 1988). These taxonomies consider the nature of the relationship of the offender to the victims as either regressed or fixated and whether they view the victim as an instrument for their gratification or as a direct expression for their emotions. The psychoanalytic model has done little to explain the biological impact of sexual abuse on the victim; rather, it assumes psychological consequences in the deviation of sexual and aggressive behaviors and relationships with others. Derived from a conflict model, the psychoanalytic assumptions do outline an important aspect of victimization—the repetition of the trauma in symbolic and/or representative terms. The psychodynamic interpretation assumes there is fixation or regression to a level of personality structure.

A second model is the *child sexual abuse accommodation syndrome* (Summit 1983). Summit argues that the negative consequences of child sexual abuse are related to conceptual shifts the child makes regarding the abuser and the actions that give the event a purulent, nefarious air. The child initially responds to the protection and nonsexual warmth of the abuser. It is the sexual connotation of the act that turns the child against his or her response and the demands for secrecy that intensifies the child's sense of shame and responsibility. The efficacy of this model is challenged when the response of children abused outside of the family are considered. Its importance is in explaining the attachment of the child to the abuser.

A third model is the *four-factor theory* of Finkelhor and Browne (1985). The first factor—sexualization—acknowledges the evocation of sexual feelings in the child under confusing circumstances resulting in disturbed sexual behavior. The second factor—stigmatization—focuses on inferred social shame that the child experiences regarding sexual activities and feelings about having participated. In part, this factor also reflects the propensity for people to deny or to blame the child. The third factor—betrayal—focuses on behaviors and symptoms attributed to the demand for secrecy and the failure of a care provider to protect. Rather, the child must deal with the fact that a trusted person exploited the relationship. The fourth factor—powerlessness—focuses on the dynamics set in motion by the child being overpowered, trapped, and unable to escape. The symptoms of helplessness, anxiety, lowered self-esteem, eating and sleeping disorder, and nightmares are acknowledged. The authors caution that this model has not been tested either through empirical or clinical methods. The categories are comprehensive, and their classification of symptoms at times is overlapping. There are no unifying assumptions addressing the categorization; nevertheless, the model does attempt to organize an array of findings of cognitive and behavioral consequences. Further, the model underscores the traumagenic dynamics in the impact of child sexual abuse.

A fourth model is derived from an *associative learning paradigm* that suggests response generalization is basic to both sexually deviant behavior and fear responses. Sexual excitation is paired with the exploitive behaviors of the offender. The abuse victim is vulnerable to future exploitive situations because of the association of physically or psychologically aggressive behavior of the offender with personal sexual arousal. The classical conditioning paradigm is used to explain sexual response dysfunctions and difficulties with intimacy. While this model does not have a particular spokesman, numerous efforts to treat victims of sexual abuse and sexual offenders use the key conditioning model premises (Abel, Blanchard, & Becker, 1978; Kilpatrick and Veronen, 1983).

What is assumed under all these models but not clearly stated is some notion of memory. The consideration of memory becomes an important point in the fifth model, the *information processing of trauma* (IPT).

INFORMATION PROCESSING OF TRAUMA MODEL

The past two decades have witnessed a phenomenal increase in research from brain science (MacLean 1976); the cognitive sciences of philosophy, psychology, artificial intelligence, linguistics, anthropology, and neuroscience (Gardner, 1985); information theory (Shannon, 1938); and stress response theory (Figley, 1984; Horowitz, 1976; van der Kolk, 1986). Contributions from the various disciplines provide the basic assumptions for the information processing of trauma (IPT).

The model assumes the basic constructs of information processing of a living system. These propositions state that experiences are processed on a sensory, perceptual, and cognitive and interpersonal level. The sensory level is the basic registrant of experience in the individual. The perceptual level is the beginning classification of the sensory processing. The cognitive and interpersonal level is the larger organization of experience into meaning systems. The effect of memory applies at each level of information processing (Hartman & Burgess, 1988).

Child sexual abuse is the psychosocial stressor under discussion. The American Psychiatric Association's *Diagnostic and Statistical Manual* lists the severity for this stressor as "extreme," thus the designation of child sexual abuse as a trauma. Horowitz (1976), researching the impact of trauma and response to stressful stimuli, identified a general response syndrome as (1) a clustering of disturbing psychological phenomena of intrusive and repetitive imagery associated with memories of the traumatic event and (2) avoidance strategies employed to keep associations to the trauma out of awareness. The presumption was made that traumatic information is kept in active awareness until it can be placed in distant memory and that trauma resolution occurs when there is sufficient processing for the information to be stored; that is, when the event is remembered, the attendant feelings are neutralized, and the anxiety generated by the event is controlled. When a traumatic event is not resolved and either remains in active memory or becomes defended by a cognitive mechanism such as denial, dissociation, or splitting, the diagnosis is generally posttraumatic stress disorder (PTSD). The central feature of PTSD, which is the stress pattern resulting from the traumatization, is that the individual experiences the original trauma both unconsciously and consciously (Hartman & Burgess, 1988).

The IPT model is concerned with how information is experienced, filtered, and related to the process of memory, retrieval, and recall. There is increasing emphasis on the limbic system as being the primary neurological system for coding of incoming information. The output of this limbic system influences basic regulatory processes of eating, sleeping, attachment, affect, sex, and aggression. The charged information is distributed to various neural maps that function in various information-processing capacities to categorize, sort, compare, and distinguish between similar and dissimilar characteristics.

When the limbic system is overwhelmed by incoming information, which occurs in most instances of child sexual abuse, there is an initial alerting response that, if unsuccessful in managing and responding to the charged information, transfers into a survival response of numbing or dissociation. Putnam (1989) through a review of literature, identified three precursors to dissociation of the nature described: (1) situations in which it is impossible to protect or release oneself through fight or flight, (2) panic over overwhelming impulses to commit suicide or homicide, and (3) loss of a loved one. Intensity of trauma, duration, and frequency play a specific role in the frequency in which one observes dissociative states in individuals.

What are the implications for this response of hyperarousal and dissociation on memory and learning in children? Basically, the major assumption is that "stress" stored in the primitive neural strata can lead to disorganized stereotypic behavior, altered affect, and neuroendocrine changes. This stored stress is distinguished from arousal (Levine 1986). Briefly, arousal is a form of stress in which activation is necessarily resolved, following termination of the stressor. Arousal is a subset of stress activation and does not impair function.

In contrast, stress occurs when there is the possibility that preactivation equilibrium will not be reestablished. There is a distinction made between resolved and unresolved stress. Resolution means some type of reorganization. This reorganization can be at the expense of organism flexibility and consequent impairment of function.

Sexual abuse has a particular probability of setting this process into motion. First, even under the ruse of the sexual abuse being a game or "play," the child's immature sexual response is easily overwhelmed. One only needs to remember being tickled and how quickly either children compensate by stating it does not bother them or they become frightened, cry, or struggle against the excessive stimulation.

This overwhelming response causes alterations in the limbic system, which interact with the prefrontal cortex (Levine, 1986). Levine further suggests that once this occurs, there is the phenomena of kindling and sensitization, e.g., a propensity to respond with intensity to stimuli that impact on the alarm system. Time does not alter this response. This propensity in part is a result of the degradation of cue discrimination because of the initial disruption basic in the trauma response. This change in the response receptivity is compounded by a lessening of counter responses that are aimed at resolving the alarm state. This unattended state of affairs leads to disorganization of responses, particularly those of arousal, including the sexual response. In turn, this dysregulation influences the elaboration of neocortical pathways, which are basic to cognitive mapping.

The limbic appraisal hypothesis is that incoming stimuli is first processed in the limbic system and then transmitted along the elaborated pathways in the neocortex, where reactions are interpreted. If the processing and routing of this information is compromised by the dysregulation in the limbic system, evolving meaning systems will be compromised.

For example, sexual thoughts and ideas can be experienced as painful and frightening, or they can be part of a redundant looping, where there is repetition of sexualized behavior, regardless of consequences to self or others. In this latter situation a pattern of minimization or denial can result with a normalization of its (sexual) expression. That is, the child accommodates the repeated behavior by developing a rationale for it that creates an illusion of control and direction. This pattern of adaptability can be found in a number of situations of severe neurological abnormalities manifested in stereotypic behavior, such as head-banging movements.

In sexual abuse some children subject themselves to the abuse even though they know that they do not want it and that it is "wrong." The children are bewildered by the behavior of the perpetrator and by their own response. In fact, they often refrain from telling a parent or another adult. The state of passivity, numbness, and automatic movement is misunderstood by the child as compliance, a thought reinforced by the perpetrator (Burgess, Hartman, McCausland, & Powers, 1984, 1985; Burgess, Hartman, & McCormack, 1987).

Recollection is fragmented. The child may be able to tell what happened but is unable to describe bodily feelings of the abuse or personal thoughts. This type of information lacks integration and breaks through in disconnected expressions, often tinged with fear and anxiety. The dissociation, as well as the hyperarousals, creates altered states of awareness of self and others that play an important role in the evolution of meaning structures. There is a fundamental disruption in the integration of experiences. Behavior is separated from affect; affect is separated from event; meaning is based on disrupted event processing. The child is confused about stimuli that elicit sexual arousal, aggression, and fear. He or she is impaired in processing sexual, aggressive, and fearful information.

The information processing of trauma model focuses on four contextual phases (Hartman & Burgess, 1986, 1988, 1989). (See Table 3–1.) Phase 1, *pretrauma*, considers the individual and social con-

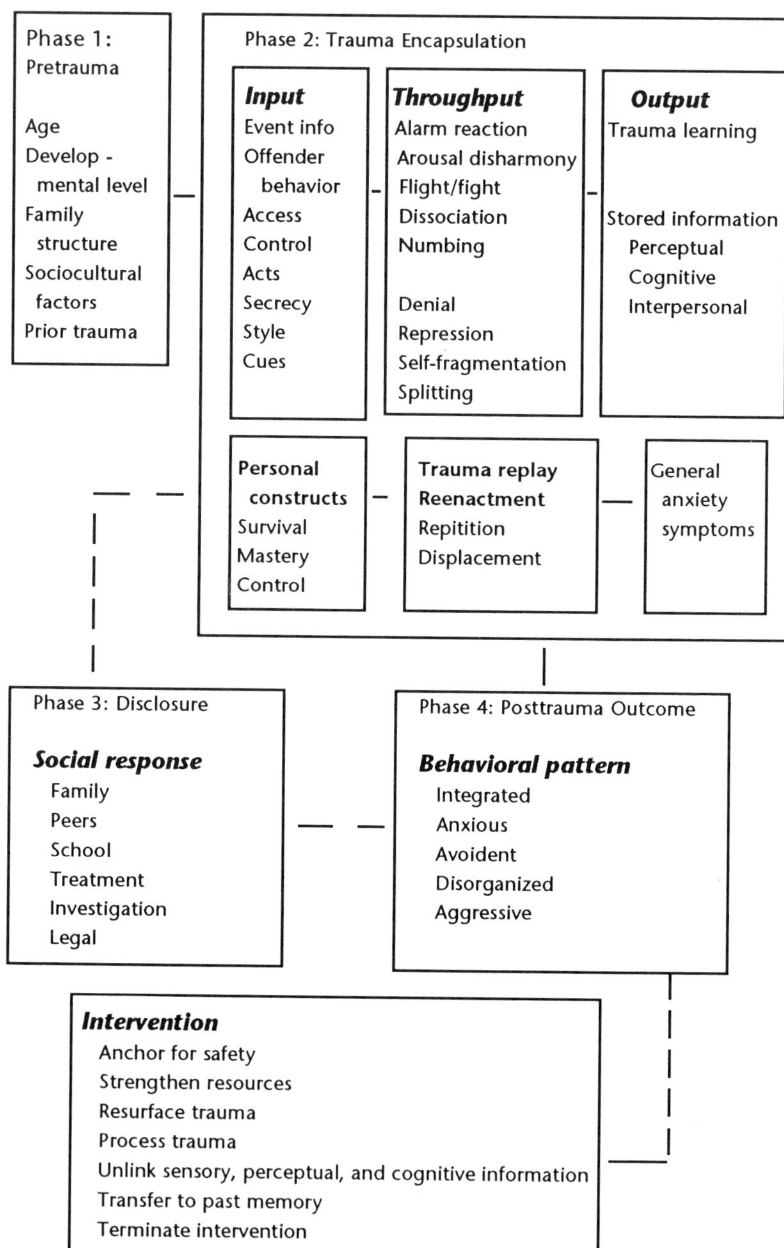

TABLE 3–1

Information Processing in Victims

Phase 1:
Pretrauma

Age
Develop -
  mental level
Family
  structure
Sociocultural
  factors
Prior trauma

Phase 2: Trauma Encapsulation

Input	***Throughput***	***Output***
Event info	Alarm reaction	Trauma learning
Offender	Arousal disharmony	
behavior	Flight/fight	
Access	Dissociation	Stored information
Control	Numbing	Perceptual
Acts		Cognitive
Secrecy	Denial	Interpersonal
Style	Repression	
Cues	Self-fragmentation	
	Splitting	

Personal	**Trauma replay**	General
constructs	**Reenactment**	anxiety
Survival	Repitition	symptoms
Mastery	Displacement	
Control		

Phase 3: Disclosure

Social response
  Family
  Peers
  School
  Treatment
  Investigation
  Legal

Phase 4: Posttrauma Outcome

Behavioral pattern
  Integrated
  Anxious
  Avoident
  Disorganized
  Aggressive

Intervention
  Anchor for safety
  Strengthen resources
  Resurface trauma
  Process trauma
  Unlink sensory, perceptual, and cognitive information
  Transfer to past memory
  Terminate intervention

Source: C.R. Hartman and A.W. Burgess, Information processing of trauma. *Journal of Interpersonal Violence* 3 (December 1988):443–457.

text prior to the victim event. Particular variables are the social economic status of the child's parents; the structure and dynamics of family life; parental attitudes toward aggression, dependency, and sexuality; prior parental abuse; mental and physical illness or criminal patterns in other family members. For the child, personal characteristics such as the age; developmental achievements; psychiatric and medical problems; quality of attachments; peer, parental sibling relationships; impulse control; and dissociative capacities.

Phase 2, *trauma encapsulation*, refers to the complex individual and contextual factors impacting on the child. Critical to the biological considerations are the biphasic alarm responses, i.e., the arousal and dissociative processes specific to survival and protection of physical and psychic integrity. These processes are basic to the defensive and coping patterns that operate on a sensory, perceptual, cognitive, behavioral, and interpersonal level. The outcome of these processes is defined as "trauma learning." This major concept is not subject to extinction and is noted in general symptoms of chronic tension, arousal, numbing, avoidance, and intrusive thoughts of the trauma itself. These are not continuous actions and thoughts; rather, they are breakthrough behaviors seen in children's play, fantasy, and nightmares. The thoughts, feelings, and behaviors of the victim are viewed as secondary, associative learned responses to both the biological disruption caused by the trauma and the ongoing contextual influences. A second major concept, trauma replay, occurs in this phase and represents the reenactment, repetition, and displacement of the sexual abuse experience. The alterations in processes in this phase operate whether the abuse is disclosed or not.

Phase 3, *disclosure*, acknowledges that for children, as well as adults, there is a potential for the family and community to have either a positive or negative effect on the victim. This occurs by the response of others either resolving the basic alarm disruption or intensifying it through further stressful encounters.

Phase 4, *posttrauma*, refers to patterns of responses that are often missed as representing a history of sexual abuse and are more likely to be labeled as a form of mental illness or character pathology. The following outcome categories were noted in clinical studies of children traumatized (Burgess, Hartman, McCausland, & Powers, 1986).

In the integrated outcome the child has mastered and processed the trauma anxiety. The child is not compelled to dwell or avoid the memory through defensive operations. Life advances, and the child is future-oriented. In the anxious outcome the child has generalized anxiety, is unable to progress in a flexible, productive manner, and remains present-oriented. There is anxious recollection of the abuse situation. Anxiety disorder, eating disorder, and phobic and obsessive compulsive disorder have been associated with children in this category. In the avoidant outcome the child will avoid, deny, or recant that the abuse has occurred. This child appears emotionally void, distant, and alienated. There is a lack of energy for living and learning as well as a preoccupation or day-dream quality to the child's existence. These children as adolescents are often seen with a substance abuse history, adjustment problem, or conduct disorder. There may be a mixture of the avoidant and anxious outcome. These children are often diagnosed as having a substance abuse problem and/or conduct disorder.

The delinquent outcome is characterized by a child who tests and breaks rules, is rebellious and impulsive and fights with peers. Anxiety is evident in fears and somatic concerns. Denial of prior abuse is typical. These children often fall under the diagnostic labels of hyperactive, learning disabled, or conduct disordered. The aggressive outcome is a child who has little or no compunction to aggress both physically and sexually against other children, usually those younger. This may be done in a bold manner or in a sneaky, secret manner. The child tends to be a loner. Denial of prior abuse is typical. These children often fall under the diagnostic label of conduct or impulse disorder.

The disorganized outcome is the child who appears fragmented and sometimes bizarre. Psychoticlike behavior is noted. Often, these children are diagnosed as psychotic. Dissociative states need to be ruled out. As with some of the other groups, there is often denial or amnesia for prior sexual abuse.

A NEUROBIOLOGY OF TRAUMA

In 1929 Cannon noted that neurobiological changes registered during acute stress were an adaptive reaction to environmental threat. Contemporary research has further advanced the biology of thought, meaning, and behavior. A precursor to this adaptive state is arousal (Levine, 1986). When the event is overwhelming and traumatic, posttraumatic stress disorder (PTSD) can occur. It is not known to what extent PTSD is composed of a prolongation of the acute stress response with the addition of other symptoms (Giller, 1990; Krystal, Kosten, Southwick, et al., 1989; Pitman, 1989). Giller (1990) considers PTSD to have specific and nonspecific symptoms. Recurrent thoughts or nightmares about the trauma are relatively specific to the traumatic event. Less specific are efforts to avoid thoughts and feelings about the trauma, and symptoms extend to psychic numbing, detachment, or a restricted range of affect.

Pitman (1989) organizes his ideas and approach to the research by noting that PTSD has a combination of tonic and phasic features. The tonic features are those that the patient manifests all or most of the time and that constitute a part of his or her baseline mental functioning. Phasic features are intermittent and apparent most often when evoked by environmental cues. Pitman summarizes symptoms as follows: intrusive symptoms are phasic; avoidant symptoms are tonic; and arousal symptoms (hyperalertness, startle reactions) are a mixture of tonic and phasic symptoms. He suggests that the PTSD symptoms might be explained by a two-type learning model—classical conditioning and operant conditioning or instrumental learning in which there is nonassociative and associative learning.

Foa and Kozak (1986) challenge the two-factor learning proposed by Pitman and others and suggest that symptoms of PTSD are best explained by fear structures in memory that take into account information about the feared stimulus situation—information about verbal, physiological, and other behavioral responses and interpretive information about the meaning of the stimulus and response elements of the structure.

Edelman (1989) does not rule out either Foa and Kozak's or Pitman's notions of learning, but he suggests that at a primary level of consciousness alterations can occur that, in fact, influence secondary meaning. Not only is nonassociative learning occurring (i.e., Krystal's theory of enhanced startle response, 1990), but also the fundamental categorizing and constructing processes can be altered. This is different than the appraisal system espoused by Foa and Kozak. Rather, restricted basic categorization can occur that is not amenable to refinement through new learning. Thus the exaggerated fear response, with its concomitant numbing, shapes the perception of environmental cues as well as the higher order cognitive structures. The prolongation of the fear reorders appraisal schema and in turn, the reordered appraisal schema sustains the fear response.

Various research models provide insight into the biological characteristics of PTSD. First is the noradrenergic-alarm model or LC model (locus cerulus). The LC is located in the pons (brain stem) and innervates discrimination, fear, and memory formation in the limbic system and cerebral cortex. LC activation has been documented in threatened monkeys, cats and rats (Krystal, 1990) and humans (Perry, Southwick, Yehuda, & Giller, 1990; Pitman, Forgue, de Jong, & Claiborn, 1987). Pitman (1989) cites studies and his own work in demonstrating that when the opiate system is blocked, there is an increase in the LC adrenergic output. There are modulating effects of the amount of adrenergic output other than the opiate. These include the corticotropin-releasing factor and the corticosterone released as part of the hypothalamus, pituitary, adrenalin-axis stress response (HPA). The second adrenergic output is the seratonergic hormones located in the raphe nucleus located in the pons brain stem (van der Kolk, 1986).

For Krystal (1990) the LC and its primary innervations with the limbic system and cerebral cortex meet the criteria for a brain "trauma center." Activation of this center can occur as a learned traumatic response, eliciting fear behaviors similar to the alarmlike symptoms of PTSD, i.e., fight/flight and numbing.

Stored and acquired information is modulated by this system. At high levels of adrenalin there is an increase in associative learning. If there is an excess of adrenalin, however, there are failures in learning and cue discrimination (McGaugh, 1990). The basic adaptive function of the LC system is to balance internal and environmental cues, priming the organism to detect danger and make appropriate responses (Krystal, 1990). Research suggests that under traumatic circumstances these interactive systems are altered and they activate when there is little valid reason for the response.

Krystal (1990) cites two important models that account for the startle and avoidant responses. The first model, the fear-enhanced startle model, is based upon a theory of neuroanatomy and development. The acoustical startle reflex is apparent at birth. This model raises the question as to whether there is a sensitization of the pathways that involve the startle response. During fear the generic startle response is increased but is not associated with an environmental cue. Thus there is a nonassociative startle response regardless of cue. The magnitude of the startle response in the presence of everyday sounds and images is an important symptom of PTSD. Pharmacological research notes that this exaggerated response is not affected by the use of traditional tricylic antidepressants; however, there is some reduction with the serotonergically selective antidepressants fluoxetine and alcohol, and opiates reduce the magnitude of the startle response (Krystal, 1990). The startle response suggests that the capacities of the individual to discriminate, codify, organize, and utilize new information is compromised greatly.

In describing the second model of avoidant learning behavior, Krystal summarized the work done by others studying the avoidant learning behavior of the aplysia snail. Experiments with the aplysia snail show that the snail learns by operating through a spectrum of intracellular processes that regulate the sensorimotor system. Through electrical and chemical changes, intracellular changes shape reactions and the structure for short-term memory. Severe or repeated exposure to aversive stimuli produces long-lasting enhanced reactivity in the snail. Under these conditions short-term memory and message coding are affected. Long-term learning depends on the specific gene products that maintain the learned response or memory trace. Evidence for the molecular change was obtained from injecting products that block gene transmission material (RNA) and gene translation material (DNA). When these products were given, long-term avoidant learning disappeared. When they were not given, long-term memory occurred under the stressful conditions outlined earlier. Further, if the gene products had appeared, the blocking agents did not work, and there was a chronic state of avoidance. Under stress there was also a proliferation of certain receptor sites and a reduction in others.

From the startle-enhancement model and these findings with the aplysia snail, Krystal suggests that there can be indelible qualities to long-term memory. Some treatments aimed at long-lasting sensitization of the alarm systems may have temporary effects. When they fade, there is a reemergence of symptoms. Krystal further suggests that this may be adaptive from an evolutionary position; from a therapeutic point of view, however, this inflexibility of memory means that periodic treatment is necessary to maintain improvement in PTSD patients.

Further models drawn from animal and human studies that focused on the impact of inescapable shock and maternal deprivation (Kosten & Krystal, 1988; Krystal, 1990; Pitman, Forgue, de Jong, & Claiborn, 1987; Sapolsky, 1990; van der Kolk, 1986) suggest that PTSD symptoms arise purely from activation-induced disturbances in homeostatic neuronal systems and not as goal-directed learned responses. Rather stress-induced dysregulation may produce learned behavioral syndromes that adaptively dampen arousal through cognitive patterns that decrease arousal or enhance phobic avoidance. For example, when animals are blocked from escape and fear or painful stimuli is introduced, animals become helpless. When the animals were taught how to escape the shock, they compulsively continued the behavior and became agitated if the stimuli were stopped. This was assumed to be a learned behavior to dampen arousal caused by the inescapable shock situation. In humans, this model has been applied to studies of Vietnam veterans. Pitman et al. (1987) found arousal levels to be higher in Vietnam vets with a diagnosis of PTSD.

Van der Kolk (1986) pays particular attention to the studies of maternal deprivation when considering victims of trauma. Not only have neuroendocrine changes been noted in maternal deprivation studies that are similar to the findings associated with inescapable shock, but the HPA axis is also activated by maternal deprivation. This activation is associated with the negative or avoidant symptoms of PTSD, such as social isolation, poor stress tolerance, and disruption of attachment.

A preliminary study carried out by Teicher, Glod, Swett, et al., (1989) explored the possible developmental changes in the limbic system as a result of abuse before age 18 and after age 18 in a sample of 254 outpatients, age range 17–69 with a mean age of 34 years. This work suggests that there are primary biological changes in the evolving attributional cognitions of abused children, in particular, sexually abused children.

The disturbance in memory suggests that sexual abuse is a contributor to dissociative processes as noted in the studies of multiple personality disorder (Kluft, 1985; Putnam, 1989) and perpetrators (Burgess, Hartman, Grant, et al., 1990; Burgess, Hartman, Ressler, et al., 1986; Friedrich, Beilke & Urquiza, 1987; Knight, 1988; Prentky & Quinsey, 1988).

Further investigation of the biology of physical and sexual trauma with regard to gender may address differences in the repetitive sexually aggressive acts of males compared to the repetitive sexual exploitations of females. One hypothesis is that sexual perpetration is associated with the dissociative effects of trauma and the interaction with levels of testosterone and cortisol, wherein males dissociate from fear with enhanced aggression and sexualization and females dissociate from aggression with enhanced fear and sexualization. Social role values may be connected to biology in ways that have not been previously acknowledged.

PRIMARY AND SECONDARY CONSCIOUSNESS

There is debate on whether memory is a status entity or whether memory is a series of processes. Edelman (1989) makes the assumption that thought and consciousness are biological with origins in brain structures. He argues that our present state of knowing arises from an ongoing, active process of memory construction. He presents two levels of consciousness as (1) primary or sensory/perceptual based and (2) secondary or language based. The theory of neuronal group selection (TNGS) accounts for perceptual categorization of an unlabeled world and certain aspects of memory and learning in terms of brain structure, development, and evolution. All cognition and consciousness rest on orderings and processes in the physical world.

Mediating this processes is a hypothesized concept of reentrant cortical integration (RCI). This model assumes that the stimulus world is distributed among multiple functionally segregated areas of the brain. Stimuli (e.g., auditory, visual, kinesthetic) are stored in various parts of the brain with neural groupings that contain value criteria. There is parallel processing of information rather than localized processing. Instead of information stored as a visual snapshot image, information is matched for similarities and differences and then organized into categories for memory recall. Consciousness is a constant construction of present memory, highly developed in humans because of language. This biological theory of consciousness assumes knowing exists prior to language and that all initial knowing (response to stimuli) is processed first through the primary consciousness (sensory system) and then to higher order consciousness (language). Because primary consciousness is rooted in the brain stem and the limbic system, alterations in these areas will have an impact on primary and secondary consciousness.

TRAUMA AND COGNITION IN CHILDREN

Clinical investigators of traumatized children, Eth and Pynoos (1985), note the following in children who have experienced and witnessed traumatic events such as murder of parents, physical or sexual abuse, or a suicide: inhibition of spontaneous thought, disruption in school performance, fixation to the trauma event noted either in incomplete or unemotional recall, new fear marked by anxious preoccupations or generalized fear to prior neutral stimuli, fear of the future, acting-out behavior either as risk taking or aggression to others, and constricted or morbid thoughts and/or fantasy.

Another effort to explore cognitive patterns in abused children was conducted by Fish-Murray, Koby, and van der Kolk (1989). Their interpretive schema was that of Piaget (1929), and they viewed the children's responses as regression or fixation to a visual representation. These researchers noted that abused children lacked empathy and were unable to shift roles. Nonabused children made more requests, told more stories, expressed pleasure, and evidenced more positive self-references in stories about themselves and what they were doing than the abused children. They noted an inconsistency in the abused group in assimilating and accommodating new people in their environment, such as the evaluators. However, when the abused children were presented with pictures of children like themselves, with parents or siblings, and were asked to associate to these images, memories of their own traumatic experiences returned and "held them captive." In addition, the evaluators noted that while these children could maintain a solid sense of conservation in the scientific-mathematical domain, this was not maintained when dealing with self or others. The strongest finding was the inflexibility in thinking. The children were frozen. Verbalization was restricted in comparison to controls, and there was an enhanced dissociative process noted in the abused children (Fish-Murray, Koby, & van der Kolk, 1989: 99–102).

Donovan and McIntyre (1990) disagree with the assumptions regarding the response patterns being observed in abused children and in particular comment on the Fish-Murray, Koby, and van der Kolk interpretations. For them, children are "slaves of logic." That is, from the earliest ages children are developing hypotheses regarding their experiences. Thus, to understand the context from which they draw their information, their reasoning about what is happening or has happened to them makes immeasurable sense. Further, they suggest that the adult demand for verbal explanations from children basically neglects how children use language. For a child, one word stands for a complex level of abstraction with regard to interactive events. The assessment of a child's understanding of causal expectancies, through verbal presentations, misses how much a child does "know." The authors demonstrate through case examples that if clinicians maintain a commitment to rigid categorical and/or epigenetic models of development, the child will be misunderstood as well as mistreated.

Miller and Aloise (1989) found that when the context of situations is taken into account, there is not the rigid evolution of reasoning suggested in the epigenetic model of Piaget. Social understanding appears much more developed in children than realized in other studies, and the reasoning characteristics suggested by Piaget may be a function of the type of questions asked.

Studies by Smetana and Kelly (1989) suggest that the type of the abuse shapes levels of moral evaluation but the arousal and numbness interferes with information formation and discrimination. This is particularly true when stimuli trigger trauma cues. Sexually abused children present confusion through perplexity as to why they remained in the abuse situation.

A study of drawings by juveniles of their memory of committing a homicide revealed fragments of their own childhood abuse and shifts in thinking where they viewed the victim in the role of the aggressor or "asking" for the violence (Burgess, Hartman, Grant, et al., 1990).

In a study on beliefs and expectations regarding reasons for running away (Janus, McCormack, Burgess, & Hartman, 1987), sexually abused youths were less likely than their nonabused counterparts to believe they could have controlled the reasons for their running, more likely to see things as unpredictable, and less likely to believe that they could have changed things. However, when the sex of the runaway was controlled, sexually abused males were more likely to blame themselves for the running than their nonabused counterparts. The opposite was found for the sexually abused females.

SUMMARY

The neurobiological basis of the altered alarm/dissociative process during and post sexual trauma impedes the development of information processing essential for the discerning of intentionality, personal responsibility (blame), sense of control over events, and trust in others. Once this imbalance occurs, the child is restricted in developing cognitive schema to deal with interpersonal intimacy. This in turn results in secondary patterns of aggression and/or avoidance. It is as if the child loses the capacity to develop the perceptual and cognitive schema to handle the nuances of interpersonal relationships. The necessary inhibition and discrimination are altered, and there is a collapsing of categories that indicate danger.

The implication of this biological understanding of trauma and information processing for treatment underscores the necessity of reducing arousal, thus lessening the dissociative processes. Once this is done, primary learning can resume. Treatment and research can now be directed to cognitive and physiological interventions as well as holding constant the social/contextual activities that support the healing potential of the therapeutic relationship.

CASE APPLICATION TO IPT MODEL

*John's memory of details of the sexual
assaults is unclear. For example, he cannot remember
the dates or year(s) the activities occurred. His
memory of grammar school is quite clear as is his
memory of his English teacher. He described his*

teacher as "popular but tough." The course was an English course that required reading books that focused on boys and their adolescent changes, for example, Lord of the Flies. The teacher had a number of activities outside his classroom that brought students into close proximity with him. He encouraged students to eat with him, first in the dining room and then in a large room in the school's basement. Boys would be invited to his home and to accompany him on summer trips to Europe. Boys at the school viewed it a "privilege" to be a favorite of this teacher. The teacher was described as fastidious and rigid in his written assignment requirements as to form, but not content. For example, papers had to be folded in a certain way and names written is a specific place. However, the student could write on any topic of his choice.

In retrospect, John remembers conversations and situations with his teacher outside the classroom to be sexually oriented and sexually tense. For example, masturbation was a frequent topic, and students were encouraged to talk about their sexual feelings and experiences. John is unclear as to the number of assaults perpetrated, the total time period, or the presence of other boys. He remembers the assaults as occurring at the teacher's home. Music played on the stereo; liquor (Scotch and bourbon) was freely available; and pornography (sexually oriented and/or fetish magazines and films) was kept in the "library" in his bedroom. Sexual activities included, but were not limited to, autoerotic acts, group masturbation, and oral sex. Vibrators were used to stimulate the genitals.

The district attorney's office began investigating allegations about the teacher, and letters were sent to parents of children who were believed to have some knowledge of the situation. John's parents talked with him about the letters, but it was two years later that John was able to disclose that he had been raped by his teacher.

Trauma Response

> *John's response to the sexual abuse was*
> *noted in his behavior by the time he was in the eighth*
> *grade. He began to drink alcohol and use drugs. He*
> *changed his appearance and dress, wearing combat*
> *boots and a mohawk hairdo and piercing his ear. He*
> *would leave school in midday, performed poorly in his*
> *studies, developed a reputation for fighting, became*
> *argumentative with his parents, particularly his*
> *mother, used sexually oriented and abusive language,*
> *and became indiscriminately sexually active. In ninth*
> *grade he was asked not to return to the private school.*
> *For his tenth grade John attended public school. His*
> *behavior continued to deteriorate. He had encounters*
> *with the police for assault and battery allegations. He*
> *was constantly angry, had violent outbursts, was bad*
> *tempered, and carried a knife. The alcohol and drug*
> *use increased. In eleventh grade John became a*
> *boarding student at another private school. When*
> *confronted by his parents with the district attorney's*
> *letter, John said he felt "shock, numb, flushed, light-*
> *headed, and physically disconnected." He denied any*
> *involvement with the teacher, feeling guilt, fear, and*
> *shame. He had an image of the teacher shooting him*
> *if he testified. Although he was able to disclose the*
> *rape in twelfth grade, John was not able to discuss it*
> *further, either with his parents or therapist.*

The information processing of trauma model is used to help explain the symptom response of John. A part of him recognized his reactions did not make sense; rather, they were frightening to him. His first line of defense was to avoid people, but that did not remove the internally experienced tension. He was unable to modulate his aggressive impulses and would verbally assault people or feel he had to defend himself physically. Whenever he was under pressure, there would be a resurrection of flashbacks, and it was disruptive to his ongoing activities. Avoidance was his main mechanism. To avoid experiences, there was an alteration of appearance and behavior and in his capacity to be engaged and attached to people. New friends were very different from childhood friends, and many were troubled adolescents. Gradually, he withdrew from school and school activities. He took alcohol and drugs, substances introduced to him by the teacher as a way to separate his mind from his body. He experienced depression, aggression, and suicidal thoughts; he felt irritable, explosive, betrayed, and lonely.

He had grave concern over his sexual identity. The numbing and tensions blocked his natural sexual development. Sexual impulses were disrupted on a sensory level; his sense of pleasure was inhibited. The only way he obtained relief was in the numb state. He induced it through substance use. The use of alcohol and drugs continues to be an attempt to handle the tonic symptoms (hyperarousal) and a way to control his internal tension.

Testing using the Derogatis SCL-90-R indicates an extremely high level of somatization. He experienced feelings of personal inadequacy and devalued self-worth; his level of anxiety is significantly elevated; he had conscious anger and hostility, and struggled with substantial levels of unresolved conflict and frustration; he had clinical levels of paranoid ideation, with evidence of suspicion, mistrust, hostility, and projection; and his thinking suggested intense confusion and a sense of marked alienation.

John was unfocused both in terms of academic pursuits and his future. He was unable to be absorbed in studies and interests as he once was. Considerable energy is exerted into efforts to maintain self-control. The excessive tense state alters neurohormones that prevent many of the above reported clinical conditions and keep mood stabilized.

The fact that John did not disclose and tried to deny the abuse for so long suggests a complicated relationship with the offender. He does not have full recollection of that involvement and the implications of that relationship. However, it can be observed that this relationship has alienated him from many meaningful relationships. There is a level of self-absorption and insensitivity that comes from his defensive stance and not having learned the give and take of relationships. All of this normal adolescent development has been circumvented by the exploitive relationship with the offender.

Trauma Therapy

Trauma therapy is very much indicated. The first phase of treatment would be for John to agree to begin treatment. This is difficult because he is at a precarious state of wanting to recover on his own. The decision for treatment needs to be his. Age 18–22 is a time of self-identification and a solidification of positive gains in life. Adolescents, in general, want to get on with their life and have little patience for reflective experiences, especially those that involve fear, sex, and aggression. Trusting someone, as structured in a therapeutic relationship, will take time. After treatment begins, the second phase would be to build his personal resources. Because he is so symptomatic, he will need personal resources to feel competent and successful before he can confront the traumatic experience that he acknowledges has torn him apart. As he gains strength, he will be able to deal with the more disruptive aspects of the trauma.

The third phase of treatment is to desensitize him to the memories. As he is successful in processing the trauma, through creative efforts and work, he will reclaim himself, his vision of life, and a positive sense of the future. Through both the constructive aspects of a therapeutic relationship and specific efforts to deal with tension, hyperarousal, and memory fragments, there should be an energy release that will strengthen his attachment to others and increase his flexibility and ability to move comfortably in the world.

REFERENCES

Abel, G.G.; Blanchard, E.B.; & Becker, J.V. (1978). An integrated treatment program for rapists. In R.T. Rada (ed.), *Clinical Aspects of the Rapist*. Pp. 161–214. New York: Grune & Stratton.

American Psychiatric Association (1987). *Diagnostic and statistical manual*, 3rd ed. rev. Washington, D.C.: The Association.

Burgess, A.W.; Hartman, C.R.; Grant, C.; et al. (1990). Juvenile murderers: assessing memory through crime scene drawings. *Journal of Psychosocial Nursing* 28 (1): 26–34.

Burgess, A.W.; Hartman, C.R.; McCausland, M.P.; & Powers, P. (1984). Impact of child pornography on the victims and families. In A.W. Burgess (ed.), *Child Pornography and Sex Ring Crimes*. Pp. 177–186. Lexington, Mass.: Lexington Books.

Burgess, A.W.; Hartman, C.R.; McClausland, M.P.; & Powers, P. (1985). Stress response patterns in children exploited through pornography. *American Journal of Psychiatry*, 141: 656–662.

Burgess, A.W.; Hartman, C.R.; & McCormack, A. (1987). Abuse to abuser: antecedents of socially deviant behaviors. *American Journal of Psychiatry* 144 (11): 1431–1436.

Burgess, A.W.; Hartman, C.R.; Ressler, R.K.; et al. (1986). Sexual homicide: a motivational model. *Journal of Interpersonal Violence* 1 (3): 251–272.

Burgess, A.W.; Hazelwood, R.; Rokous, F.; et al. (1988). Serial rapists and their victims: reenactment and repetition. In R. Prentky & V. Quinsey (eds.). *Human Sexual Aggression: Current Perspectives.* Annals of the New York Academy of Sciences, Vol. 528, pp. 277–295. New York: The Academy.

Cannon, W.B. (1929). *Bodily Changes in Pain, Hunger, Fear and Rage.* New York: Appleton.

Donovan, D., & McIntyre, D. (1990). *Healing the Hurt Child.* New York: Norton.

Edelman, G. (1989). *The Remembered Present: A Biological Theory of Consciousness.* New York: Basic Books.

Eth, S., & Pynoos, R. (eds.) (1985). *Post-Traumatic Stress Disorder in Children.* Washington, D.C.: American Psychiatric Press.

Ferenczi, S. (1949). Confusion of tongues between the adult and the child. *International Journal of Psychoanalysis* 30: 225–231.

Figley, C.R. (1984). *Trauma and Its Wake,* New York: Brunner/Mazel.

Finkelhor, D., & Browne, A. (1985). The traumatic impact of child sexual abuse. *American Journal of Orthopsychiatry* 55: 530–541.

Fish-Murray, C.; Koby, E.; & van der Kolk, B. (1986). Evolving ideas: the effects of abuse on children's thought. In B. van der Kolk (ed.), *Psychological Trauma.* Pp. 89–110. Washington, D.C.: American Psychiatric Press.

Foa, E.B., & Kozak, M.J. (1986). Emotional processing of fear: exposure to corrective information. *Psychological Bulletin* 99: 20–35.

Friedrich, W.; Beilke, R.; & Urquiza, A. (1987). Children from sexually abusive families: a behavioral comparison. *Journal of Interpersonal Violence.* 2 (4): 391–402.

Freud, S. (1920). *Beyond the Pleasure Principle.* Trans. and ed. J. Strachey (1961). Paperback. New York: Liveright (1970).

Gardner, H. (1985). *The Mind's New Science.* New York: Basic Books.

Giller, E. (ed.) (1990). *Biological Assessment and Treatment of Posttraumatic Stress Disorder.* Progress in Psychiatry Series. Washington, D.C.: American Psychiatric Press.

Hartman, C.R., & Burgess, A.W. (1986). Child sexual abuse: generic roots of the victim experience. *Journal of Psychotherapy and the Family* 2: 83–92.

Hartman, C.R., & Burgess, A.W. (1988). Information processing of trauma: case application of a model. *Journal of Interpersonal Violence* 3 (4): 443–457.

Hartman C.R., & Burgess, A.W. (1989). Sexual abuse of children: causes and consequences. In D. Cicchetti & V. Carlson (eds.), *Child Maltreatment.* Pp. 95–128. New York: Cambridge University Press.

Horowitz, M.J. (1976). *Stress Response Syndromes.* New York: Aronson.

Janus, M.; McCormack, A.; Burgess, A.; & Hartman, C. (1987). *Adolescent Runaways.* Lexington, Mass.: Lexington Books.

Kilpatrick, D., & Veronen, L. (1983). Stress management for rape victims. In D. Meichenbaum & M. E. Jaremko (eds.), *Stress Reduction and Prevention.* Pp. 341–374. New York: Plenum Press.

Kluft, R. (ed.) (1985). Childhood antecedents of multiple personality. *Monograph Series of the American Psychiatric Press.* Washington, D.C.: American Psychiatric Press.

Knight, R. (1988). A taxonomic analysis of child molesters. In R. Prentky & V. Quinsey (eds.), *Human Sexual Aggression: Current Perspectives.* Annals of the New York Academy of Sciences, Vol. 528, pp. 2–20. New York: The Academy.

Kosten, T., & Krystal, J. (1988). Biological mechanisms in posttraumatic stress disorder: relevance for substance abuse. In M. Galanter (ed.), *Recent Advances in Alcoholism.* Vol. 6, pp. 49–68. New York: Plenum Press.

Krystal, J. (1990). Animal models for posttraumatic stress disorder. In E. Giller (ed.), *Biological Assessment of Posttraumatic Stress.* Pp. 1–26. Washington, D.C.: American Psychiatric Press.

Krystal, J; Kosten, T.; Southwick, S.; et al. (1989). Neurobiological aspects of PTSD: review of clinical and preclinical studies. *Behavior Therapy* 20: 177–198.

Levine, P. (1986). Stress. In M. Coles, E. Donchin, & S. Porges, (eds.), *Psychophysiology, Systems, Processes and Applications.* New York: Guilford Press.

Lewis, M., & Sarrel, P. (1969). Some psychological aspects of seduction, incest and rape in childhood. *Journal of the American Academy of Child Psychiatry* 8: 606–619.

MacLean, P. (1976). *A Triune Concept of Brain and Behavior.* Toronto: Toronto Press.

McGaugh, J.L. (1990). Significance and Remembrance : The Role of Neuromodulatory Systems. *Psychological Science* 1 (1): 15–25.

Miller, P., & Aloise, P. (1989). Young children's understanding of the psychological causes of behavior: a review. *Child Development* 60: 257–285.

Perry, B.; Southwick, S.; Yehuda, R.; & Giller, E. (1990). Adrenergic receptor regulation in posttraumatic stress disorder. In E. Giller (ed.), *Biological Assessment of Posttraumatic Stress Disorder.* Pp. 87–114. Washington, D.C.: American Psychiatric Press.

Piaget, J. (1929). *The Child's Conception of the World.* New York: Harcourt Brace.

Pitman, R. (1989). Biological findings in PTS: Implications for DSM-IV Classification. Unpublished position paper. NH Veterans Administration Medical Center/Dept. of Psychiatry, Harvard Medical School Research Services, 151a.

Pitman, R.; Forgue, D; de Jong, J; & Claiborn, J. (1987). Psychophysiologic assessment of posttraumatic stress disorder imagery in Vietnam combat veterans. *Archives of General Psychiatry* 44: 970–975.

Prentky, R.; Knight, R.; & Rosenberg, R. (1988). Validation analyses on a taxonomic system for rapists: disconfirmation and reconceptualization. In R. Prentky & V. Quinsey (eds.), *Human Sexual Aggression: Current Perspectives.* Annals of the New York Academy of Sciences. Vol 528, pp. 21–40. New York: The Academy.

Prentky, R., & Quinsey, V. (eds.) (1988). *Human Sexual Aggression: Current Perspectives.* Annals of the New York Academy of Sciences, Vol. 528. New York: The Academy.

Putnam, F.W. (1989). *Diagnosis and Treatment of Multiple Personality Disorder.* New York: Guilford Press.

Putnam, F.W. (1989). Pierre Janet and modern views of dissociation. *Journal of Traumatic Stress* 2: 413–429.

Pynoos, R., & Eth, S. (1985). Children traumatized by witnessing acts of personal violence: homicide, rape, or suicidal behavior. In S. Eth and R. Pynoos (eds.) *Posttraumatic Stress Disorder in Children.* Washington, D.C.: American Psychiatric Press.

Sapolsky, R.M. (1990). Stress in the wild, *Scientific America*: 116–123.

Shannon, C. E. (1938). Symbolic analysis of relay and switching circuits. *Transactions of the American Institute of Electrical Engineers* 57: 1–11.

Smetana, J., & Kelly, M. (1989). Social cognition in maltreated children. In D. Cicchetti & V. Carlson (ed), *Child Maltreatment.* Pp. 620–646. New York: Cambridge University Press.

Sugar, M. (1983). Sexual abuse of children and adolescents. *Adolescent Psychiatry* 11: 199–211.

Summit, R. (1983). The child sexual abuse accommodation syndrome. *Child Abuse and Neglect,* 7: 177–193.

Teicher, M.; Glod, C.; Swett, C., Jr.; et al. (1989). *Childhood Abuse and Limbic System Dysfunction.* American Psychiatric Association Abstract 142: 212. Washington, D.C.: The Association.

van der Kolk, B. (ed.) (1986). *Psychological Trauma.* Washington D.C.: American Psychiatric Press.

Sexually Abused Children's Symptoms and Disorders of Extreme Stress Not Otherwise Specified: Does This Proposed Psychiatric Diagnosis Fit?

David L. Corwin
The author wishes to acknowledge the
assistance of Michael Grogan, Ph.D., and Erna
Olafson, Ph.D., in the preparation of this review

INTRODUCTION

This chapter reviews the literature on the emotional and behavioral effects of sexual abuse on children and adolescents in relation to a recently proposed psychiatric diagnostic category—Disorders of Extreme Stress Not Otherwise Specified (van der Kolk, Pelcovitz, Herman, et al., 1991). Relevant works have been divided into three categories and compared to a 1984 review of the short-term symptoms of child sexual abuse completed by Gomes-Schwartz, Horowitz, and Sauzier (1984). This comparison serves as a reliability check for the current review in that it represents independent determinations of whether particular symptoms are reported in the individual references. The present analysis and that review share five references in common (Adams-Tucker, 1982; Bender & Blau, 1937; Browning & Boatman, 1977; Lewis & Sorrel, 1969; Peters, 1976). Gomes-Schwartz and her associates examined another 28 clinically based works. This review includes 22 such references under the category of Uncontrolled Studies and Case Reports, see Table 4–2. However, priority for inclusion in this critique was given to those studies that utilized comparison groups or standardized assessment instruments. Thirty-three such investigations are reviewed, as shown in Table 4–1 entitled Controlled Studies. The final category of references covers consensus, guidelines, reviews, and surveys as listed in Table 4–3. Although this category is to some degree dependent upon the first two, it adds the dimension of agreement among various groups of experienced clinicians.

References for this review were obtained from a variety of sources, including the National Resource Center on Child Sexual Abuse, the Family Violence Research Program at the University of New Hampshire, the Crime Victims Research and Treatment Center at the Medical College of South Carolina, and the National Clearinghouse for Child Abuse and Neglect. Two computerized bibliographies—REFLINE at the National Library of Medicine and Dialog File 64, Spring 1989 from the Clearinghouse—were reviewed for recent works. Articles in press were obtained from two journals that focus on child abuse or interpersonal violence, the *Journal of Interpersonal Violence* and *Child Abuse and Neglect*. The child sexual abuse bibliographies from the spring and summer issues of the *Family Violence Bulletin* from the University of Texas at Tyler were also reviewed. Several researchers in this area of inquiry, including Lucy Berliner, Jon Conte, David Finkelhor, William Friedrich, Benjamin Saunders, and Jill Waterman, were contacted by phone. They provided several articles in press and other recent references as well as their viewpoints on the proposed Disorders of Extreme Stress Not Otherwise Specified. In addition to the two journals contacted, whose past issues were also directly reviewed, particular attention was given to articles appearing in the *American Journal of Psychiatry* and the *Journal of the American Academy of Child and Adolescent Psychiatry*. The reference list of each citation was reviewed as were those from a recent chapter by Green (1988) and a book by Haugaard and Reppucci (1988).

OVERVIEW OF LITERATURE

Anecdotal case reports describing the adverse effects of child sexual abuse began to appear in the late 1800s and early 1900s. Freud (1962) and Ferenczi (1932) both contributed major works on this topic that were received by their peers with considerable condemnation and disbelief (Masson, 1984). In 1937 Bender and Blau (1937) published their report of 16 cases involving adult-child sexual contact. Despite occasional study and publication, it was not until the mid-1970s that significant professional attention and publication began to focus on child sexual victimization (Brant & Tisza, 1977; Browning & Boatman, 1977; Peters, 1976; Shengold, 1977).

During the 1980s there has been a very significant increase in both the number and quality of studies and publications on child sexual abuse. In 1985 studies began to appear in print that compared sexually abused children and adolescents to various comparison groups or normative groups on standardized measures (Table 4–1). In response to appropriate criticism of earlier uncontrolled studies and case reports, most recent studies utilize standardized assessment instruments and comparison groups. The process of professional consensus development and publication of diagnostic and treatment guidelines also surfaced in 1985 with the publication of the American Medical Association's Diagnostic and Treatment Guidelines Concerning Child Abuse and Neglect.

In late 1985 a National Summit Conference on Diagnosing Child Sexual Abuse was held in Los Angeles. This meeting examined the developing consensus among an interdisciplinary group of professionals with significant experience in addressing child sexual victimization. This process ultimately led to the founding of the American Professional Society on the Abuse of Children (APSAC). The participating professionals from the health care, law enforcement, legal, mental health, and social welfare fields agreed that such an interdisciplinary professional society was needed to work alongside existing single discipline professional societies to improve the standards, research, and professional practice encompassing the problems of child abuse and neglect (Corwin, 1988).

One of the strongest areas of agreement among the 30 to 40 mental health experts on child sexual abuse who participated in the Summit Conference was that none of the currently existing diagnostic categories in DSM-III really fit many of the sexually abused children and adolescents whom they were encountering. In addition, even though these victims did not meet the criteria of any DSM-III disorder, many of them were symptomatic and deserving of mental health care. There was a consensus that although PTSD is an

TABLE 4–1

CONTROLLED STUDIES (N = 33)[A]

Author Year	Abused No. Ages	Source of Subjects	Controls	Measures	Criteria Supported
Aiosa-Karpas et al. 1991	31G 13–18	inpat & clin tx	NA clin & NA notx	CBCL YSR GRAS DE GICS	3, 4, 13
Basta & Peterson 1990	32 6–10	sex abuse Tx program school	clin + WISC–R	CPQ	1, 2, 7, 14, 19
Burgess et al. 1987	34 14–21	prior study follow-up	NA sibs+ school	Int PHCSCS MFES	3, 4, 13, 19
Caviola & Schiff 1988	150 13–18	drug tx program (N = SA + PA)	NA clin + school	RecRev Int controls	13, 19, 20
Caviola & Schiff 1989	150 13–18	drug tx program (N = SA + PA)	NA clinc + school	TSCS	2
Cohen & Mannarino 1988	24G 6–12	rape crisis centers	test norms clin & not	Int CDI PHCSCS STASC CBCL	1, 3, 13, 14, 19
Conte & Schuerman 1988	369 4–17	sex assault center	community	Sx ChLst CBP	1, 2, 3, 14, 19, 20
Deblinger et al. 1989	58 3–13	psych unit (N = 29 SA + 29 PA)	NA in-pat	RecRev PTSD ChLst	13
DiPietro 1987	15G 11–21 & sibs	social service agencies	NA G sibs NA school	EPI BAI–RSF IE, TSCS VV-SHQ	None
Einbender & Friedrich 1989	46G 6–14	CPS agency & therapist ref	school	WISC–R WRAT–R RATC, LE ChLst CDI, CBCL Rorschach PHCSCS, FES:C,E,C	3, 13, 14, 19
Friedrich 1988	155 3–12	social service & mental health ref	well peds & conduct D & Psych Clinic	CBCL	13, 14, 19
Friedrich et al. 1988	31B 3–8	clinical ref	Conduct + oppositional dis	CBCL	13, 19
Friedrich et al. 1989	155 2–12 Clin	social service & mental health ref	880 NA peds	CBCL CSBI	13
Gale et al. 1988	72 2–7	men health center (N = 37 SA + 35 PA)	NA center Patients	RecRev	3, 13, 14, 19
Gomez-Schwartz et al. 1985	156 1–18	sex abuse tx Program	test norms	LBCL	1, 3, 13, 14, 19
Grogan 1988	12G 8–10	sex abuse tx program	school & prob ref RATC	FACES CBCL	3, 13, 14, 19
Jampole & Weber 1987	10 3–8	in-state custody due to sex abuse	state empl children & wards	SAC Doll Int	13

Author Year	Abused No. Ages	Source of Subjects	Controls	Measures	Criteria Supported
Janus et al. 1987	89 12–18	Canadian runaways (N = SA + PA + NA)	NA runaways	Int	3
Kolko et al. 1988	59 5–14	Psych unit	NA peers on unit	SASx Chlst RecRev	3, 13, 14
Lipovsky et al. 1989	88 x = 11.2	ref via Fa's NA sibs tx program		RCMAS CDI ISE CBCL	2, 14
Livingston 1987	28 6–12	psych unit	NA psych patients	DICA	4, 13, 14, 19, 20
McLeer et al. 1988	31 3–16	psych clinic	test norms	Int SEI STAIC CDI CBCL	2, 14
Mannarino et al. 1989	94G 6–12	ref rape crisis centers	clinical & school	CDI STAIC PHCSCS CBCL	1, 3, 5, 13, 14, 19
Orr & Downes 1985	20 9–15	child sex abuse clin	NA peds clin + NA acute ill	OSIQ	1, 3, 13
Rimsza & Berg 1988	72 2–17	county hospital	general peds clin	RecRev	3, 14, 19, 20
Sansonnet- Hayden et al. 1987	17 12–18	psych unit patients	NA psych	DISC	13, 14, 19, 20
Scott & Stone 1986	22 15–20	CSA tx program	NA	MMPI DQ	3, 4, 13, 19
Stiffman 1989	141 12–18	shelter homes for runaway youth (N = 28 SA + 128 PA)	NA runaways	CBCL BDI, Int, PMS, ALCEQ, RSES	2
Tong et al. 1987	49 5–19	prior evaluation by CSA team	school	Int PHCSCS CBCL, TRF, YSR	1, 2, 3, 5, 13, 19, 20
Waterman et al. 1990	97 5–14	ref from therapists (N = 82 alleged ritual/ SA + 15 confirmed SA by teacher)	community source of controls	CBCL WISC-R PIAT Harter LFS TRF DAP KFD ISB Rorschach	1,2,13
White et al. 1986	25 2–5.6 Int	ref to CSA eval program	NA pre- schoolers	SAC Doll	13
White et al. 1988	17 2–7	hosp sex abuse tx program neglect tx program	hosp staff	MCDI SAS kids +	1,2,3,4, 13,20
Yates et al. 1985	18G 3–17	psych clinic ref	NA non	DAP	13

[a] For abbreviations, see Appendix at the end of the chapter.

TABLE 4–2

UNCONTROLLED STUDIES AND CASE REPORTS[A]

(N = 22)

Author Year	Abused No. Ages	Source of Subjects	Measures	Criteria Supported
Adams-Tucker 1982	28 2–15	child guidance clinic	clin eval LBCL	1, 3, 13, 19, 20
Becker 1988	27 12–19	sex offender tx program	clin int	13
Bender & Blau 1937	16 5–12	child psych	clin eval unit	1, 3, 4, 9, 13, 19
Brant & Tisza 1977		hosp ER & peds gynecology clin	clin eval	13
Browning & Boatman 1977	14 4–15	child psychiatry clin	clin eval	4, 13, 14
Burgess & Hartman 1987	12 6–9	eval for civil suit questions	drawings	1, 6, 14
Burns et al. 1988	87 2–5	national study of molest in preschools	ChList	3, 4, 13, 14
Ferenczi 1932	adults	psychoanalytic practice	Tx	1, 4, 7, 11, 13
Fisher 1983	26 13–18	clin sample included committed for crimes	ISE Behav Sx ChLst	2, 3, 4, 5, 7, 13, 14, 19, 20
Freud 1896	18 adults	psychoanalytic practice	Tx	
Johnson 1988	47 4–13	child perpetrator Tx group	Eval tx	13, 19
Kiser et al. 1988	10 2–10	child psych clin	VidFamInt FES, FILEC, DAS, MCMI, MCDI, PIC, CBCL	1, 3, 4, 13, 14, 19

Author Year	Abused No. Ages	Source of Subjects	Measures	Criteria Supported
Lewis & Sarrel 1969	2–18	child psych practice	clin eval Tx	2, 3, 13, 14, 19
Lindberg & Distad 1985	27 12–18	placement for dependent children	Tx	1, 2, 3, 7, 13, 14, 20
Mannarino & Cohen 1986	45 3–16 Clin eval	child welfare ref Sx due to sex abuse	ChLst IQ test	2, 3, 4, 13, 14
McLeer et al. 1988	31 3–16	child psych clinic	structured int SEI, STAIC, CDI, CBCL	2, 14
Mian et al. 1985	125 0–6	hospital sex abuse team	medical RecRev	13
Peters 1976	64 2–12	rape crisis centers	clin eval	3
Shengold 1979	2	psychoanalytic adultspractice	psych tx	4, 5, 7, 19
Sirles et al. 1989	207 2–17	intrafamilial sex abuse tx program	clin eval RecRev	4, 14, 19
Summit 1983	2,000+ all	varied as consult to many programs	consult Tx	1, 4, 5, 7, 10, 13, 19, 20
Yates et al. 1985	40 children	child psych practice	clin eval	13, 14

[a]For abbreviations, see Appendix at the end of the chapter.

TABLE 4–3
CONSENSUS, GUIDELINES, REVIEWS, AND SURVEYS

Author	Source of Subjects	Criteria Supported	Year
AMA	Council on Scientific Affairs, Advisory Panel on Child Abuse	2, 3, 11, 13, 20	1985
Boat & Everson	295 police, CPS, physicians, & mental health professionals	13	1988
Conte et al.	212 recognized experts of eval of suspected child sexual abuse	3, 13, 14, 19, 20	1988
Corwin	two interdisciplinary consensus meetings on diagnosing CSA, 1985–1986	3, 4, 5, 6, 7, 13, 19, 20	1988
Finkelhor & Browne	review of the literature & conceptualization of types of effects	1, 2, 3, 4, 7, 8, 9, 13, 14, 19, 20	1985
Kohan et al.	110 child & adolescent psych hosp comparing 325 SA patients to NA	3, 13, 19, 20	1987

appropriate diagnosis for some sexually abused children, there remains a need for development of a diagnostic category that more specifically encompasses the behavioral and emotional difficulties commonly found among sexually abused children and adolescents (Corwin, 1988).

The increasingly sophisticated research into the effects of sexual abuse on children and adolescents provides much new and relevant information for this review. Although these studies raise new questions, the exploration of which will require more years of specific inquiry, a number of important facts are currently well established. It is now clear that sexual victimization is associated with significant detrimental effects. It has also been empirically demonstrated that these effects differentiate some groups of sexually abused children from those with no known history of sexual abuse, including groups of nonreferred, neglected, physically abused, and other clinically referred children (see Table 4–1). This analysis focuses on the clinical, empirical, and consensus support for the various symptoms found among different groups of sexually abused young

TABLE 4–4

SUPPORT FROM 33 CONTROLLED STUDIES

Proposed symptoms[a]	Number of Studies
(1) Ineffectiveness	10
(2) Damaged for good	9
(3) Distrust	16
(4) Anger disharmony	7
(5) Minimizing	2
(6) Amnesia for victim	—
(7) Responsible for	1
(8) Revictimization	—
(9) Perpetrator beliefs	—
(10) Idealization of perpetrator	—
(11) Shame & stigma	—
(12) Revenge on perpetrator	—
(13) Sexual disharmony	25
(14) Despair & hopeless	15
(15) Disillusionment	—
(16) Preoccupation	—
(17) Invulnerability	—
(18) None understand	—
(19) Victimize others	16
(20) Self-destructive	8

Other Reported Symptoms

Anxiety, fears, phobias	11
Attention problems	3x
Cross-dressing	1
Eating disturbances	—
Encopresis/enuresis	—
Delinquency	2
Difficulty with parents	3
Dissociation	1
Emotional inhibition	1
Friendly toward strangers	1
Hyperactivity	5
Identity confusion	1
Lower verbal IQ	1
Nightmares	2
Obsessions	2
Psychosis	4
Psychosomatic concerns	13
Regressive behavior	2
Running away	1
School problems	3
Sleep problems	2
Substance abuse	—
Underachievement	4

[a]Proposed symptoms of the Disorders of Extreme Distress Not Otherwise Specified psychiatric category.

people and the degree to which this data suggests that the proposed Disorder of Extreme Stress Not Otherwise Specified would provide a suitable diagnostic category for symptomatic victims of such abuse.

SYMPTOMS AMONG SEXUALLY ABUSED CHILDREN AND ADOLESCENTS AND THE PROPOSED DISORDERS

Table 4–4 summarizes the number of comparative studies listed in Table 4–1 that support each of the 20 proposed symptoms of the Disorders of Extreme Stress Not Otherwise Specified. Symptoms found among sexually abused children and adolescents that are not among those 20 are also included. Table 4–5 provides a similar analysis of the uncontrolled studies and case reports listed in Table 4–2, and Table 4–6 does the same for Table 4–3, the consensus, guideline, survey, or review references. Table 4–7 condenses the information on the proximate symptoms of child sexual abuse from that compiled in 1984 by Gomes-Schwartz et al. Review of these tables demonstrates a very similar pattern of support for a number of symptoms.

Of the 20 proposed symptoms, 10 receive at least some support from comparative studies. In order of decreasing support followed by the percentage of references supporting each symptom, they are:

1.   #13—overinhibition or excessive expression of sexual drive (e.g., lack of sexual drive following rape, promiscuity following sexual abuse) 76%

2.   #3—inability to trust or to be intimate with others 48%

3.   #19—victimizing others in the same way that one was victimized (e.g., adult victim of child abuse abuses own child) 48%

4.   #14—despair and hopelessness about future 45%

5.   #1—a generalized sense of being ineffective in dealing with one's environment that is not limited to the victimization experience, ranging from lack of confidence in one's own judgment to total immobilization 30%

TABLE 4–5

SUPPORT FROM 22 UNCONTROLLED STUDIES OR CASE REPORTS

Proposed Symptoms[a]	Number of Studies
(1) Ineffectiveness	7
(2) Damaged for good	4
(3) Distrust	8
(4) Anger disharmony	7
(5) Minimization	2
(6) Amnesia for victim	1
(7) Responsible for	4
(8) Revictimization	—
(9) Perpetrator beliefs	—
(10) Idealization of perpetrator	1
(11) Shame and stigma	1
(12) Revenge on perpetrator	—
(13) Sexual disharmony	15
(14) Despair & hopeless	9
(15) Disillusionment	—
(16) Preoccupation	—
(17) Invulnerability	—
(18) None understand	—
(19) Victimize others	7
(20) Self-destructive	3

Other Reported Symptoms

Anxiety, fears, phobias	12
Attention problems	2
Delinquency	2
Denial	1
Difficulty with parents	1
Dissociation	3
Disruptive behavior	1
Eating disturbances	3
Encopresis/enuresis	4
Homosexuality	1
Hyperactivity	2
Hysterical symptoms	2
Impulsivity	2
Learning disabilities	1
Low frustration tolerance	1
Lying	1
Nail biting	1
Nightmares	5
Obsessions	1
Perfectionism	1
Precocious Maturity	2
Psychosis	2
Psychosomatic complaints	5
Regressive behavior	3
Role reversal	1
Running away	4
School problems	6
Sleep problems	7
Speech problems	1
Splitting	2
Substance abuse	4
Tics	1
Toilet training problems	1

[a]Proposed symptoms of the Disorders of Extreme Distress Not Otherwise Specified psychiatric category.

6.   #2—the belief that one has been permanently damaged by the victimization experience (e.g., a sexually abused child or rape victim believing that he or she will never be attractive to others) 27%

7.   #20—physically self-destructive acts (e.g., self-mutilation) 24%

8   #4—overinhibition of anger or excessive expression of anger 21%

9   #5—inappropriate minimizing of the injuries that were inflicted 6%

10.   #7—exaggerated sense of responsibility for the victimization experience (e.g., belief that one could have prevented the victimization despite obvious evidence to the contrary) 3%

The uncontrolled studies and case reports, Table 4–5, provide additional support for these 10 symptoms in slightly different order of percentages: #13 (68%); #14 (40%); #3 (36%); #1, #4, and #19 (31%); #2 and #7 (18%); #20 (13%); #5 (9%). This category also includes one reference supporting 3 more of the 20 original criteria:

11.   #6—amnesia for the victimization experiences 4%

12.   #10—inappropriate idealization of the perpetrator or paradoxical gratitude (e.g., hostage victim feels gratitude for not having been killed) 4%

13.   #11—persistent shame, embarrassment, or humiliation regarding others' knowledge of the victimization experience 4%

Table 4–6 demonstrates further support for those symptoms listed above in the following order and percentages: #13 (100%); #3 and #20 (83%); #19 (67%); #2, #4, #7, and #14 (33%); #1, #5, #6, and #11 (17%). Two more symptoms found the support of one reference from this group of works:

14.   #8—increased vulnerability to being revictimized by a different perpetrator 17%

15.   #9—adopting the distorted beliefs of the perpetrator with regard to interpersonal behavior (e.g., believing that it is okay for parents to have sex with their children or that it is okay for a husband to beat his wife to keep her obedient) 17%

TABLE 4–6
SUPPORT FROM SIX CONSENSUS, GUIDELINE,
SURVEY OR REVIEW REFERENCES

Proposed Symptoms[a]	Number of References
(1) Ineffectiveness	1
(2) Damaged for good	2
(3) Distrust	5
(4) Anger disharmony	2
(5) Minimization	1
(6) Amnesia for victim	1
(7) Responsible for	2
(8) Revictimization	1
(9) Perpetrator beliefs	1
(10) Idealization of perpetrator	—
(11) Shame and stigma	1
(12) Revenge on perpetrator	—
(13) Sexual disharmony	6
(14) Despair & hopeless	2
(15) Disillusionment	—
(16) Preoccupation	—
(17) Invulnerability	—
(18) None understand	—
(19) Victimize others	4
(20) Self-destructive	5

Other Reported Symptoms

Anxiety, fears, phobias	5
Aggression disharmony	1
Compliant	1
Cross-dressing	1
Cruel	1
Delinquency	1
Denial	1
Dependency	1
Dissociation	2
Eating disturbances	1
Encopresis/enuresis	2
Hyperactivity	1
Lying	1
Nightmares	2
Precocious maturity	2
Psychosomatic complaints	3
Regressive behavior	3
Running away	2
School problems	2
Sleep problems	2
Speech problems	1
Substance abuse	2

[a]Proposed symptoms of the Disorders of Extreme Distress Not Otherwise Specified psychiatric category.

Findings from the 1984 review by Gomes-Schwartz are summarized in Table 4–7 for comparison to the preceding tables. This earlier review reinforces eight of the above symptoms in the following order and percentages: #13 (55%); #14 (48%); #7 (45%); #3 (39%); #19 (36%); #20 (30%); #4 (24%); #2 (5%).

Tables 4–4 through 4–7 also show that a number of other symptoms have support from the literature:

Percentages of References Supporting

	Table 4–4	Table 4–5	Table 4–6	Table 4–7
Anxiety, fears, and phobias	33	54	83	23
Delinquency	6	9	16	10
Dissociation	3	13	33	0
Eating disturbances	0	9	16	15
Hyperactivity	15	9	16	9
Nightmares	6	22	33	0
Psychosis	12	9	0	9
Psychosomatic concerns	39	22	50	9
Regressive behavior	6	13	50	27
Running away	3	18	33	48
School problems	9	27	33	39
Sleep problems	6	31	33	11
Substance abuse	0	18	33	21

OTHER FINDINGS

Cohen and Mannarino (1988) and Tong, Oates, and McDowell (1987) included parent and/or teacher ratings as well as self-report from the sexually abused children and adolescents whom they studied. Both of these investigations found that the victims tend to deny or minimize problems that are clearly noted by parents or teachers. This observation may help explain the lack of any significant findings in DiPietro's study (1987), which used siblings and matched sibling pairs as comparisons but did not obtain parental or teacher reports.

Two investigations confirm that the most discriminating effect of child sexual victimization is its impact on sexual behavior. Friedrich, Beilke, and Urquiza (1988) and Kolko, Moser, and Weldy (1988) found that 49% of the variance between the sexually abused and nonabused children they studied was explained by sexual behavior. In the Friedrich study an additional 10% of the variance was accounted for by another factor the authors called Gender Issues. Kolko's study found another 5% was associated with a fear/mistrust factor.

TABLE 4–7

SUPPORT FROM 1984 REVIEW OF SHORT-TERM SYMPTOMS OF CHILD
SEXUAL ABUSE IN 33 REFERENCES BY GOMES-SCHWARTZ ET AL.

Proposed Symptoms[a]	Number of References
(1) Ineffectiveness	—
(2) Damaged for good	5
(3) Distrust	13
(4) Anger disharmony	8
(5) Minimization	—
(6) Amnesia for victim	—
(7) Responsible for	15
(8) Revictimization	—
(9) Perpetrator beliefs	—
(10) Idealization of perpetrator	—
(11) Shame and stigma	—
(12) Revenge on perpetrator	—
(13) Sexual disharmony	18
(14) Despair & hopeless	16
(15) Disillusionment	—
(16) Preoccupation	—
(17) Invulnerability	—
(18) None understand	—
(19) Victimize others	12
(20) Self-destructive	10

Other Reported Symptoms

Anxiety, fears, phobias	23
Delinquency	10
Eating disturbances	5
Encopresis/enuresis	1
Hyperactivity	3
Hysterical symptoms	7
Psychosis	3
Psychosomatic complaints	3
Regressive behavior	9
Running away	16
School problems	13
Sleep problems	11
Substance abuse	7

[a]Proposed symptoms of the Disorders of Extreme Distress Not Otherwise
Specified psychiatric category.

Both of these findings are consistent with the majority of studies cited that found clear differences in these areas. Aiosa-Karpas, Pelcovitz, et al. (1991) also found significant gender identity conflict among the female incest victims they studied.

One of the nine comparative studies that found lower self-esteem among sexually abused children and adolescents was also able to identify accurately a high percentage of abused subjects from nonabused controls with self-esteem-related factors. Cavaiola and Schiff (1989) compared 150 chemically dependent adolescent victims of physical and/or sexual abuse to 60 randomly selected chemically dependent youths treated at the same residential drug treatment program but who denied any history of abuse and 60 randomly selected nonchemically dependent nonabused students from nine suburban, urban, and rural high schools in the same general geographic area as the treatment center. On the Tennessee Self-Concept Scale the authors found significantly lower scores for the abused subjects on each of the instrument's eight subscales (p <.001). With discriminant function analysis the authors were able to develop a formula that successfully classified 88.7% of the abused subjects. The Identity and Moral-Ethical subscales were the best predictors for this purpose.

Three articles specifically addressed the relationship between PTSD and child sexual abuse (Deblinger, McLeer, Atkins, et al., 1989); Kiser, Ackerman, Brown, et al., 1988; McLeer, Deblinger, Atkins, et al., 1988). McLeer et al. (1988) found that 48.4% of 31 sexually abused children being seen in a psychiatric outpatient clinic met DSM-III-R criteria for PTSD. This same group of researchers report in an article by Deblinger et al. (1989) that in a retrospective blind chart review of 29 sexually abused child psychiatric inpatients, 20 of whom were also physically abused, only 20.7% met PTSD criteria compared to 6.9% of 29 matched physically abused and 10.3% matched nonabused children. In Deblinger et al., the authors point out a significant limitation of their chart review being that it is subject to the record keeping and diagnostic biases of the original clinicians. Finkelhor (1987) discusses, from a theoretical perspective the limitations of using PTSD to describe the psychological injury to sexually abused children.

Contrary to the frequent assumption that intrafamilial child sexual abuse is more harmful to its victims than extrafamilial sexual abuse due to the increased sense of betrayal in the victims and or distortions in the dynamics of incestuous families, Basta and Peterson (1990) and Mannarino, Cohen, and Gregor (1989) found no significant difference between these two groups of victims. Based on these findings, Mannarino et al. assert that the pathological effect of child sexual victimization may be more related to the sexual abuse itself than to the family dynamics surrounding it.

Friedrich (1988) and White and her associates (1988) compared the effect of sexual victimization on boys to its effect on girls. Both studies found significant differences in symptoms between boys and girls as well as between abused and nonabused children. For example, as girls approach adolescence, both sexually abused and nonabused obtain similar scores on Friedrich's Child Sexual Behavior inventory. Sexually abused boys in the Friedrich sample showed a different pattern of symptom evolution scoring significantly higher on the inventory at all ages from 2–12 years except for age 6. White and her co-workers found numerous significant differences between the sexually abused male and female preschoolers they studied. In view of these findings, White et al. suggest that studies that do not analyze data separately for each sex may well miss significant findings because effects in one gender can obscure findings in the other.

DISCUSSION

One readily apparent observation in comparing Tables 4–4 through 4–7 is the similarity in the pattern of symptoms reported in the various literatures on sexually abused children and adolescents. The comparative studies support many of the clinical observations of earlier references, and the consensus, guidelines, and survey findings provide a measure of present agreement among experienced clinicians. Each of these categories of information provide a particular perspective on the effects of sexual victimization on children and adolescents. Although comparative studies offer the most statistically validated information, they are more restricted in their view. Not all aspects of young victims' psychological and behavioral reactions to sexual abuse are equally amenable to comparative research. Negative symptoms, such as denial or minimizing and internal processes such as thoughts and feelings, are more difficult to study than are behaviors. Developmental limitations and changes provide additional complexity when attempting to formulate a category that is useful for all age groups including adults. Justifiable concerns regarding possible adverse effects on human subjects preclude many inquiries. Critical consideration of clinical observations, statistical analyses, and professional consensus provides the most balanced and comprehensive understanding of current knowledge on the effects of sexual abuse on children and adolescents.

Of particular relevance to the proposed Disorders of Extreme Stress Not Otherwise Specified is the "fit" between the known effects of sexual victimization on children and adolescents and the proposed symptoms for the disorder. This review suggests that a few changes in the wording of several proposed symptoms for the Disorders of Extreme Stress Not Otherwise Specified would increase its "fit" for sexually abused children and adolescents. Criteria that warrant this "fine tuning" include:

#2 Children and adolescents rarely acknowledge feeling permanently damaged by sexual abuse. What clinicians and researchers frequently observe is lower self-esteem in these victims. In preparing this review, findings of low self-esteem were reported as supportive of this particular criteria.

#3 In this review, the most frequent clinical and psychometric finding related to this criteria is "social withdrawal." This symptom should include those words.

#13 There are other effects in this area related to the premature and distorted sexualization associated with child sexual abuse. In addition to overinhibition or excessive expression of sexual behavior, other cognitive changes such as gender identity conflict and sexual preoccupation may occur that may not be manifested directly in sexual behavior during any particular time frame.

#14 The most frequently noted clinical or psychometric finding related to this symptom is "depression." Perhaps this symptom should include the words "sadness and depression."

#19 This criteria should be "victimizing others" without specification of "as victimized." There is a pattern of some victimized children becoming victimizers but not always in the same way that they were victimized, e.g., Seghorn et al. (1987) found more than twice (58% vs. 23%) as much physical abuse as sexual abuse in the background of a group of incarcerated rapists.

Another refinement that would increase the "fit" of the proposed disorder with this group of victims would be the inclusion of some of the symptoms shown above that are often reported among sexually abused children and adolescents but are not included among the 20 original suggested criteria. Leading contenders for addition are:

anxiety, fear and phobias	school problems
dissociative symptoms	substance abuse
nightmares and sleep disorders	regressive behaviors
psychosomatic symptoms	

Perhaps aggression should be included in the same manner as anger and sexual behavior, which would allow for inclusion with either inhibition or excessive expression. On Tables 4–4 through 4–7 the word "disharmony" is used to describe this polarization of affect or behavior toward opposite ends of a continuum.

When considering cases in which PTSD may overlap with the proposed Disorders of Extreme Stress Not Otherwise Specified, sexual behavior deserves further examination. Are the various sexual behaviors noted among sexually abused children always reenactments of the sexual abuse, or are they in some instances the result of premature and distorted activation of sexual capacities? Ferenczi (1932) wrote of a "traumatic progression, of a precocious maturity" as a consequence of sexual victimization during childhood. The answer to this question may, in some cases, determine which diagnostic criteria are met. Judgments on whether particular sexualized behavior is a reenactment or a prematurely awakened capacity might yield considerably different results in research that attempts to examine the overlap between PTSD and the proposed Disorders of Extreme Stress Not Otherwise Specified.

Clinical work and research on syndromes is often confronted with the challenge of discriminating those symptoms that are a product of the condition from those which antedated it. There are, as yet, no longitudinal studies of sexually abused children and adolescents to provide a definitive answer to this dilemma. It is easier in individual clinical evaluations to explore this problem through comprehensive history taking and review of pertinent information, such as school records, than to prove it empirically. The number and diversity of well-designed studies of sexually abused children that have found very similar effects showing significant differences between abused and nonabused groups certainly suggests that the differences are associated with the sexual abuse, but more research on this question is warranted.

A significant weakness in most of the existing studies on the effects of sexual victimization on children and adolescents is the use of relatively small numbers of clinically referred subjects. At this time several large studies are underway, and more will certainly follow. The results of these and other such extensive investigations will increase our understanding of this kind of victimization. The use of clinically referred victims of child sexual abuse may diminish the generalizability of findings to all sexually victimized children and adolescents, but it may also be the most appropriate method for learning about those victims who are most adversely affected by these experiences.

CONCLUSION

This review demonstrates that sexually abused children and adolescents commonly demonstrate a cluster of symptoms, some of which discriminate groups of sexually victimized from physically abused children and from nonabused children. There now exists a significant and rapidly growing body of research that substantiates many earlier clinical reports and impressions. These findings fit many of the proposed criteria for the Disorders of Extreme Stress Not Otherwise Specified. A number of refinements and possible additions are suggested.

That a diagnosis should suggest a treatment is an important organizing principle in medicine. Summit (1989) asserts the importance for therapists who treat child sexual abuse survivors to recognize the "centrality of victimization" in order to focus the patient's treatment and recovery. The development of a diagnostic category suitable for survivors of victimization including sexually abused children and adolescents would help educate therapists to recognize the psychological effects of victimization. Such a category would also validate victims' access to mental health care and help focus their treatment. Improved access to appropriate treatment will, hopefully, increase the number of victimized children, adolescents, and adults, who truly become survivors.

REFERENCES

Adams-Tucker, C. (1982). Proximate effects of sexual abuse in child-hood: a report on 28 children. *American Journal of Psychiatry* 139:1252–1256.

Aiosa-Karpas C.; Karpas, R.; Pelcovitz, D.; Kaplan S.; (1991). Gender identification and sex role attribution in sexually abused adolescent females. *Journal of the American Academy of Child Adolescent Psychiatry* 30: 266–271.

American Medical Association (1985). AMA Diagnostic and Treatment Guidelines Concerning Child Abuse and Neglect. *JAMA* 254:796–800.

Basta, S.M., & Peterson, R.F. (1990). Perpetrator status and the person-ality characteristics of molested children. *Child Abuse and Neglect* 14: 555–566.

Becker, J.J. (1988). The effects of child sexual abuse on adolescent sexual offenders. In G.E. Wyatt & G.J. Powell (eds.), *Lasting Effects of Child Sexual Abuse*. Newbury Park, Calif.: Sage.

Bender, L., & Blau, A. (1937). The reaction of children to sexual relations with adults. *American Journal of Orthopsychiatry* 7:500–518.

Boat, B., & Everson, M. (1988). Use of anatomical dolls among professionals in sexual abuse evaluations. *Child Abuse and Neglect* 12: 171–179.

Brant, R.S.T., & Tisza, V.B. (1977). The sexually misused child. *American Journal of Orthopsychiatry* 47:80–90.

Browne, A., & Finkelhor, D. (1986). Initial and long-term effects: a review of the research. In D. Finkelhor (ed.), *Sourcebook of Child Sexual Abuse*. Newbury Park, Calif.: Sage.

Browning, D.H., & Boatman, B. (1977). Incest: Children at risk. *American Journal Psychiatry* 134: 69–72.

Burgess, A.W.; Hartman, C.R.; & McCormack, A. (1987). Abused to abuser: antecedents of socially deviant behaviors. *American Journal of Psychiatry* 144:1431–1436.

Burgess, A.W.; Hartman, C.R.; Wolbert, W.A.; & Grant, C.A. (1987). Child molestation: assessing impact in multiple victims. *Archives of Psychiatric Nursing* 1(1):33–39.

Burns, N.; Williams, L.M.; & Finkelhor, D. (1988). Victim impact. In D. Finkelhor & L.M. Williams (eds.), *Nursery Crimes: Sexual Abuse in Day Care*. Newbury Park, Calif.: Sage.

Cavaiola, A.A., & Schiff, M. (1988). Behavioral sequelae of physical and/or sexual abuse in adolescents. *Child Abuse and Neglect* 12:181–188.

Cavaiola, A.A., & Schiff, M, (1989). Self-esteem in abused chemically dependent adolescents. *Child Abuse and Neglect* 13:327–334.

Cohen, J.A., & Mannarino, A.P. (1988). Psychological symptoms in sexually abused girls. *Child Abuse and Neglect* 12:571–577.

Conte, J.R., & Schuerman, J.R. (1988). The effects of sexual abuse on children: a multidimensional view. In G.E. Wyatt & G.J. Powell (eds.), *Lasting Effects of Child Sexual Abuse*. Newbury Park, Calif.: Sage.

Conte, J.[R.]; Sorenson, E.; & Fogarty, L.; et al. (1988). Evaluating children's reports of sexual abuse: results from a survey of professionals. Report of project funded by the U.S. Department of Health and Human Services and the Illinois Department of Children and Family Services.

Corwin, D.L. (1988). Early diagnosis of child sexual abuse: diminishing the lasting effects. In G.E. Wyatt & G.J. Powell, (eds.), *Lasting Effects of Child Sexual Abuse*. Newbury Park, Calif.: Sage.

Deblinger, E.; McLeer, S.V.; & Atkins, M.S.; et al. (1989). Post-traumatic stress in sexually abused and non-abused children. *Child Abuse and Neglect* 13:403–408.

DiPietro, S.B. (1987). The effects of intrafamilial child sexual abuse on the adjustment and attitudes of adolescents. *Violence and Victims* 2:59–78.

Einbender, A.J., & Friedrich, W.N. (1989). Psychological functioning and behavior of sexually abused girls. *Journal of Consulting and Clinical Psychology* 57:155–157.

Ferenczi, S. (1932). Confusion of tongues between adults and the child: the language of tenderness and of passion. In M. Balint (ed.) & E. Mosbacher (ed.), *Final Contributions to the Problems and Methods of Psycho-Analysis*. New York: Basic Books.

Finkelhor, D. (1987). The trauma of child sexual abuse: two models. *Journal of Interpersonal Violence* 2:348–366.

Finkelhor, D., & Browne A. (1985). The traumatic impact of child sexual abuse: a conceptualization. *American Journal of Orthopsychiatry* 55:530–541.

Fischer, M. (1983). Adolescent adjustment after incest. *School Psychology International* 4:217–222.

Freud, S. (1962).The etiology of hysteria. In *The Standard Edition of the Complete Psychological Works of Sigmund Freud*. Ed. & trans. J. Strachey. London: Hogarth. Originally published 1896.

Friedrich, W.N. (1988). Behavior problems in sexually abused children: an adaptational perspective. In G.E. Wyatt & G.J. Powell (eds.), *Lasting Effects of Child Sexual Abuse*. Newbury Park, Calif.: Sage.

Friedrich, W.N.; Beilke, R.L.; & Urquiza, A.J. (1988). Behavior problems in young sexually abused boys. *Journal of Interpersonal Violence* 3:21–27.

Friedrich, W.N.; Grambsch, P.; & Broughton, D.; et al. (1991). Normative sexual behavior in children. *Pediatrics* 88:456–464.

Gale, J.; Thompson, R.J.; Moran, T.; & Sack, W.H. (1988). Sexual abuse in young children: its clinical presentation and characteristic patterns. *Child Abuse and Neglect* 12:163–170.

Gomes-Schwartz, B.; Horowitz, J.; & Sauzier, M. (1985). Severity of emotional distress among sexually abused preschool, school age, and adolescent children. *Hospital and Community Psychiatry* 36:503–508.

Gomes-Schwartz, B.; Horwitz, J.; & Sauzier, M. (1984). Sexually abused children: service and research project. Office of Juvenile Justice and Delinquency Prevention, Washington, D.C.: U.S. Government Printing Office.

Green, A.H. (1988). Child maltreatment and its victims: a comparison of physical and sexual abuse. *Psychiatric Clinics of North America* 11 (4): 591–610.

Grogan, M.C. (1988). A comparative investigation of the behavioral and projective patterns of three groups of latency age females. Doctoral dissertation, California Graduate School of Family Psychology, San Rafael.

Haugaard, J.J., & Reppucci, N.D. (1988). *The Sexual Abuse of Children*. San Francisco: Jossey-Bass.

Jampole, L., & Weber, M.K. (1987). An assessment of the behavior of sexually abused and nonsexually abused children with anatomically correct dolls. *Child Abuse and Neglect* 11:182–187.

Janus, M.D.; Burgess, A.W.; & McCormack. A. (1987). Histories of sexual abuse in adolescent male runaways. *Adolescence* 22:405–417.

Johnson, T.C. (1988). Child perpetrators—children who molest other children: preliminary findings. *Child Abuse and Neglect* 12:219–229.

Kiser, L.J.; Ackerman, B.J.; Brown, E.; et al. (1988). Post-traumatic stress disorder in young children: a reaction to purported sexual abuse. *Journal of the American Academy of Child & Adolescent Psychiatry* 27:645–649.

Kohan, M.J.; Pothier, P.; & Norbeck, J.S. (1987). Hospitalized children with history of sexual abuse: incidence and care issues. *American Journal of Orthopsychiatry* 67:258–264.

Kolko, D.J.; & Moser, T.M.; Weldy, S.R. (1988). Behavioral/emotional indicators of sexual abuse in child psychiatric inpatients: a controlled comparison with physical abuse. *Child Abuse and Neglect* 12:529–541.

Lewis, M., & Sarrel, P.M. (1969). Some psychological aspects of seduction, incest, and rape in childhood. *Journal of the American Academy of Child and Adolescent Psychiatry* 8:606–619.

Lindberg, F.H., & Distad, L.J. (1985). Survival responses to incest: adolescents in crisis. *Child Abuse and Neglect* 9:521–526.

Lipovsky, J.A.; Saunders, B.E.; & Murphy, S.M. (1989). Depression, anxiety, and behavioral problems among victims of father-child sexual assault and nonabused siblings. *Journal of Interpersonal Violence* 4:452–468.

Livingston, R. (1987). Sexually and physically abused children. *Journal of the American Academy of Child and Adolescent Psychiatry* 26:413–415.

McLeer, S.V.; Deblinger, E.; & Atkins, M.S.; et al. (1988). Post-traumatic stress disorder in sexually abused children. *Journal of the American Academy of Child and Adolescent Psychiatry* 27:650–654.

Mannarino, A.P., & Cohen, J.A. (1986). A clinical-demographic study of sexually abused children. *Child Abuse and Neglect* 10:17–23.

Mannarino, A.P.; Cohen, J.A.; & Gregor, M. (1989). Emotional and behavioral difficulties in sexually abused girls. *Journal of Interpersonal Violence* 4:437–451.

Masson, J.M. (1984). *The Assault on Truth: Freud's Suppression of the Seduction Theory*. New York: Penguin.

Mian, M.; Wehrnspann, W.; & Klajner-Diamond, H., et al. (1985). Review of 125 children 6 years of age and under who were sexually abused. *Child Abuse and Neglect* 10:223–229.

Orr, D.P., & Downes, M.C. (1985). Self-concept of adolescent sexual abuse victims. *Journal of Youth and Adolescence* 14:401–410.

Peters, J.J. (1976). Children who are victims of sexual assault and the psychology of offenders. *American Journal of Psychotherapy* 30 (5):398–421.

Rimsza, M.E., & Berg, R.A. (1988). Sexual abuse: somatic and emotional reactions. *Child Abuse and Neglect* 12:201–208.

Sansonnet-Hayden, H.; Haley, G., & Marriage, K., et al. (1987). Sexual abuse and psychopathology in hospitalized adolescents. *Journal of the American Academy of Child and Adolescent Psychiatry* 26:753–757.

Scott, L.R., & Stone, D.A. (1986). MMPI profile constellations in incest families. *Journal of Consulting and Clinical Psychology* 54 (3):364–368.

Seghorn, T.K.; Prentky, R.A.; & Boucher, R.J. (1987). Childhood sexual abuse in the lives of sexually aggressive offenders. *Journal of the American Academy of Child and Adolescent Psychiatry* 26:262–267.

Shengold, L.L. (1979). Child abuse and deprivation: soul murder. *Journal of the American Psychoanalytic Association* 27 (3):533–559.

Sirles, E.A.; Smith, J.A.; & Kusama, H. (1989). Psychiatric status of intrafamilial child sexual abuse victims. *Journal of the American Academy of Child and Adolescent Psychiatry* 28:225–229.

Sivan, A.B.; Schor, D.P.; & Koeppl, G.K.; et al. (1988). Interaction of normal children with anatomical dolls. *Child Abuse and Neglect* 12:295–304.

Sloane, P., & Karpinski, E. (1942). Effects of incest on the participants. *American Journal of Orthopsychiatry*, 1942; 12:666–673.

Stiffman, A.R. (1989). Physical and sexual abuse in runaway youths. *Child Abuse and Neglect* 13:417–426.

Summit, R.C. (1989). The centrality of victimization: regaining the focal point of recovery for survivors of child sexual abuse. *Psychiatric Clinics of North America* 12:413–430.

Summit, R.C. (1983). The child sexual abuse accommodation syndrome. *Child Abuse and Neglect* 7:177–193.

Tong, L.; Oates, K.; & McDowell, M. (1987). Personality development following sexual abuse. *Child Abuse and Neglect* 11:371–383.

van der Kolk, B.; Pelcovitz, D.; & Herman, J.; et al. (1991). Structured interview for Disorders of Extreme Stress—Not Otherwise Specified. (Available from first author.) Massachusetts Mental Health Center, Boston, February 10.

Waterman, J.; Kelly, R.; & Oliveri, M.K.; et al. (1989). Manhattan Beach molestation study. Summary for NCCAN grantees meeting, Washington, D.C.: March.

White, S.; Halpin, B.M.; & Strom, G.A.; et al. (1988). Behavioral comparisons of young sexually abused, neglected, and nonreferred children. *Journal of Clinical Child Psychology* 17:53–61.

White, S.; Strom, G.A.; & Santilli, G. et al. (1986). Interviewing young sexual abuse victims with anatomically correct dolls. *Child Abuse and Neglect* 10:519–529.

Yates, A. (1982). Children eroticized by incest. *American Journal of Psychiatry* 139:482–485.

Yates, A.; Beutler, L.E.; & Crago, M. (1985). Drawings by child victims of incest. *Child Abuse and Neglect* 9:183–189.

APPENDIX

A glossary of the abbreviations used.

Adol	Adolescent
ALCEQ	Adolescent Life Change Events Questionnaire
B	Boys
BAI-RSF	Bell Adjustment Inventory–Revised, Student Form
BDI	Beck's Depression Inventory
BEHAV	Behavior
CBCL	Children's Behavior Checklist
CBP	Children's Behavior Profile
CDI	Children's Depression Inventory
ChLst	Checklist
Clin	Clinic, clinical
CPQ	Children's Personality Questionnaire
CPS	Children's protective services
CSA	Child Sexual Abuse
CSBI	Child Sexual Behavior Inventory
D, Ds	Disorder, disorders
DAP	Draw A Person
DE	Deprivation-enhancement fantasy patterns
DICA	Diagnostic Inventory for Children and Adolescents

DISC	Diagnostic Inventory Schedule for Children
DQ	Demographic questionnaire
Empl	Employee
EPI	Eysenck Personality Inventory
ER	Emergency Room
Eval	Evaluation
FACES	Family Adaptability and Cohesion Evaluation Scales
FES: C,E,C	Family Environmental Scale: Conflict, Expressiveness, and Cohesion
G	Girls
GRAS	Gender Role Assessment Schedule
GICS	Gender Identity Conflict Scale
Hosp	Hospital
IE	Internal-External Scale
Inpat	Inpatient
Int	Interview
ISB	Incomplete Sentences Blank
ISE	Index of Self-esteem
KFD	Kinetic Family Drawing
LBCL	Louisville Behavior Checklist
LE	Life events
LFS	Louisville Fear Survey
MCDI	Minnesota Child Development Inventory

Men	Mental
MFES	Moos Family Environmental Scale
MMPI	Minnesota Multiphasic Personality Inventory
NA	Nonabused
OSIQ	Offer Self-Image Questionnaire for Adolescents
PA	Physically abused
Peds	Pediatrics
PHCSCS	Piers-Harris Children's Self-Concept Scale
PIAT	Peabody Individual Achievement Test
PIC	Personality Inventory for Children
PMS	Perlin's Mastery Scale
Prob	Probation
Psych	Psychiatric, psychiatry
PTSD	Posttraumatic Stress Disorder
RATC	Roberts Apperception Test for Children
RCMAS	Revised Children's Manifest Anxiety Scale
RecRev	Record review
Ref	Referred
RSES	Rosenberg Self-Esteem Scale
SA	Sexually abused
SAC	Sexually anatomically correct
SAS	Sexual abuse sensitive
SEI	Self-Esteem Inventory
Sibs	Siblings
STAIC	State-Trait Anxiety Inventory for Children
STASC	State-Trait Anxiety Scale for Children
Sx	Symptom

TRF	Teacher report form
TSCS	Tennessee Self-Concept Scale
Tx	Treatment
Vid Fam Int	Videotape Recorded Family Interview
VV-SHQ	Victim and victim-sister history questionnaire
WISC-R	Wechsler Intelligence Scale for Children–Revised
WRAT-R	Wide Range Achievement Test–Revised
YSR	Youth self-report

CHAPTER
5

Juvenile Prostitution:
Profile of Recruitment

Evelina Giobbe

The average age of entry into prostitution is estimated to be 14 (Enablers, 1978; Gray-Hilton, 1971; James, 1980). The vast majority of juveniles used in prostitution are initially recruited by a pimp or subsequently fall under the control of a pimp (Satterfield, 1981; Silbert & Pine, 1982). While some studies report that very few adolescents have pimps (James, 1978; Newman & Caplan, 1981), this data may be misleading as many women and girls are reticent to, or do not, recognize their present partner as a pimp in spite of objective evidence to the contrary (Enablers, 1978).

Procuring is a tactic for acquiring juveniles and turning them into prostitution. Pimping keeps them there. Procuring, according to Barry, involves convincing a person to be a prostitute through cunning, fraud, and/or physical force, taking her against her will or knowledge, and putting her into prostitution (Barry, 1979:86).

A primary method of procuring a juvenile is befriending or the use of feigned friendship and love. A combination of seduction and terrorism appears to be the most common approach used by pimps to recruit girls into prostitution. In these situations pimps will typically frequent areas where juveniles are apt to congregate, such as shopping malls, video game arcades, bus stations, etc., and target isolated young girls.

In phase one of this approach, a pimp's initial conversation with a girl is essentially an information-gathering mission where he attempts to identify her vulnerabilities. He is friendly or flirtatious, depending on which approach he believes she will respond to. It is during this initial conversation that he encourages her to tell him information about herself that he will subsequently use to seduce her. Is she a runaway? Why? Is she window shopping, looking at clothing that she cannot afford? Is she a truant, tired of the restrictions of school and her parent's rules? Does she perceive herself as gawky, unattractive, unpopular? The pimp then uses the information that she so naively provides him to tailor his recruitment strategy—or rap—to meet what he perceives her needs to be. If she is a runaway, he will offer her food and shelter and vaguely hint at the possibility of a job. Are her parents too strict? He will commiserate with her, tell her she is too smart, too mature, to have all of those restrictions. Is she lonely? Does she consider herself undesirable? Then he will fawn over her. Pimps then use a combination of flattery and charm, the promise of money, protection, companionship, and intimacy to con or "sweet-talk" a young girl into prostitution (Barry, 1979; James, 1978).

Although it is acknowledged that juvenile prostitution triggers a wide range of legal, health, and social concerns, the major impact of such work rests with the young person. The advent of the human immunodeficiency virus (HIV) and the spread of sexually transmitted diseases among the adolescent population in general has heightened concern for the life of the juvenile prostitute. It becomes critical that people whose work brings them into contact with neglected children, runaways, sexually abused victims, and distressed and emotionally disturbed adolescents gain an understanding of procuring and pimping from the life histories of juvenile prostitutes. The following case describes a pimp's procurement strategy using feigned friendship and love and illustrates how Karen, at age 13, was recruited into prostitution (Giobbe, 1988).

KAREN

At the time of interview for the Oral History Project (Giobbe, 1988), Karen was a 31-year-old Caucasian woman who had completed the sixth grade. She had been in prostitution for 13 years between the ages of 13 and 26. Her only paid employment prior to entry into prostitution was babysitting. Karen is currently separated from her husband (who was also her pimp), and she has custody of their five children, ages 6 through 13. At the time of the interview

Karen was in hiding from her pimp, working as a bookkeeper for a small nonprofit agency in a rural area, where she and her children lived in subsidized housing.

Family Background

Karen was raised by her natural parents in the suburbs of a moderate-sized mid-western city. She is one of eight children. Karen describes her family as "upper-middle class." They owned their own home, each of the children went to parochial school, and the children had their basic needs met.

Karen described her father as a strict authoritarian, who often frightened her by "yelling." Although she describes her mother as "real supportive, " she complained that she often unfavorably compared her to her sisters. There was no history of alcoholism or drug abuse in the family, nor any criminal activity. Karen never experienced or witnessed any physical or sexual abuse in her home. According to her account, the two biggest problems in her family were that her parents compared her siblings to each other and that they were not physically demonstrative. Karen said:

> *They never expressed their love. . . . I never saw*
> *any affection. They always compared everyone to*
> *everyone else, and I was always the one that didn't—*
> *that did wrong. I could never—be up to their. . . .*
> *[M]aybe it wasn't their standards, what I'm trying to*
> *say is that all my sisters had a talent. One could do*
> *real good art work, another one could crochet, another*
> *one could sew, another one could bake, and one was*
> *real good in sports. And I always tried to do all them*
> *things, and be just like them, but I was never good*
> *enough.*

Karen stated that she suffered from performance anxiety in school, freezing up during exams. She also said that she was unpopular with her peers and attributed this to her feelings of unattractiveness.

> *I was the tallest girl in the school, and my class, so*
> *I mean all the boys were shorter than me and I had*
> *big ears, and I had red hair, and I had freckles, and I*
> *wasn't one of the perfect people. You know, I just*
> *never believed I would ever get anybody.*

Recruitment

Karen was 13 when she met Mark. He was 18 and fresh out of prison. Mark had been involved with the juvenile courts from age 7 and had been arrested for numerous offenses, including car theft, simple assault, robbery, assault with a deadly weapon, and assault on a police officer. Karen was playing hooky that day—she had never "ditched school" before—when he approached her at a bus stop where she was standing with her schoolmate.

> *He had this kind of trench coat on and this hat*
> *and then he had a beard and the hat was tilted to the*
> *side. I mean pimp written all over him. . . . I says,*
> *"God, this man is gorgeous," but I know he'd never*
> *come talk to me. So we ran across the street, you*
> *know, and you know we're talking, and all of a*
> *sudden he came up behind me and he says, "Hello.*
> *What's your name?"*

Mark was the first "boy" to pay attention to Karen. She left her friend and went to a local ice cream parlor with him, where he subsequently invited her to his (brother's) apartment. On the bus ride over he pointed out the prostitutes on the local stroll and told Karen that "these women really cared about their man. That's the kind of woman I want." Karen was confused by his remark; she thought the women were waiting for a bus. Karen was also intrigued by Mark.

> *I always wanted a different life. I wanted some*
> *excitement out of my life. . . . I think the biggest thing*
> *why I went with Mark was because he looked*
> *"gangsterous," and my family always told me about*
> *these black people are real bad, and it was like I have*
> *to find this out for myself.*

When they arrived at the apartment, Mark left Karen under the watchful eye of an older woman with two black eyes. At this point Karen began to feel a bit frightened.

> *I remember looking out the window and thinking,*
> *"How am I going to get out of here?" We're on the*
> *third floor, and he left me there. He said he'd be right*
> *back. And it's like I didn't know this woman. I didn't*

> *know what was going on, what was going to happen*
> *to me, or anything. . . . And he had made this*
> *comment to her about, make sure I don't leave. So it*
> *was like, so, God, you know "Where am I going to go*
> *now?"*

When Mark returned a half hour later, he seduced Karen. She was a virgin at the time. Afterward he attempted to persuade her to engage in prostitution.

> *[W]e decided, and did "it." And then he's talking*
> *about making him some money. And just for me—*
> *because he's just out he doesn't have a place of his*
> *own—[we] could get our own place . . . he says he*
> *wanted me for his girlfriend and that's all it took. So I*
> *went out and did my first trick.*

Prostitution

Mark arranged Karen's first "date." She was so nervous that she forgot to get the money.

> *He told me everything I had to do. There was three*
> *Rules: one was get the money first; another one [was]*
> *only take less than 10 minutes; and third, you don't*
> *tell him [the customer] anything. He says, "I'll go in*
> *there and make all the arrangements. All you got to*
> *do is just fuck him and leave him," he said. That's*
> *what I did, but I forgot to get the money. I told him*
> *my name [and] he wouldn't let me go after 10*
> *minutes. Mark didn't get his money. [I] got slapped*
> *across the face because I told him I didn't want to do*
> *it ever again.*

Karen believed that this was going to be a "one time thing," but the next day Mark put her out on the street and told her to "just stand there . . . people will stop . . . all you gotta do is ask them. Just don't talk to anybody. Just go with the white guys. Don't talk to anybody that you think is gonna harm you or anything, and I'll be right there and you can just give me your money when you're done, and that way nobody will rip you off."

When Karen was about 14 or 15, she told Mark that she wanted to leave prostitution.

> *He laughed at me. He asked me what else I was*
> *good for? One time when I refused to go out to work,*
> *but I'll never do that again. He went crazy, he took a*
> *two by four and just continued to bang my head in.*

The Abusive Relationship

Mark subjected Karen to emotional and physical battering throughout their relationship.

> *I remember him filling up the bathtub with hot,*
> *warm water and putting his gin into it and I had open*
> *sores and he made me sit in this bathtub.*

Mark was also sexually abusive to Karen.

> *I was his property. Do what he wanted. A lot of*
> *times it was just pleasing him. A lot of times, he held*
> *a gun to my head, tell me I had to continue sucking*
> *. . . that if I didn't make him come by sucking him—*
> *which you very seldom could do—that if I fell asleep,*
> *or if I bit him—if my teeth touched him—he'd blow*
> *my head off.*

Karen and Mark lived a transitory life during the 13 years they were together, moving from place to place to avoid the police or being evicted for not paying their rent. Although they occasionally rented an apartment or lived in motels, most of the time they, and their children, lived at Mark's grandmother's home. Karen idealized the older woman in spite of the fact that she must have been aware of the nature of her grandson's relationship to the girl.

> *She was almost like a mother to me. She took care*
> *of my kids she took care of me. She used to tell me*
> *some stories about her life. I knew she was a really*
> *wise woman. She always understood where I was*
> *coming from because she would tell me, why do I let*
> *him beat me and all this, [that] I deserve more than*
> *that. [She was] just someone I could talk to.*

Karen had little contact with her children, who were usually under the watchful eye of Mark or one of his female relatives. She attempted to leave Mark on several occasions over the years. Mark used a combination of emotional manipulation and terrorism to get

Karen to return home, often using her children to lure her back or
threatening her family.

> *He threatened to take [the children] from me and
> keep them away from me. . . . He threatened . . . if I
> didn't come back that he would go to my family's
> house; he would rape my little sister, he would fuck
> my mother . . . .*

When she was 19, Mark devised a "punishment" that was to keep
her bound to him for the next seven years.

> *I had taken off and came back to him, and I
> always knew that there was a punishment coming for
> taking off. . . . [O]ne day after work he just took me to
> this one apartment building . . . he was talking real
> quiet about me taking off and all this, so I knew it
> must be coming. So I had a kind of warning of it. He
> just told me that the reason he has to do this is to
> teach me a lesson, because he loves me and I really
> hurt him and he doesn't want to hurt me but if he
> didn't do anything to make me pay for what I did that
> I would call him a wimp and wouldn't have any
> respect for him. . . .*

> *We went into the bedroom after he first said
> that he wasn't going to do nothing. He just decided
> that he wasn't going to hurt me because he loved me
> so much, and we started making love, and [I'm] really
> feeling like he's treating me to this night off, and then
> he gets up and he leaves the room and comes back
> and he ties me up. Once in a while he'd get into this
> real shit of tying me up and making love to me and
> that's what I though he was going to do. This time he
> tied me tighter where I really couldn't get loose, and I
> didn't know if I was going to get beat or what, but he
> told me he wasn't going to hurt me so I believed him.
> And he took this belt and he starts whipping me.*

> *I don't know how long that went on. [After a
> while] he says, "You think that's all you deserve?"*

> *And I said, "No." He says, "This hurts me more than*
> *it hurts you," which is a typical line he always used,*
> *and he grabbed the dog and the dog knew just what to*
> *do. And he said, "This just shows how worthless you*
> *are." Just continued to put me down. I lost a lot of*
> *respect that day. He took pictures of it, and he told me*
> *that if I ever left him again, that these would be*
> *mailed to my family. I stayed with him for almost*
> *seven more years after that.*

Prostitution History

Karen primarily solicited her customers on the street and occasionally in adult bookstores (peep show booths) and in pornographic movie theaters. Over the years she collected the names of steady customers and called on them during her pregnancies when it was more difficult to solicit out-of-doors. During her first pregnancy she turned tricks through her ninth month.

> *A lot of it was hand jobs; a lot of times it was just*
> *sucking my breasts so they could get milk.*

On rare occasions her pimp would arrange "dates" for her. The actual sex acts she engaged in with her customers took place in any available place, including cars, motels, her (or her customer's) apartment, hallways, alleyways, public bathrooms, and secluded beaches. She also had sex with johns in the aisles of pornographic movie theaters and in peep show booths.

Karen "worked" every day after her first date. In the beginning she saw two customers per day, but by time she was 16 her pimp raised her quota, forcing her to have contact with as many as 15 to 20 men per day. She was paid between $15 and $25 per customer, occasionally as little as $5. The actual sex act took approximately 10 minutes. The most common acts she engaged in were masturbation, intercourse, and fellatio. She tried to avoid anal intercourse and being tied up when possible. However, Karen rarely refused any requests (some of which were photographed or filmed), including acts involving urination and defecation, "lesbian shows" with other children, sadomasochism (S&M), bondage, and discipline.

> *This guy used to dress me up as—didn't have to*
> *really dress up, I was—this little girl: had pigtails in*
> *my hair, blowing bubbles. And he would spank me.*

She absolutely refused however, to allow her customers to kiss her on her mouth.

Karen states that she did not enjoy sex with her customers, and if her body occasionally responded to their physical manipulations, she was unaware of it. She said that she particularly hated having to engage in any conversation at all with her customers, including "sex talk," and coped with their sexual demands by dissociating herself from the events.

> *I left my body. Very seldom I was ever there. I had*
> *a good technique for leaving. I knew where I was at, I*
> *mean I knew what they were doing, but it was like I*
> *have no feeling. . . . It was my survival. That was a*
> *way of knowing that they might have my body, but*
> *they're not going to get me.*

Customer Violence

Karen estimates that she was raped by a customer on approximately 15 to 20 occasions. She defined rape as a situation in which a customer had sex with her and then refused to pay or took back their money after the act. These situations commonly entailed a customer driving her to a deserted area, forcing sex by knife point, and abandoning her there. Karen also described being literally forced to engage in sex acts by her customers that she defined as assaultive or abusive in spite of the fact that she was paid. On one occasion she was forcibly sodomized. On other occasions customers would ejaculate in her mouth against her expressed wishes, then force her to swallow their semen. Other times they would force intercourse a second time against her wishes. Karen expressed an extremely negative response to the sex she was compelled to engage in as a prostitute emphatically stating that she was "raped by all of them. Anytime someone did it and I didn't want to do it [which was] every time I turned a trick."

Karen estimated that she was beaten up by a customer on approximately 30 separate occasions—usually within the context of a robbery or a sexual assault. After one such assault she required medical attention for a knife wound. She was also the victim of kidnapping by customers on three occasions where she was held against her will for "a couple hours" and sexually assaulted.

Health Implications

Over the years Karen has sustained numerous injuries by both her pimp and johns, some of which have had a long-term impact on her health.

> *I've had three broken arms, nose broken twice, [and] I'm partially deaf in one ear. . . . I have a small fragment of a bone floating in my head that gives me migraines. I've had a fractured skull. My legs ain't worth shit no more; my toes have been broken. My feet, bottom of my feet, have been burned; they've been whopped with a hot iron and clothes hanger . . . the hair on my pussy had been burned off at one time . . . I have scars. I've been cut with a knife, beat with guns, two by fours. There hasn't been a place on my body that hasn't been bruised somehow, some way, some big, some small.*

There are many emotional effects to prostituting.

> *I quit feeling, I think . . . I don't cry anymore. I wasn't allowed to cry, so I quit crying and that's what I miss most because there's times I just want to sit down and cry, and there's no tears anymore.*

Pseudoidentities in Prostitution

At one point during her life in prostitution, Karen was diagnosed as a multiple personality. This is believed to be a misdiagnosis based on her therapist's lack of knowledge about the dynamics of prostitution. It is typical for women to assume different identities (appearance and name) while in prostitution. There are two practical reasons for this: the first is to attract customers, who are always looking for someone new; the second reason is that women assume a string of aliases when arrested to avoid building a long criminal record. On a psychological level, compartmentalization and dissociation techniques are typical survival mechanism used by women in prostitution in an attempt to cope with ongoing sexual use and abuse by customers. For women like Karen who did not have the benefit of drugs or alcohol (which act like a "psychological buffer" for many prostitutes), such coping mechanisms may reach extreme proportions, causing a form of self-alienation that may subsequently lead to a hasty diagnosis of multiple personality disorder by a mental health professional.

> *When I would work the street, I wasn't "Karen."*
> *Karen's this person that cares about people, that has*
> *feelings. . . . When I was on the street, "Candy"*
> *would come out, and Candy didn't give a fuck. Candy*
> *didn't care about no one but herself. Candy was*
> *tough, Candy was a survivor. Karen is a real mild,*
> *meek person that people could destroy easily. Karen*
> *was 13 years old. Karen didn't know nothing. Karen*
> *still has me today. Karen has come a long ways.*
> *Karen had quit growing at 13. Candy took over, or*
> *"Randi," or "Susie," or how many others all took*
> *over. Those are the ones that survived that life. Karen*
> *would not have survived it.*

When asked how she felt about being diagnosed a multiple, she replied:

> *What I think is that was my survival technique.*
> *That's how I survived. . . . I stopped growing at age*
> *13. . . . I did what I had to do to survive. . . . There's*
> *times that I believe I have a split personality, but*
> *that's okay. It's not this split, split personality that*
> *people [would say] "God, this woman's crazy!" It's a*
> *split personality that can make me survive.*

Vocabulary of Motivation

Karen was ambivalent about her motivation to become a prostitute. Although she said that her initial motivation to became a prostitute was to have a relationship with her former husband, her loneliness, low self-esteem, and needs for attention were striking as she perceived herself as a young teenager.

> *I wanted to please him. I wanted him to want me,*
> *and I knew if I didn't be a prostitute, that he wouldn't*
> *want me and I didn't want to be alone. . . . [H]e's the*
> *only one that ever paid attention to me. He's the only*
> *one that ever told me he loved me. And everything*
> *that I thought was bad about me, he said was good.*

Adolescent attachment to persons outside of the family is often a response to lack of attention in the home rather than an attraction to the individual. Karen's unhappy home situation, not unlike that of many other women and girls used in prostitution, left her vulnerable to the recruitment tactics of a pimp. Karen, however, also appeared to be motivated, in part, by fear.

> *I believed my only choice was not to tell him no. [If*
> *I did, I'd] get beat up, killed because I'd seen the*
> *violent side of him. I mean I knew he was in prison*
> *for cutting this man's throat.*

Whereas both seduction and fear were factors in her recruitment, it was ultimately blackmail coupled with other tactics of power and control that prevented Karen from escaping her pimp. In a short time, she felt that she could not turn back.

> *By the time I got into it, when it had been a*
> *month. . . . I knew that no one else would ever want*
> *me now that I had turned all these tricks. . . . And I*
> *was scared he was going to tell my mother . . . he*
> *knew everything about me. I told him everything, and*
> *I didn't know too much about him at all. . . . I didn't*
> *tell my family because they would look down on me*
> *then . . . that it was my choice or it was my fault. . . .*
> *I didn't tell the police because . . . when they arrested*
> *me for the first time for prostitution, I gave them my*
> *false name and I was young, and I had to act tough*
> *and I was scared, and then I had a police record. And*
> *because he told me not to tell anybody. And I did*
> *everything he told me. He told me that he'd be*
> *watching me. He was always there. . . . He told me*
> *from day one that he would always know where I was*
> *at, he'd know when I was messing up, and I would*
> *pay for it.*

In spite of the emotional and psychological manipulation she was subjected to by her pimp beginning at the age of 13, and the overt violence he used to control her over the following 13 years, Karen still felt that she had somewhat made a choice to engage in prostitution.

> *In a sense I made a choice. But I didn't have much*
> *of, there wasn't much of choice there, because it was,*
> *I don't believe it was a choice. I could have left. But I*
> *knew that if I left that I don't know what would've*
> *happened to me . . . if he would've killed me. I didn't*
> *think I could survive on my own, and I couldn't go*
> *back home. I didn't have anywhere to go, so at first,*
> *when he first brought it up to me, I had a choice. I*
> *feel I could've said "no" and walked home. But I don't*
> *know, after seeing the beating that I went through,*
> *and maybe not. Maybe he wouldn't have given me a*
> *choice. I don't know.*

Yet she expressed regret at "not having a childhood, [losing] 13 years of my life that I'll never be able to get back again . . . never, ever feeling like I'm a clean person."

Mode of Exit

After 13 years in prostitution Karen found herself homeless and impoverished at age 26.

> *I came in with nothing and left with nothing.*
> *Came in with the clothes on my back and left with*
> *the clothes on my back and five kids. And the clothes*
> *on their backs.*

She was only to escape prostitution through the help of a battered women's shelter.

REFERENCES

Barry, K. (1979). *Female Sexual Slavery*. New York: Avon Books.

Enablers (1978). *Juvenile prostitution in Minnesota: the report of a research project*. P. 52. St. Paul, Minn.

Giobbe, E. (1988). WHISPER oral history project. Unpublished interviews with 19 survivors of prostitution. Minneapolis.

Gray-Hilton, D. (1971). Turning-out: a study of teenage prostitution. Unpublished master's thesis, University of Washington, Seattle.

James, J. (1980). *Entrance into Prostitution*. P. 29. Washington, D.C.: National Institute of Mental Health.

Newman, F., & Caplan, P.J. (1981). Juvenile female prostitution as a gender consistent response to early deprivation. *International Journal of Womens Studies* 5 (2):133.

Satterfield, S.B. (1981). Clinical aspects of juvenile prostitution. *Medical Aspects of Human Sexuality* 15 (9):126–132.

Silbert, M., & Pine, A.M. (1982). Entrance into prostitution. *Youth and Society* 13 (4):481–496.

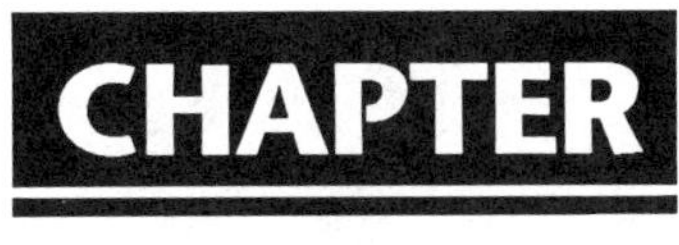

CHAPTER 6

Children as Witnesses in Court: The Influence of Expert Psychological Testimony

Eugene Borgida, April W. Gresham, Margaret Bull Kovera, and Pamela C. Regan

The research reported in this chapter was supported by a subcontract to the first author from the National Council of Jewish Women's Center for the Child, and by Grant No. 90-CA1273 from the National Center on Child Abuse and Neglect to the NCJW's Center for the Child.

THE INFLUENCE OF EXPERT PSYCHOLOGICAL TESTIMONY

Psychologists and other mental health professionals have contributed their expertise to court proceedings for many years on such topics as insanity and competency to stand trial. Both the frequency of the use of expert psychological testimony and the types of issues about which psychologists testify have increased in recent years. Controversy surrounding the admissibility and ethics of such testimony also have escalated (see, e.g., Elliott, 1991; Ellsworth, 1991; McCloskey, Egeth, & McKenna, 1986; Saks, 1990).

The professional controversy generated by the admission of expert psychological testimony in child sexual abuse cases, fueled by extensive media coverage of divorce and custody disputes involving allegations of child sexual abuse, has become particularly heated within the psychological and legal communities (Kovera, Borgida, Gresham, et al., 1991). As the number of child sexual abuse cases reaching the courtroom has increased, legal scholars have begun to examine the legal and scientific status of expert testimony in these cases. While there is no uniformly accepted standard by which courts evaluate expert testimony, there are a few basic requirements that must be met in order for expert testimony to be admissible. First, the expert must be qualified "by knowledge, skill, experience, training, or education" (Rule 702, Federal Rules of Evidence, 1984). Second, the evidence must assist the trier of fact (i.e., be helpful to jurors in their decision making). Third, the evidence must be scientifically reliable. In determining reliability, some courts rely on *Frye v. United States* (1923), which requires that scientific evidence be "generally accepted" within the relevant scientific community in order to be admissible. Other courts rely on the Federal Rules of Evidence, which do not require "general acceptance." The final criterion for admissibility is that the expert testimony be probative and not unfairly prejudicial to the defendant.

Legal scholars have begun to scrutinize case law involving the admission of expert psychological testimony in child sexual abuse trials. For example, McCord (1986) has classified the prosecutorial use of expert testimony in such cases into four categories. One type of expert testimony involves the diagnosis of sexual abuse to prove that abuse occurred. A second category involves cases wherein an expert directly vouches for the complainant's credibility as a witness to the alleged sexual abuse. Third, expert testimony has also been introduced to enhance the credibility of the child witness by explaining any "unusual" behavior questioned by the defense. The fourth type of expert psychological testimony involves expert testimony about the cognitive capabilities of child witnesses, testimony that indirectly enhances the credibility of the child witness. The courts, according to McCord, have been divided in their rulings to date on which type of expert testimony to admit.

Serrato (1988) also divides expert psychological testimony into a continuum of categories ranging from testimony resulting in minor impact on the ultimate issue in the trial to high impact on the ultimate issue. The lesser impact categories in her "spectrum model" of expert testimony include expert psychological testimony constituting a denial of defense claims, more general testimony on common characteristics of sexually abused children, testimony about the general veracity of child sexual abuse allegations, and expert opinion on the veracity of a particular child witness. Higher impact categories include testimony by the expert linking general characteristics of sexually abused children with the particular child witness, general testimony on characteristics of child sexual abusers, and expert testimony on the abuser's identity. Serrato discusses case law on each type of testimony and weighs factors such as the need for expert testimony in dispelling common myths about child sexual abuse against the likelihood of unfairly biasing the jury against the defendant.

As the use of expert psychological testimony in child sexual abuse cases has increased in recent years, various empirical questions associated with the admission of expert psychological testimony in such cases have assumed greater importance in legal decision making (see, e.g., APA amicus brief filed in *Maryland v. Craig,* 1990). To what extent, for example, are children competent courtroom witnesses? What do we know about the cognitive and memorial abilities of children as witnesses that may bear on the admissibility of expert testimony in such cases? What are jurors' beliefs and expectations about children as witnesses in court? And how do these beliefs and expectations influence jurors' perceptions of child witnesses, particularly in child sexual abuse cases? Finally, to what extent does expert psychological testimony influence jury decision making in criminal trials involving allegations of child sexual abuse? These kinds of questions represent the foci of our chapter. In the first section of the chapter, therefore, we review some of the research conducted to date on the nature of children's cognitive abilities as well as research that examines jurors' perceptions of child witnesses. In the second section of the chapter we review the influence of expert psychological testimony on jury decision making in two different contexts—in cases involving expert testimony on eyewitness identification and in cases involving expert testimony on rape trauma syndrome. With this work in mind, the final section of the chapter presents some of our own research on the influence of expert psychological testimony on juror decision making in a simulated child sexual abuse trial.

CHILDREN AS WITNESSES

One empirical question that must be considered when thinking about children as witnesses in court is, What do we know about the cognitive and memorial abilities of children as witnesses? In a recent and comprehensive review by Penrod, Bull, and Lengnick (1989), research on adults' and children's memory was examined from an information-processing perspective. According to these investigators, the process of perception, the first stage in information processing, is similar in children and adults. In order to be perceived, an event must occur in close enough proximity to be sensed. Because it is impossible for adults or children to sense all of the attributes of an event, it is therefore necessary to select certain attributes to which to pay attention. This selective attention to the stimulus may introduce distortion into the process of perception. Some research suggests that the ability to attend selectively to information improves with age (Enns & Girgus, 1985). However, the Penrod review (1989) suggests that because past research has primarily focused on children's passive observation of events, it is unclear whether the same deficiencies in selective attention would be present when the child is the object of criminal activity such as sexual abuse.

The next step in the child's processing of information is the entry of information into the memory system, or encoding. Encoding can be affected by characteristics of the event and characteristics of the witness. For example, the complexity of a stimulus is one of the event characteristics that differentially affects the encoding of adults and children. Although the complexity of a stimulus can introduce distortion in what is perceived, complex stimuli are more likely to be recognized by adults than less complex stimuli. It appears that a child's ability to recognize complex stimuli (such as faces) improves with age (Carey & Diamond, 1977; Mandler & Robinson, 1978; Newcombe, Rogoff, & Kagan, 1977). Encoding can also be affected by the stressfulness of the event. However, research by Goodman, Aman, and Hirschman (1989) examining the memories of children of various ages for the events surrounding a venipuncture or inoculation procedure under varying levels of stress has failed to discover any significant age differences. Even more interesting is that children were able to respond accurately to questions that might be asked in child sexual abuse investigations. Specifically, the children were generally able to declare whether or not the nurse kissed them, hit them, touched them on the arm or the thigh, or put anything in their mouths. When children were mistaken in their responses, they tended to make errors of omission rather than commission (e.g., a child who had been given a shot in the arm claimed that she had not been touched on that part of her body).

There are several witness characteristics, such as expectations held by the witness, that also affect the encoding processes of both adults and children. Prior expectations often result in information being encoded that is consistent with those expectancies. However, at least one study suggests that children are no more susceptible to this error than are adults (List, 1986). Rehearsal also affects encoding, and the likelihood that children will rehearse (as well as engage in other memory strategies) increases with age (Brown, 1979). Once information has been perceived and encoded, it must be stored in memory for later use. The length of time and the interference of other information affects the information that is stored. However, the length of the retention interval does not appear to affect adults and children differentially (Nigro & Gudatis, 1987).

The final stage of information processing involves the retrieval of information from storage. Many factors may affect a child's retrieval of information. The type of question is a factor known to affect recall in both children and adults. For example, the use of definite versus indefinite articles increases inaccuracies in responding (Dale, Loftus, & Rathbun, 1978), and free recall produces more accurate but less detailed memories for children (Marquis, Marshall, & Oskamp, 1972). Children and adults possess similar retrieval abilities in photo lineup studies except when the child is very young, i.e., 3 years old (Goodman & Reed, 1986), and except when disguises are employed that impair the abilities of both children and adults to recognize faces (although the abilities of children to decipher disguises appear to improve with age; Diamond & Carey, 1977). Finally, there is no evidence for the benefits of context reinstatement in children despite the evidence for this effect in adults (Nigro & Gudatis, 1987).

The belief that children are more suggestible (more likely to incorporate misleading information into their accounts of an event) has spawned an abundance of research on the topic. The findings of these studies, according to Penrod, Bull, and Lengnick (1989) are equivocal. Some studies contend that children are more suggestible than adults (Cohen & Harnick, 1980; King & Yuille, 1987); some maintain that adults are more suggestible than children (Duncan, Whitney, & Kunen, 1982); and still others find no differences (Marin, Holmes, Guth, & Kovac, 1979; Saywitz, 1987). Penrod et al. (1989) suggest that a problem in this area of research is that most studies have introduced only a single piece of misleading or suggestive information at one point in time and, therefore, the procedures employed in these studies fail to resemble the repeated questioning of a child that would be typical, for instance, in a child sexual abuse investigation. Although Poole and White (1990) have recently attempted to rectify this inadequacy by conducting research on the effects of repeated questioning on the accuracy of adults and children, Penrod et al. (1989) justifiably argue that more research is required to clarify the issue of whether the suggestibility of children and adults differs.

The research, however, is more conclusive in its findings that *both* children and adults are susceptible to suggestions. Additionally, the research indicates that children are more likely to respond to social influence or demand characteristics and that the inaccuracies in their testimony merely reflect their incorporation of information they believe the researcher wants to hear (Ceci, Ross, & Toglia, 1987). Penrod et al. (1989) conclude that the above findings support the need for carefully conducted interviews that incorporate nonleading questions and introduce new information in a neutral manner so that the child does not feel that the researcher wishes him or her to endorse the information. In addition, they also assert that the use of suggestive questions will make it impossible to determine whether the child's statements are true, are solely attempts to please the interviewer, or contain some misleading information that has been incorporated into memory as the result of the suggestive questioning.

Although it is important to assess the scientific status of research on the actual capabilities of children in order to determine what experts may ethically testify about in court, it is equally, if not more, important to determine how people perceive children and the testimony they offer. For example, it may be very informative to know that the research indicates that individuals are not differentially affected by the length of the retention interval as a function of age. However, it is also important to know what jurors think about children's capabilities. If jurors do not perceive that children's capabilities are equivalent to the abilities of adults in this regard, this perception may negatively affect their evaluation of the child's testimony. Some research, reviewed in the next section, has attempted to assess the beliefs that people hold about children's mental abilities.

Juror perceptions of child witnesses. A few researchers have conducted survey research to examine the beliefs that individuals hold about the capabilities of child witnesses. Yarmey and Jones (1983) surveyed potential jurors, law students, psycholegal researchers, and legal professionals in order to examine their beliefs about the capabilities of a hypothetical 8-year-old witness. In general, the child was believed to be an unreliable, inaccurate witness who could be easily manipulated by any investigator. Psycholegal researchers were more likely to support this position than lay persons. However, one must keep in mind that these responses reflect perceptions of a hypothetical, average 8-year-old child and that in the context of a trial, jurors' perceptions of a child witness who has been prepared for the courtroom experience might be very different.

Similarly, respondents to a survey conducted by Leippe and Romanczyck (1987) held unfavorable beliefs about the capabilities of child witnesses. Subjects were presented with descriptions of the conditions in the study by Marin, Holmes, Guth, and Kovac (1979) and, subsequently, were asked to estimate the number of accurate eyewitness identifications made in a group of 100 witnesses. Leippe and Romanczyck found that subjects consistently underestimated the accuracy of the subjects in the Marin et al. study. Taken together with the research by Yarmey and Jones (1983), this study suggests that jurors believe that children are less accurate and more suggestible than older witnesses.

Conversely, young children who testify in child sexual abuse cases may appear to be more credible than their older counterparts. Corder and Whiteside (1988) conducted a survey of actual jurors in North Carolina to determine whether beliefs about children's abilities and issues related to child sexual abuse differed as a function of the age of the child victim. These individuals felt that most children

3 years of age or older are capable of providing accurate testimony about sexual abuse. Respondents were also asked whether they felt that a child was capable of lying about being sexually abused. Older children were viewed as being more capable of lying than children under 5, although 55% of the respondents thought that children as young as 3 years of age were capable of fabricating a sexual abuse allegation. Of all jurors polled, 98% believed that a mental health professional can determine whether a child's allegations of sexual abuse are false. While this finding suggests that jurors might be unduly biased by the testimony of an expert psychologist, it is quite possible that jurors, when faced with evaluating testimony in an actual trial, would not place as much weight on an expert's testimony as they indicate in self-reports.

Although the results of these surveys are informative, it is unclear whether jurors would respond similarly when presented with the live testimony of a child in the context of a trial. Several experimental studies have attempted to bridge this gap. For example, Goodman and her colleagues have conducted a series of experiments that examine jurors' reactions to a child's testimony. Results from their study in which participants viewed a videotaped trial in which the eyewitness was either 6, 10, or 30 years old showed that jurors perceive children as less credible than older witnesses (Goodman, Golding, & Haith, 1984). Specifically, the 6-year-old witness was seen as less perceptive, less accurate, and more easily manipulated than the adult. The child's testimony, in conjunction with other evidence, did lead, however, to the same conviction rates as were found in conditions with an adult eyewitness. Therefore, Goodman et al. (1984) concluded that children's testimony is not disregarded but rather given less weight in decision making. An identical pattern of results was found for college undergraduates and a more representative sample of potential jurors from the community. Results also converged whether the trial was a vehicular homicide or murder (Goodman, Golding, Helgeson, et al., 1987).

In a series of experiments conducted by Leippe and Romanczyck (1989) jurors indicated their beliefs that children make unreliable witnesses. The first of these studies varied the age of the eyewitness in a description of a robbery trial and replicated Goodman et al.'s findings (1984, 1987) that children are perceived to be less credible than adults. Furthermore, Leippe and Romanczyck found that the age of the eyewitness does affect the number of guilty verdicts, particularly when the other evidence in the case is strong. Specifically, there were more convictions when an adult eyewitness testified than when either a 6- or a 10-year-old testified when the case for the prosecution was strong. There were no differences in the number of guilty verdicts rendered when the strength of the prosecution's case was moderate or weak.

The second study varied age as well as the consistency of the testimony provided by the eyewitness. Leippe and Romanczyck (1989) failed to find a main effect of age on credibility ratings, yet there was a main effect for eyewitness consistency such that the consistent witness was viewed as more credible. There was also an interesting two-way interaction between witness age and consistency such that inconsistency negatively affected the credibility ratings of the 6-year-old but had no effect on the credibility of the 10- or 30-year-old.

The third and final study by Leippe and Romanczyck (1989), in which participants were provided with a transcript of the eyewitness's testimony rather than a mere description of the trial, demonstrated that jurors perceived a 6-year-old child as more credible than an adult witness before and after jury deliberations. Leippe and Romanczyck (1987) suggest that these contradictory results were obtained because jurors typically underestimate the abilities of child witnesses and therefore were impressed with the relative coherence and quality of the child's testimony. It is important to note, however, that the average juror estimate of the child's age was slightly over 9 years old. Perhaps jurors overestimated her age because, despite efforts to the contrary, the testimony of the 6-year-old was written in a more powerful speech style (i.e., contained fewer pauses, hedges, and nonfluencies) than is appropriate for a child of that age. This powerful speech style enhances the perceived credibility of child witnesses because it is contrary to the expectations that people have of a child's abilities. However, it does not produce a corresponding increase in credibility for an adult witness and, therefore, might explain the discrepancy of these results from earlier findings (Nigro, Buckley, Hill, & Nelson, 1989).

This effect of speech style might also explain the results found by Ross, Dunning, Toglia, and Ceci (1990). When they examined jurors' perceptions of a child witness in comparison to a young adult and an elderly witness, they utilized identical testimony in all three conditions. Therefore, it is not surprising that subjects rated the child witness as more credible than either the 21- or the 74-year-old witness who gave the identical testimony because the powerfulness of an adult's style of speech would increase the credibility of a young child's testimony but should have less effect on the credibility ratings of an adult witness. These findings on jurors' expectations of children's consistency and speech style have interesting implications for the practice of preparing a child for the experience of testifying in a court of law. One would expect that a child who has become comfortable with the courtroom would appear more confident and composed on the witness stand and would provide testimony with fewer hesitations and hedges. According to these studies, such demeanor should result in a more credible witness.

It is also entirely possible that child witnesses in sexual abuse cases are scrutinized with regard to a different set of criteria than are young eyewitnesses in other types of trials. For example, an average child's knowledge of sexual details at a particular age may play an important role in jurors' evaluations of whether the child has the ability to fabricate the allegation and thereby will affect jurors' ratings of the child's credibility. Or, jurors may question the child's ability to differentiate between fantasy and reality, an ability that is rarely at issue with older witnesses. Therefore, it is necessary to examine jurors' perceptions of child witnesses within the context of child sexual abuse cases in order to determine the factors that might affect a child's credibility in that particular type of case. Witness credibility is especially important in child sexual abuse trials. Due to the nature of child sexual abuse, material evidence is seldom found. Because it is a secretive crime, there are often only two key witnesses: the child and the alleged perpetrator. Thus the child witness's credibility becomes a key aspect of the prosecution's case. Jurors' standards for the child witness's demeanor and their expectations about how a child witness should talk and act when on the stand should strongly influence assessments of the credibility of a child witness.

At least two studies have examined factors that affect the perception of a child witness's credibility in child sexual abuse case. Goodman, Bottoms, Herscovici, and Shaver (1989) had subjects read a one-page description of an alleged sexual assault case. The victim alleged that her teacher had called her into the classroom after school to discuss class grades and forced her to perform an act of oral copulation. The primary independent variable was the victim's age (6, 14, or 22 years). The results showed that the 6-year-old victim was perceived as significantly more credible than the 22-year-old victim. Also, the defendant was viewed as more likely to be guilty when the victim was a 6-year-old. The credibility of the 14-year-old did not differ from the credibility of either of the other two witnesses. However, it is impossible to determine if jurors would react differently to an actual child witness within the context of a trial than they would to an abbreviated written description of the trial facts (see Konecni & Ebbesen, 1979).

In a more externally valid study Duggan, Aubrey, Doherty, et al. (1989) presented potential jurors, who had been randomly sampled from voter-registration rolls, with a videotaped simulated child sexual abuse trial. The jurors deliberated and then provided ratings of their perceptions of the trial. Duggan et al. examined the effects of the age of the victim/witness (either 5, 9, or 13) and the strength of an adult's versus a child's corroborative testimony on jurors' perceptions of the child witness's credibility. Jurors who viewed the 9-year-old victim were more likely to convict the defendant than jurors who viewed the 5- or 13-year-old victim. The jurors who viewed the 13-year-old victim were the least likely to render a guilty verdict. Jurors' ratings of the credibility of the victim/witness followed the same pattern found in their verdicts. Corroboration of the child witness's testimony by another child resulted in a higher proportion of guilty verdicts than did either corroboration by an adult or no corroboration, and adult corroboration produced more convictions than the no corroboration condition.

While there indeed have been studies that examine juror perceptions of child witnesses and the factors that influence credibility inferences, research to date has neglected to examine the effects of one potentially powerful variable, namely, expert psychological testimony, that may influence jurors' perceptions of the credibility of a child witness in a child sexual abuse trial. In the next section of this chapter, therefore, we first examine research on the effects of expert psychological testimony in two legal domains other than child sexual abuse (eyewitness identification and rape trauma syndrome), domains wherein researchers have begun to examine the effects of expert testimony on juror and jury decision making. We then discuss some of the key findings from our own research with regard to expert psychological testimony in child sexual abuse trials.

EXPERT TESTIMONY ON EYEWITNESS IDENTIFICATION

A large body of empirical research indicates that many individuals are unaware of the manner in which certain psychological factors influence eyewitness memory (e.g., Brigham & Bothwell, 1983; Deffenbacher & Loftus, 1982; Loftus & Burns, 1982). As a result of this lack of common understanding, jurors and prospective jurors may not possess the knowledge or skills necessary to assess adequately the reliability of eyewitness identifications (Brigham & Bothwell, 1983). For example, student jurors often ignore factors that have been shown to affect identification accuracy (such as disguise, weapon focus, presence of violence, length of retention interval, exposure to mug shots, biased lineup instructions, lineup size, and fairness of lineup) when arriving at their individual verdicts and when rating the perceived probability that an eyewitness identification was correct (Cutler, Penrod, & Stuve, 1988).

Jurors may also tend to overbelieve eyewitnesses, endowing their testimony with a credibility that may not be warranted (Ellison & Buckhout, 1981; Lindsay, Wells, & Rumpel, 1981; Loftus, 1974, 1979; Loftus & Monahan, 1980; Wall, 1965; Wells, Lindsay, & Tousignant, 1980). In addition, jurors do not appear able to distinguish well between accurate and inaccurate eyewitnesses (Lindsay, Wells, & Rumpel, 1981; Loftus, 1974, 1979, 1983; Loftus & Monahan, 1980; Wells, Lindsay, & Ferguson, 1979; Wells, Lindsay, & Tousignant, 1980). They often assign disproportionate weight to eyewitness confidence (i.e., jurors tend to believe that a confident witness is a truthful and accurate witness; Cutler, Penrod, & Stuve, 1988). This assumption that eyewitness confidence is highly related to accuracy has not been supported by research conducted in the area (Fox & Walters, 1986). Indeed, the correlation between eyewitness confidence and accuracy has often been demonstrated to be at or near zero (Buckhout, 1974; Buckhout, Alper, Chern, et al., 1974; Deffenbacher, 1980; Loftus, Miller, & Burns, 1978; Yarmey, 1979).

In view of the above findings, individual psychologists and members of the legal system have proposed the use of expert psychological testimony on the unreliability of eyewitness identification as an educative aid to jurors (Loftus, 1983). Such testimony, it is argued, would provide the jury with relevant information about basic memory processes (e.g., perception, encoding, storage, and retrieval stages of memory) and factors that potentially influence eyewitness accounts (e.g., weapon focus, lineup procedures, stress, etc.). Though a recent survey of psychological experts on eyewitness testimony indicates that a substantial majority believe that juries are more competent with the aid of experts than without (Kassin, Ellsworth, & Smith, 1989), the use of expert testimony remains a matter of considerable debate among psychologists and jurists alike (see, e.g., Loftus, 1983; McCloskey & Egeth, 1983; McCloskey, Egeth, & McKenna, 1986).

A large portion of the debate surrounding expert testimony centers around the empirical question of what, if any, effects expert testimony has on jury judgment and decision-making processes. Recent jury simulation experiments suggest that the inclusion of expert psychological testimony regarding the unreliability of eyewitness identification may affect juror judgments and decision-making processes in beneficial ways. Specifically, expert testimony has been found to result in lower ratings of defendant guilt or lower conviction rates (Fox & Walters, 1986; Loftus, 1980; Maass, Brigham, & West, 1985), increased discussion of eyewitness accounts during deliberation (Hosch, Beck, & McIntyre, 1980; Loftus, 1980), and reduced reliance on eyewitness confidence as a reliable indicator of accuracy (Fox & Walters, 1986; Wells, Lindsay, & Tousignant, 1980). On the other hand, some researchers propose that expert testimony may serve to increase jurors' skepticism toward eyewitness accounts rather than to increase their sensitivity to potential biases inherent within such accounts (McCloskey & Egeth, 1983; Wells, 1978; Wells & Turtle, 1987). For example, jurors exposed to expert testimony often exhibit a decreased tendency to believe that the eyewitness has made an accurate identification (Fox & Walters, 1986; Hosch, Beck, & McIntyre, 1980; Wells, Lindsay, & Tousignant, 1980), lending credence to the supposition that expert testimony merely contributes to a general suspicion toward eyewitness identifications or an inappropriate tendency to dismiss eyewitness testimony (McCloskey & Egeth, 1983).

Cutler and his colleagues (Cutler, Dexter, & Penrod, 1989; Cutler, Penrod, & Dexter, 1989) have conducted a series of studies specifically designed to determine whether expert testimony biases jurors rather than sensitizing them to the nature of eyewitness testimony. Cutler, Dexter, and Penrod, for example, exposed experienced jurors and student mock jurors to versions of a videotaped trial in which three factors were manipulated: witnessing and identification conditions (poor or good), witness confidence (80% or 100%), and expert testimony (present or control). In the "poor" witnessing identification condition the perpetrator was disguised and brandished a weapon; there was a two-week retention interval between the crime and the identification; and the eyewitness received suggestive lineup instructions. In the "good" witnessing identification condition the perpetrator was not disguised and hid the weapon; there was a two-day retention interval between the crime and identification; and the eyewitness received fair lineup instructions. In addition, the eyewitness testified that she was either 80% or 100% confident that she had correctly identified the perpetrator. In the no-expert conditions the prosecution and defense attorneys reiterated the conditions surrounding the eyewitness identification. Subjects in the expert conditions subsequently heard the expert give testimony on the reconstructive nature of memory; identify the factors that affect memory at perception, encoding, storage, and retrieval stages; and discuss the ways in which aspects of the crime and identification procedure might have impaired the witness's memory for the perpetrator and the effects of various specific factors such as stress, violence, weapon focus, passage of time, and relations between confidence and identification accuracy. During rigorous cross-examination by the prosecuting attorney, the expert qualified various research findings and admitted that he was paid for his testimony.

The results of this study provided scant evidence for the hypothesis that expert testimony influences jurors to be more skeptical. Expert testimony yielded no main effects on eyewitness credibility ratings, ratings of strength of prosecution case, or verdicts. Expert testimony did, however, appear to sensitize jurors to witnessing and identification conditions and witness confidence. Specifically, jurors exposed to expert testimony gave less weight to eyewitness confidence when rating eyewitness credibility and defense case strength than did jurors who were not exposed to expert testimony. In addition, jurors who heard expert testimony gave more weight to the witnessing and identification conditions when rating the strength of both the prosecution's and the defense's cases.

In general, then, it appears that expert testimony improves juror sensitivity to the factors that influence eyewitness memory without causing them to be skeptical of eyewitness testimony in general. Without such testimony jurors appear to rely upon inappropriate cues in assessing witness accuracy and to ignore factors that do influence accuracy when forming their judgments. Thus, this influence of expert psychological testimony on juror decision making is consistent with the rationale for admitting such testimony, namely, to educate jurors and sensitize them to factors that may be important to consider in their deliberations.

EXPERT TESTIMONY ON RAPE TRAUMA SYNDROME

A second area in which research has begun to examine expert testimony is particularly relevant to child sexual abuse cases. It has been argued that societal attitudes and stereotypes regarding rape, rape victims, and rapists may prejudice jurors from reaching a fair verdict in rape trials. The prevalence of certain rape myths, such as the belief that women secretly want to be raped (Bond & Mosher, 1986), that rape victims provoke rape by their manner of dress or behavior (Abbey, Cozzarelli, McLaughlin, & Harnish, 1987) and are more likely to make false reports than victims of other crimes (Frazier & Borgida, 1988), and that rape is a crime of sex or passion rather than of violence (Tetreault, 1989) often contribute to or result in a pro-defense bias that may influence jurors' verdicts (Tetreault, 1989).

The inclusion of expert testimony in rape trials may counteract these misconceptions by providing jurors with information that will help them reach an informed verdict (Borgida & Brekke, 1985; Frazier & Borgida, 1985; Frazier & Borgida, in press). A key objection to expert testimony in such trials has been that the testimony is not helpful to the triers of fact (Frazier & Borgida, 1985). That is, judges have often assumed that jurors are adequately informed about rape and rape victim behavior and that testimony offered on these topics would merely reiterate what is already common knowledge to jurors. To test this assumption, Frazier and Borgida (1988) administered a Sexual Assault Questionnaire (SAQ) to experts on rape and posttraumatic stress disorder (PTSD) and to two nonexpert comparison groups. Contrary to the opinions of several courts, the results of this study supported the conclusion that nonexperts were poorly informed on many rape-related issues. Results indicated that both nonexpert groups scored significantly lower on the SAQ than the experts. The two nonexpert groups answered at almost chance levels. For example, the nonexperts did not appear aware of the frequency of multiple victimization experiences or the behavioral changes often apparent following a rape. Both of these could be important factors in jurors' assessments of the credibility of a complainant. That is, jurors may perceive a complainant who has made a number of life changes as unstable rather than as exhibiting a normal reaction to a crisis situation.

In addition to completing the SAQ, both expert groups were asked for their opinions about the admissibility of rape trauma syndrome evidence and its helpfulness to jurors. There was almost complete agreement among the experts that jurors are not sufficiently knowledgeable about rape and its aftereffects. Thus, both the responses to the SAQ and the experts' opinions about juror knowledge suggest that expert testimony on rape trauma could be helpful in educating jurors and that the judicial assumption that jurors *are* adequately informed about rape victim behavior may not be well founded.

Social psychological studies have also utilized mock jury trials to investigate whether such testimony is indeed helpful and nonprejudicial to the jury. Brekke and Borgida (1988) examined juror use of expert psychological testimony by exposing student jurors to an audiotaped reenactment of a rape trial with a consent defense. In the first study mock juries of balanced sex composition were randomly assigned to one of five versions of the trial: a no-expert-testimony control; standard or specific hypothetical expert testimony presented early in the trial; and standard or specific hypothetical expert testimony presented late in the trial. The standard expert testimony addressed the low level of public awareness regarding sexual assault and contained empirical evidence designed to refute a number of widely held misconceptions about rape and rape victim behavior. The specific hypothetical testimony consisted of the standard expert testimony followed by an explicit link between the expert testimony and the case under consideration via a hypothetical example. Significant differences were found between the no-expert-testimony control and the expert-testimony conditions, indicating that the inclusion of expert testimony affects juror judgments and decision-making. The expert testimony with the greatest impact on juror perception and judgment was always the specific hypothetical version when it was presented early in the trial. Jurors exposed to the specific hypothetical expert testimony were more likely to vote for conviction and to recommend harsher sentences for the defendant, considered it less likely that the victim consented to have sexual intercourse with the defendant, and viewed the victim as being more credible than jurors who received standard expert testimony or those who did not hear any expert.

Brekke and Borgida (1988) further examined the effect of expert testimony on jury decision making by analyzing the content of audiotaped jury deliberations from the aforementioned study. Not surprisingly, jurors were more likely to use expert testimony to support the prosecution's arguments. Jurors in the specific hypothetical-expert first condition were also significantly more likely to discuss the expert's helpfulness than were jurors in the other conditions. In discussing other, nonexpert issues, expert testimony did not appear to influence the tone of jury discussion about victim credibility, to facilitate juror empathy with the victim, or to affect the way in which juries discussed the defendant or the amount of time spent discussing him. Rather, the results suggested that the most substantial change in interpretation of case facts resulting from the inclusion of expert testimony concerned the issue of resistance. Without expert testimony juries spent approximately 15% of the deliberation discussing victim resistance in a primarily defense-oriented manner (i.e., the victim did not resist enough). Jurors in the specific hypothetical-expert first condition, by contrast, discussed victim resistance less than 2% of the time, and their discussion was generally prosecution-oriented. Brekke and Borgida (1988) concluded that expert testimony, if presented strategically (i.e., linked directly to the case at hand by means of a hypothetical example and presented early in the trial), may counteract the otherwise pervasive effects of rape myths on juror judgments.

Though the existing research is provocative, it fails to provide a complete picture of the effect of expert testimony on jury decision making. Brekke (in press) conducted a study designed to examine not only the potential negative effects of expert testimony, but also the possibility that jurors respond differentially to various types of expert testimony. Mock jurors were exposed to an audiotaped reenactment of a sexual assault trial with a consent defense. Juries were randomly assigned to one of five conditions: a no-expert-testimony control; expert testimony about polygraphy presented by one or two experts; and expert testimony about rape trauma syndrome presented by one or two experts. In the single-expert versions of the trial, the expert testified on behalf of the prosecution, providing evidence based upon a polygraph test or rape trauma syndrome examination that corroborated the claims of the victim. The two-expert versions contained the testimony of the first expert and also the testimony of a second expert testifying for the defense regarding problems associated with polygraph tests or rape trauma syndrome diagnoses. Analyses of both a postdeliberation questionnaire and jury deliberations provided scant support for the notion that jurors exposed to expert scientific testimony will fall prey to inferential errors and biases and therefore fail to process information in a systematic and logical manner. On the contrary, jurors in the one- and two-expert conditions did not seem to accept blindly the testimony of expert witnesses in forming their verdicts; deliberation concerning the expert testimony was neither consistently nor overwhelmingly positive in tone; the seemingly more "scientific" results of a polygraph test did not influence jurors any more than did reports of a psychiatric interview and corresponding diagnosis; and the presence of expert testimony did not encourage the discussion of issues of dubious legal relevance or diminish the extent to which other relevant aspects of the case were discussed during deliberation. In addition, jurors exposed to conflicting evidence by two experts did not engage in a "battle" about the experts during deliberation.

The introduction of expert testimony did result in an increase in deliberation time. Jurors exposed to the experts also reported that they gave more consideration to issues of force and defendant credibility, their deliberations focused on these issues more than on the victim herself, and they used evidence presented by the experts to make inferences about the victim but not to infer negative defendant characteristics. In sum, Brekke's (in press) results suggest that many fears about the detrimental, biasing, prejudicial effects of expert testimony on juror judgment and decision making are not well founded.

EXPERT TESTIMONY IN CHILD SEXUAL ABUSE TRIALS

Many of the psycholegal research issues that have been raised and empirically examined with regard to the effects of expert testimony on eyewitness identification and rape trauma syndrome on jury decision making are clearly applicable to understanding the effects of expert testimony in child sexual abuse trials. In theory, the prescribed function of expert testimony in child sexual abuse cases is to educate the jury, either by adding new information about child sexual abuse and child memory or by addressing certain "myths" that jurors may hold about child sexual abuse (McCord, 1986; Roe, 1985; Serrato, 1988). As discussed in an earlier section of this chapter, jurors have a tendency to disbelieve young children and thus are likely to overlook the testimony of one who is usually the only eyewitness to the sexual abuse (e.g., Ross, Dunning, Toglia, & Ceci, 1989). The introduction of expert testimony could lead to a more balanced comparison of the testimony of a "young, traumatized child against [that of] a seemingly respectable adult" (Roe, 1985: 97). Thus, while expert testimony is introduced to educate the jury, expert testimony also may enhance the child witness's credibility by leading jurors to have a more informed set of expectations for children as witnesses. According to Leippe and Romanczyk (1987), jurors rely greatly upon their beliefs about how a trustworthy person acts when evaluating the credibility of witness testimony; so, expert testimony affecting these beliefs should indirectly affect juror assessment of the child witness. In particular, jurors may be more sensitive to the demeanor of a child witness to the extent that expert testimony enables them to understand important aspects of the child's testimony. For example, they may judge a nervous and hesitant child witness more leniently to the extent that they realize from expert testimony that the child witness could be hesitant for reasons other than deception. On the other hand, uninformed jurors may have a narrower range of "acceptable behaviors" that they expect a child witness to exhibit, and when children's testimony violates these expectations, children are judged as less credible (Leippe & Romanczyk, 1989).

Also, expert testimony may increase the credibility of the child witness by linking the *content* of his or her testimony to the "unusual behaviors" and reactions that children in general have to sexual abuse (McCord, 1986; Serrato, 1988). That is, jurors may judge the child's credibility by determining how well the child's description of the defendant's behavior and her reactions "match" expectations about how "this kind of thing" occurs (Leippe & Romanczyk, 1987). Since expert testimony may broaden jurors' understanding about abuse and reactions to abuse, jurors hearing expert testimony should be better able to match the reactions of a particular child witness with an understandable (and believable) sexual abuse scenario. In fact, the tendency for expert testimony to increase the favorableness of jurors' evaluations of victims' credibility has been shown in adult sexual assault cases (Brekke & Borgida, 1988).

While these hypotheses are plausible, we know surprisingly little about whether and how expert testimony may affect jurors' perceptions of child witnesses in child sexual abuse cases. In the remainder of this chapter, therefore, we generally discuss one of our own jury simulation studies that investigated the influence of expert testimony and child witness preparation on jurors' verdicts and impressions in a child sexual abuse trial. Gresham, Bull, Regan, and Borgida (1991) examined two types of expert psychological testimony: (1) the *standard* summary of symptoms of child sexual abuse victims and (2) the summary heightened by the diagnosis of a *hypothetical* case described as identical to the case in question. This study also examined the effect of child witness preparation by varying the demeanor of the child witness. Based on the Brekke and Borgida

(1988) study, Gresham and her associates expected that the hypothetical expert testimony would be more persuasive than standard expert testimony based on its explicit linking of aggregate-level scientific testimony to the case at hand. They also predicted that, given previous findings related to the demeanor of the child witness, a prepared child witness would be more persuasive and more credible as he or she would act with more consistency and confidence than an unprepared child witness.

In the Gresham research, two key independent variables were experimentally manipulated in a fully crossed factorial design: expert testimony (none, standard, hypothetical) and witness demeanor (prepared, unprepared).

Standard

Standard expert testimony described the research on relationships within a family system in which a child is being sexually abused and research on children's typical emotional and behavioral reactions to sexual abuse. Here, the prosecution asked the expert leading questions that allowed her to detail the research in a basically "lecture-style format" and to "debunk" several typical myths about child sexual abuse. However, the expert did not describe the reactions as a "syndrome."

In particular, the expert testified about her qualifications (she was a clinical psychologist) and described typical characteristics of a young sexual abuse victim. These included several fears: of telling, of being blamed, of men, of being alone, and other emotions such as confusion, shame, and guilt. Common results, according to the expert, include nightmares with assaultative content, delays in reporting, and unusual sexual knowledge. The expert described a sexually abusive family as typically including the abuser in a parenting role (though not necessarily biologically related), poor mother-daughter communication, and denial on the mother's part.

Hypothetical Testimony

Hypothetical expert testimony differed from standard testimony in its application to the case. In hypothetical testimony the expert explicitly made the link between general research and the case at hand (Brekke & Borgida, 1988). The attorney usually describes a "hypothetical" example to the expert that closely parallels the case at hand and then asks that the expert give an opinion about whether sexual abuse occurred in this particular "hypothetical" case. In this case, the hypothetical was taken directly from a key abusive incident discussed during the trial. The attorney described this "hypothetical example" to the expert and she pointed out the commonalities between it and typical incest cases.

WITNESS DEMEANOR

As discussed earlier, whether a child witness has been prepared for courtroom testimony should influence jury decision making insofar as witness credibility is affected. Gresham, Kovera, Regan, and Borgida (1991) asked 14 assistant county attorneys who often prosecute child sexual abuse cases to describe how they would prepare a child witness for court and, in their opinion, what kinds of behaviors appear to be affected by this preparation. All questions were rated on 7-point Likert scales. The attorneys agreed that court preparation greatly affects a child (M = 6.2), has a positive effect on their case (M = 6.5), and that child witnesses are almost always prepared for their time on the witness stand (M = 6.5). They next rated the frequency of typical behaviors of a prepared child witness when testifying from 1 (hardly ever) to 7 (almost always). Based on their experience, they feel that a prepared child is still somewhat upset (M = 4.6) but is less confused and uncertain (M = 3.2) and not very hesitant (M = 3.5). She also tends to be somewhat confident (M = 4.9) and to have her emotions under control (M = 4.1).

According to these experts, preparedness directly affects the child witness's demeanor during testimony. A prepared child witness should be *more* likely to look at the attorney and have her emotions under control but should be *less* likely to appear nervous, to fidget or hesitate when answering, or to appear upset. Thus, in the Gresham jury simulation study (1991), the same child actress was videotaped twice: once with specific instructions to appear nervous, upset, hesitant, and fidgety while testifying and once with instructions to appear calm, under control, reliable, and less upset. The verbal content of the testimony was virtually identical, with the exception of a few more "I don't know" answers to minor questions in the unprepared condition.

Both females (n = 122) and males (n = 104) participated in five-hour group sessions for either money or credit. In each session undergraduate college students viewed the trial together and then were divided into separate juries. After the trial these jurors deliberated in juries of either five or six members for up to 45 minutes, recorded their verdicts, and filled out several questionnaires. Data were collected from six or seven juries in each experimental condition.

JURY SIMULATION

Jurors viewed a highly involving and realistic 3.5 hour videotape of a simulated child sexual abuse case recorded by a professional camera crew in a courtroom setting. In the trial the defendant was charged with first-degree criminal sexual conduct, attempted first-degree criminal sexual conduct, and second-degree criminal sexual conduct. Professional actors played the parts of the witnesses, practicing attorneys played the parts of the legal advocates, and a retired judge played the role of the judge. The simulation was based on a 1987 Minnesota Supreme Court case, but it was modified somewhat for research purposes. The witnesses, in order of presentation, were the clinical psychology expert on child sexual abuse (in the conditions with expert testimony), the 8-year-old female victim, the social worker (the first professional to interact with the child), the child's mother, the obstetrician/gynecologist, and the child's stepfather (the defendant). The testimony of the child sexual abuse expert always came first to maximize its impact (Brekke & Borgida, 1988).

Several different versions of witnesses' testimony were filmed and edited to form the six experimental conditions. In the basic version, the abuse was reported when a 5-year-old girl described to a social worker how her stepfather had sexually abused her. The social worker testified about the initial encounter with the girl. The child witness's testimony covered such issues as what specific abuse occurred, where and when such incidents happened, and focused on a key abuse incident that appeared to lead to the actual reporting. The mother's testimony primarily described typical interactions between family members, and she was portrayed as ambivalent and confused. The doctor's testimony stated that a vaginal exam could neither confirm nor rule out penile penetration. The defendant's testimony contradicted much of the child's testimony, particularly in the area of the key abuse incident, and offered the alternative explanation of jealousy for her accusations.

After viewing the trial version for that condition, jurors recorded their verdicts for the three counts on an initial straw vote before deliberations began and then recorded them a second time either after reaching a verdict or after 45 minutes of audiotaped deliberation. Jurors rated the defendant as either guilty or innocent on three possible charges: first-degree criminal sexual conduct (CSC), attempted first-degree CSC, and second-degree CSC. After deliberations each juror received and individually completed a questionnaire. First, they recorded verdicts and rated the defendant's guilt for each of the three separate charges in the case.

Jurors also rated the importance of witnesses and several key aspects of testimony in determining verdicts for each of the three separate counts. Thus, they rated the items three separate times, once for each charge. Then, jurors gave semantic differential ratings of the characters assessing impressions of credibility, veracity, and likeability, or (in the case of the attorneys) likeability and competence. Jurors next reported how strongly they felt during the child witness's testimony. Finally, jurors' memories for the evidence and judge's instructions were tested in a free-recall format focusing on criteria differentiating various charges and factual points made in the child's testimony and the expert's testimony.

According to previous research on expert testimony concerning adult sexual assault (Brekke & Borgida, 1988), the hypothetical expert condition should lead to significantly more favorable evaluations of the victim and guilty verdicts than either the standard expert testimony or no expert testimony. The second experimental factor examined by Gresham, et al.—witness preparedness—should affect credibility perceptions of the child witness and, in turn, influence juror verdicts. A child witness who has been prepared for the courtroom experience should be more likely to give calm, less hysterical and confused testimony on the stand. The research on children's speech styles of power, powerlessness, and witness credibility, reviewed earlier in this chapter, suggests that a calmer, less hesitant delivery should lead to more favorable evaluations of the child's credibility and to a greater tendency to convict the defendant in a child sexual abuse case.

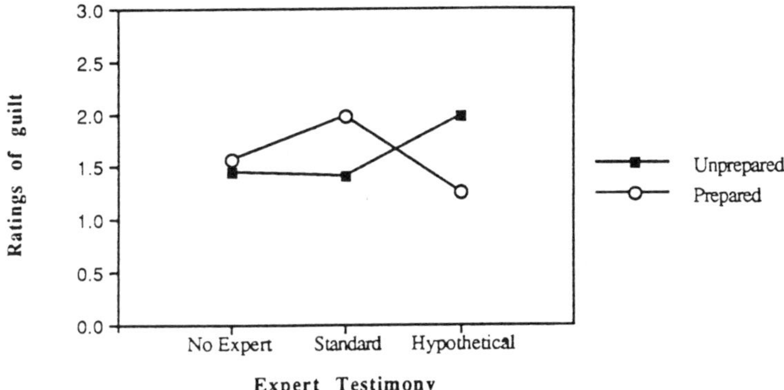

Figure 6.1: Jurors' combined ratings of guilt on three charges.

Juror Verdicts

It will be recalled that jurors rated the defendant as either guilty or innocent on three possible charges. These three dichotomous measures were then combined into a scale ranging from 0 (not guilty on all charges) to 3 (guilty on all charges). An analysis of variance on this scale (expert testimony x child witness demeanor) revealed no main effects but a reliable two-way interaction, $F (2,219) = 5.65$, $p < .01$, such that child witness demeanor did not have a strong effect in the no-expert condition but showed an interesting crossover interaction in the other two conditions. It may be seen in Figure 6–1 that when jurors listened to *standard* expert testimony and viewed the prepared child witness, they tended to judge the defendant as somewhat more guilty than those viewing the unprepared child witness. In contrast, jurors who listened to the *hypothetical* expert and viewed the unprepared child judged the defendant as more guilty than those who viewed the prepared child witness.

Juror Ratings of the Child Witness

Jurors rated the child witness on several semantic differential items related to both credibility (credible-not credible; certain-uncertain; convincing-unconvincing) and to likeability (like-dislike; attractive-unattractive; good-bad). The interaction between type of expert testimony and child witness demeanor, however, was not found in the semantic differential ratings of the child's credibility. Some main effects were found for expert testimony on jurors' ratings of the child witness's likeability, F (2,220) = 3.00, p = .05. Jurors seem to view the child witness as more attractive in the standard expert condition. This main effect, however, was subsumed by a reliable interaction between expert testimony and child demeanor, F (2,220) = 3.18 p < .05. As seen in Figure 6–2, this interaction was similar to the one described above in that jurors in the *hypothetical* expert condition viewed the unprepared child witness as more likeable, attractive, and good than the prepared child. Jurors in both the other two expert conditions, however, viewed the prepared child as more likeable.

Juror Ratings of the Defendant

Analysis of variance again revealed a significant expert testimony by child demeanor interaction on the defendant's likeability ratings, F (2,220) = 6.37, p < .01. As may be seen in Figure 6–3, jurors who viewed *hypothetical* expert testimony were consistent with their previous ratings, such that those who viewed the unprepared child witness disliked the defendant more than those viewing a prepared witness. However, the other expert conditions were less clear: jurors hearing the standard expert testimony showed little differentiation between prepared and unprepared witnesses, whereas jurors in the no-expert-control condition showed the least favorability to the

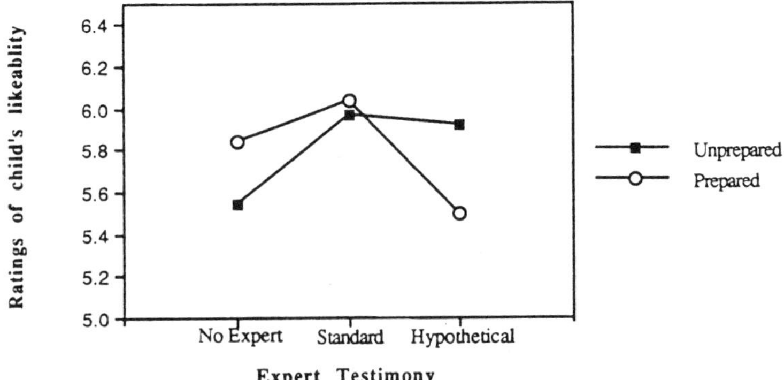

Figure 6.2: Likeability ratings of child witness as a function of child witness demeanor and expert testimony.

defendant when viewing a prepared child witness. In addition, juror ratings revealed a main effect for expert testimony on the defendant's credibility, $F (2,220) = 4.82$, $p = .009$, such that the defendant was perceived as less credible in the standard expert condition.

In conclusion, jurors in the Gresham study who heard hypothetical expert testimony viewed the courtroom testimony of a nervous, hesitant, unprepared child witness as *more* credible and were more likely to convict the defendant than jurors who heard comparable testimony from a prepared child witness. In child sexual abuse cases, then, witness demeanor represents one important psychological variable that interacts with and qualifies the effects of expert psychological testimony on jury decision making. To the extent that expert testimony sensitizes jurors to use certain features of the evidence (e.g., the child's courtroom demeanor) to evaluate the overall strength of evidence in a given case, one would expect hypothetical expert testimony to demonstrate the most inferential impact when jurors evaluate a nervous, hesitant child witness. By allowing the expert to link explicitly the nervous and hesitant reactions of child sexual abuse victims in general directly to the case at hand, the expert hypothetical may influence jurors' typical expectations of how the child witness would be expected to behave. Thus, jurors may come to expect a confused, hesitant demeanor from more credible child witnesses. When these beliefs are disconfirmed (e.g., by a prepared child witness), in fact jurors may be more likely to evaluate negatively the child witness.

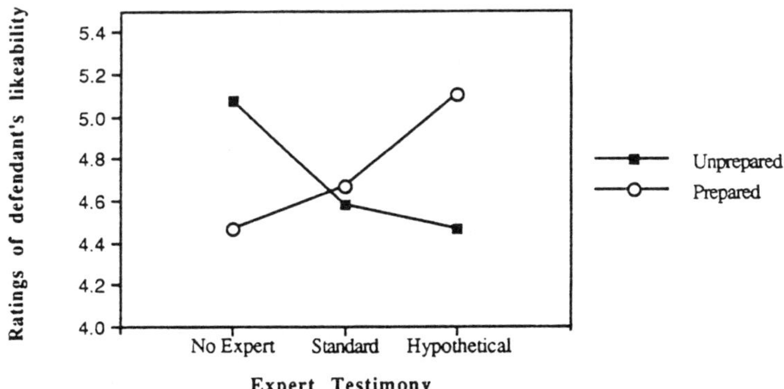

Figure 6.3: Likeability ratings of defendant as a function of child witness demeanor and expert testimony.

CONCLUSIONS

In this chapter we discussed some of the research issues raised by the expanded prosecutorial use of expert psychological testimony in child sexual abuse cases. Research on the nature of children's cognitive abilities and studies from psychology that examine jurors' perceptions of child witnesses were overviewed, and our own research on the influence of expert testimony on juror decision making in a simulated child sexual abuse trial was presented. A consideration of the legal and scientific status of expert testimony in child sexual abuse cases, however, must conclude with an acknowledgement of two more general issues that pertain to the analysis of *any* type of expert psychological testimony. First, as psychology and social science become increasingly prevalent in the legal system, including appellate decisions, there will always be questions about the adequacy of the scientific database (Fiske, Bersoff, Borgida, et al., in press). How perfect does the database have to be for psychologists to render expert opinions in court?

Whereas (arguably) the sufficiency of the scientific databases with regard to eyewitness identification (e.g., Kassin, Ellsworth, & Smith, 1989), death qualified juries (e.g., Elliott, 1991; Ellsworth, 1991), and sex stereotyping (e.g., Fiske, Bersoff, Borgida, et al, in press) are now reasonably well established; to date, only a few aspects of the scientific database on child sexual abuse have achieved the level of convergent validity that characterizes these other more scientifically mature databases (e.g., see APA amicus brief in *Maryland v. Craig*, 1990). Presumably, as the scientific research literature on child sexual abuse expands, and is deemed more adequate by the application of generally accepted peer review standards, the use of expert psychological testimony in child sexual abuse cases will become less controversial.

Finally, it is important to note that the ethical issues that arise in the child sexual abuse context are the same as those that arise in regard to other types of expert psychological testimony (Frazier & Borgida, in press). Which victim behaviors have been reliably established, of course, is open to interpretation, and experts are bound to disagree. Thus, it is the ethical responsibility of each expert to be familiar with the existing research database and only to describe victim behaviors that have been reliably established in the literature.

REFERENCES

Abbey, A.; Cozzarelli, C.; McLaughlin, K.; & Harnish, R. (1987). The effects of clothing and dyad sex composition on perceptions of sexual intent: do women and men evaluate these cues differently? *Journal of Applied Social Psychology* 17: 108–126.

American Psychological Association (1990). Motion for leave to file brief amicus curiae and brief for amicus curiae to the U.S. Supreme Court in *Maryland v. Craig*. No. 89–478.

Bond, S.B., & Mosher, D.L. (1986). Guided imagery of rape: fantasy, reality, and the willing victim myth. *Journal of Sex Research* 22: 162–183.

Borgida, E. (1981). Legal reform of rape laws. In L. Bickman (ed.), *Applied Social Psychology Annual*. Vol. 2, pp. 211–241. Newbury Park, Calif.: Sage.

Borgida, E., & Brekke, N. (1985). Psycholegal research on rape trials. In A. Burgess (ed.), *Rape and Sexual Assault: A Research Handbook*. Pp. 313–324. New York: Garland.

Borgida, E.; Gresham, A.W.; Swim, J.; et al. (1989). Expert testimony in child sexual abuse cases: an empirical investigation of partisan orientation. *Family Law Quarterly* 23: 433–449.

Brekke, N. (in press). Expert psychological testimony: are we underestimating the average juror? *Law and Human Behavior*.

Brekke, N., & Borgida, E. (1988). Expert psychological testimony in rape trials: a social-cognitive analysis. *Journal of Personality and Social Psychology* 55: 372–386.

Brigham, J.C., & Bothwell, R.K. (1983). The ability of prospective jurors to estimate the accuracy of eyewitness identifications. *Law and Human Behavior* 7: 19–30.

Brown, A.L. (1979). Theories of memory and the problem of development: activity, growth and knowledge. In L. Cermak & F.I.M. Craik (eds.), *Levels of Processing in Memory*. Pp. 225–258. Hillsdale, N.J.: Erlbaum.

Buckhout, R. (1974). Eyewitness testimony. *Scientific American* 231: 23–31.

Buckhout, R.; Alper, A.; Chern, S.; et al. (1974). Determinants of eyewitness performance on a lineup. *Bulletin of the Psychonomic Society* 4: 191–192.

Carey, S., & Diamond, R. (1977). From piecemeal to configurational representation of faces. *Science* 195: 312–314.

Ceci, S.J.; Ross, D.F.; & Toglia, M.P. (1987). Age differences in suggestibility: narrowing the uncertainties. In S.J. Ceci, M.P. Toglia, & D.F. Ross (eds.), *Children's eyewitness memory*. Pp. 79–91. New York: Springer-Verlag.

Cohen, J., & Cohen, P. (1975). *Applied multiple regression/correlation analysis for the behavioral sciences*. Hillsdale, N.J.: Erlbaum.

Cohen, R.L., & Harnick, M.A. (1980). The susceptibility of child witnesses to suggestion: an empirical study. *Law and Human Behavior* 4: 201–21.

Corder, B.F., & Whiteside, R. (1988). A survey of jurors' perception of issues related to child sexual abuse. *American Journal of Forensic Psychology* 6: 37–43.

Cutler, B.L.; Dexter, H.R.; & Penrod, S.D. (1989). Expert testimony and jury decision making: an empirical analysis. *Behavioral Sciences and the Law* 7: 215–225.

Cutler, B.L.; Penrod, S.D.; & Dexter, H.R. (1989). The eyewitness, the expert psychologist, and the jury. *Law and Human Behavior* 13: 311–322.

Cutler, B.L.; Penrod, S.D.; & Dexter, H.R. (1990). Juror sensitivity to eyewitness identification evidence. *Law and Human Behavior* 14: 185–191.

Cutler, B.L.; Penrod, S.D.; & Stuve, T.E. (1988). Juror decision making in eyewitness identification cases. *Law and Human Behavior* 12: 41–55.

Dale, P.S.; Loftus, E.F.; & Rathbun, L. (1978). The influence of the form of the question on the eyewitness testimony of preschool children. *Journal of Psycholinguistic Research* 7: 269–277.

Deffenbacher, K.A. (1980). Eyewitness accuracy and confidence: can we infer anything about their relationship? *Law and Human Behavior* 4: 243–260.

Deffenbacher, K.A., & Loftus, E.F. (1982). Do jurors share a common understanding concerning eyewitness behavior? *Law and Human Behavior* 6: 15–30.

Diamond, R., & Carey, S. (1977). Developmental changes in the representation of faces. *Journal of Experimental Child Psychology* 23: 1–22.

Duggan, III, L.M.; Aubrey, M.; Doherty, E.; et al. (1989). The credibility of children as witnesses in a simulated child sexual abuse trial. In S.J. Ceci, D.F. Ross, & M.P. Toglia (eds.), *Perspectives on Children's Testimony*. Pp. 71–99. New York: Springer-Verlag.

Duncan, E.M.; Whitney, P.; & Kunen, S. (1982). Integration of visual and verbal information in children's memories. *Child Development* 53: 1215–1223.

Elliott, R. (1991). Social science data and the APA: the *Lockhart* brief as a case in point. *Law and Human Behavior* 15: 59–76.

Ellison, K.W., & Buckhout, R. (1981). *Psychology and Criminal Justice.* New York: Harper & Row.

Ellsworth, P. (1991). To tell what we know or wait for Godot? *Law and Human Behavior* 15: 77–90.

Enns, J.T., & Girgus, J.S. (1985). Developmental changes in selective and integrative visual attention. *Journal of Experimental Child Psychology* 40: 319–337.

Fiske, S.T.; Bersoff, D.N.; Borgida, E.; et al. (in press). Social science research on trial: the use of sex stereotyping research in *Price Waterhouse v. Hopkins. American Psychologist.*

Fox, S. G., & Walters, H. A. (1986). The impact of general versus specific expert testimony and eyewitness confidence upon mock juror judgment. *Law and Human Behavior* 10: 215–228.

Frazier, P., & Borgida, E. (1985). Rape trauma syndrome evidence in court. *American Psychologist* 40: 984–993.

Frazier, P., & Borgida, E. (1988). Juror common understanding and the admissibility of rape trauma syndrome evidence in court. *Law and Human Behavior* 12: 101–122.

Frazier, P., & Borgida, E. (in press). Rape trauma syndrome: a review of case law and psychological research. *Law and Human Behavior.*

Frye v. United States, 293 F. 1013 (1923).

Goodman, G.S.; Aman, C.; & Hirschman, J. (1987). Child sexual and physical abuse: children's testimony. In S.J. Ceci, M.P. Toglia, & D.F. Ross (eds.), *Children's Eyewitness Memory.* Pp. 1–23. New York: Springer-Verlag.

Goodman, G.S.; Bottoms, B.L.; Herscovici, B.B.; & Shaver, P. (1989). Determinants of the child victim's perceived credibility. In S.J. Ceci, D.F. Ross, & M.P. Toglia (eds.), *Perspectives on Children's Testimony.* Pp. 1–22. New York: Springer–Verlag.

Goodman, G.S.; Golding, J.M.; & Haith, M.M. (1984). Jurors' reactions to child eyewitnesses. *Journal of Social Issues* 40: 139–156.

Goodman, G.S.; Golding, J.M.; Helgeson, V.S.; et al. (1987). When a child takes the stand: jurors' perceptions of children's eyewitness testimony. *Law and Human Behavior* 11: 27–40.

Goodman, G.S., & Reed, R.S. (1986). Age differences in eyewitness testimony. *Law and Human Behavior* 10: 317–332.

Gresham, A.W.; Bull, M.A.; Regan, P.C.; & Borgida, E. (1991). The influence of expert testimony and child witness demeanor on jury decision making. Paper presented at the annual meeting of the American Psychological Society, Washington, D.C.

Hosch, H.M.; Beck, E.L.; & McIntyre, P. (1980). Influence of expert testimony regarding eyewitness accuracy on jury decisions. *Law and Human Behavior* 4: 287–296.

Kassin, S.M.; Ellsworth, P.C.; & Smith, V.L. (1989). The "general acceptance" of psychological research on eyewitness testimony: a survey of the experts. *American Psychologist* 44: 1089–1098.

King, M.A., & Yuille, J.C. (1987). Suggestibility and the child witness. In S.J. Ceci, M.P. Toglia, & D.F. Ross (eds.), *Children's Eyewitness Testimony*. Pp. 24–35. New York: Springer-Verlag.

Konecni, V.J., & Ebbesen, E.B. (1979). External validity of research in legal psychology. *Law and Human Behavior* 3: 39–70.

Kovera, M.B.; Borgida, E.; Gresham, A.W.; et al. (1991). Do child sexual abuse experts hold partisan beliefs?: a national survey of the Society for Traumatic Stress Studies. Unpublished manuscript, University of Minnesota, Minneapolis.

Leippe, M.R., & Romanczyk, A. (1987). Children on the witness stand: a communication/persuasion analysis of jurors' reactions to child witnesses. In S.J. Ceci, M.P. Toglia, & D.F. Ross (eds.), *Children's Eyewitness Memory*. New York: Springer-Verlag.

Leippe, M.R., & Romanczyck, A. (1989). Reactions to child (versus adult) eyewitness: the influence of jurors' preconceptions and witness behavior. *Law and Human Behavior* 13: 103–132.

Lindsay, R.C.L.; Wells, G.L.; & Rumpel, C.M. (1981). Can people detect eyewitness-identification accuracy within and across situations? *Journal of Applied Psychology* 66: 79–89.

List, J.A. (1986). Age and schematic differences in the reliability of eyewitness testimony. *Developmental Psychology* 22: 50–57.

Loftus, E.F. (1974). Reconstructing memory: the incredible eyewitness. *Psychology Today* 8: 116–119.

Loftus, E.F. (1979). *Eyewitness Testimony*. Cambridge: Harvard University Press.

Loftus, E.F. (1980). Impact of expert psychological testimony on the unreliability of eyewitness identification. *Journal of Applied Psychology* 65: 9–15.

Loftus, E.F. (1983). Silence is not golden. *American Psychologist* 38: 564–572.

Loftus, E.F., & Burns, T. (1982). Mental shock can produce retrograde amnesia. *Memory and Cognition* 10: 318–323.

Loftus, E.F.; Miller, D.G.; & Burns, H.J. (1978). Semantic integration of verbal information into a visual memory. *Journal of Experimental Psychology: Human Learning and Memory* 4: 19–31.

Loftus, E. F., & Monahan, J. (1980). Trial by data: psychological research as legal evidence. *American Psychologist* 35: 270–283.

Maass, A.; Brigham, J.C.; & West, S.G. (1985). Testifying on eyewitness reliability: expert advice is not always persuasive. *Journal of Applied Social Psychology* 15: 207–229.

McCloskey, M., & Egeth, H. (1983). Eyewitness identification: what can a psychologist tell a jury? *American Psychologist* 38: 550–563.

McCloskey, M.; Egeth, H.; & McKenna, J. (1986). The ethics of expert testimony. *Law and Human Behavior* (special issue) 10: (12).

McCord, D. (1986). Expert psychological testimony about child complainants in sexual abuse prosecutions: a foray into the admissibility of novel psychological evidence. *Journal of Criminal Law and Criminology* 77: 1– 67.

Mandler, J.M., & Robinson, C.A. (1978). Developmental changes in picture recognition. *Journal of Experimental Child Psychology* 26: 122–136.

Marin, B.V.; Holmes, D.L.; Guth, M.; & Kovac, P. (1979). The potential of children as eyewitnesses: a comparison of children and adults on eyewitness tasks. *Law and Human Behavior* 3: 295–305.

Marquis, K.H.; Marshall, J.; & Oskamp, S. (1972). Testimony validity as a function of question form, atmosphere, and item difficulty. *Journal of Applied Social Psychology* 2: 167–186.

Newcombe, N.; Rogoff, B.; & Kagan, J. (1977). Developmental changes in recognition memory for pictures of objects and scenes. *Developmental Psychology* 13: 337–341.

Nigro, G.N.; Buckley, M.A.; Hill, D.E.; & Nelson, J. (1989). When juries "hear" children testify: the effects of eyewitness age and speech style on jurors' perceptions of testimony. In S.J. Ceci, D.F. Ross, & M.P. Toglia (eds.), *Perspectives on Children's Testimony.* Pp. 57–70. New York: Springer-Verlag.

Nigro, G.N., & Gudatis, R. (April 1987). The effects of age, context, and retention interval on memory for a single event. Paper presented at the Biennial Meetings of the Society for Research in Child Development, Baltimore.

Penrod, S.; Bull, M. A.; & Lengnick, S. (1989). Children as observers and witnesses: the empirical data. *Family Law Quarterly* 23: 411–431.

Poole, D.A., & White, L.T. (May 1990). The effects of repeated questioning on the eyewitness testimony of children and adults. Paper presented at the meetings of the Midwestern Psychological Association, Chicago.

Roe, R. (1985). Expert testimony in child sexual abuse cases. *University of Miami Law Review* 40: 97–113.

Ross, D.F.; Dunning, D.; Toglia, M.P.; & Ceci, S.J. (1989). Age stereotypes, communication modality, and mock jurors' perceptions of the child witness. In S.J. Ceci, D.F. Ross, & M.P. Toglia (eds.), *Perspectives on Children's Testimony.* Pp. 37–56. New York: Springer-Verlag.

Ross, D.F.; Dunning, D.; Toglia, M.P.; & Ceci, S.J. (1990). The child in the eyes of the jury: assessing mock jurors' perceptions of the child witness. *Law and Human Behavior* 14: 5–24.

Ross, D.F.; Miller, B.S.; & Moran, P.B. (1987). The child in the eyes of the jury: assessing mock jurors' perceptions of the child witness. In S.J. Ceci, M.P. Toglia, & D.F. Ross (eds.), *Children's Eyewitness Memory.* Pp. 142–154. New York: Springer-Verlag.

Saks, M. (1990). Expert witnesses, nonexpert witnesses, and nonwitness experts. *Law and Human Behavior* 14: 291–314.

Saywitz, K.J. (1987). Children's testimony: age-related patterns of memory errors. In S.J. Ceci, M.P. Toglia, & D.F. Ross (eds.), *Children's Eyewitness Memory.* Pp. 36–52. New York: Springer-Verlag.

Serrato, V. (1988). Expert testimony in child sexual abuse prosecutions: a spectrum of uses. *Boston University Law Review* 68: 155–192.

Summit, R.C. (1983). The child sexual abuse accommodation syndrome. *Child Abuse and Neglect* 7: 177–193.

Tetreault, P. (1989). Rape myth acceptance: a case for providing educational expert testimony in rape jury trials. *Behavioral Sciences and the Law* 7: 243–257.

Wall, P.M. (1965). *Eyewitness Identification in Criminal Cases.* Springfield, Ill.: Thomas.

Wells, G.L. (1978). Applied eyewitness testimony research: system variables and estimator variables. *Journal of Personality and Social Psychology* 36: 1546–1557.

Wells, G.L.; Lindsay, R.C.L.; & Ferguson, T.J. (1979). Accuracy, confidence, and juror perceptions in eyewitness identification. *Journal of Applied Psychology* 64: 440–448.

Wells, G.L.; Lindsay, R.C.L.; & Tousignant, J.P. (1980). Effects of expert psychological advice on human performance in judging the validity of eyewitness testimony. *Law and Human Behavior* 4: 275–285.

Wells, G.L.; & Turtle, J.W. (1987). Eyewitness testimony research: current knowledge and emergent controversies. *Canadian Journal of Behavioural Science* 19: 363–388.

Yarmey, A.D. (1979). *The Psychology of Eyewitness Testimony*. New York: Free Press.

Yarmey, A.D., & Jones, H.P.T. (1983). Is the psychology of eyewitness identification a matter of common sense? In S.M.A. Lloyd-Bostock & B.R. Clifford (eds.), *Evaluating Witness Evidence: Recent psychological research and new perspectives*. Pp. 13–40. Chichester, England: Wiley.

CHAPTER 7

The Child Witness in Florida

Garrett J. McAvoy

Data collection and analysis were supported by a
U.S. Department of Justice, Office of Juvenile
Justice and Delinquency Prevention grant
(MC-CX-K001).

THE CHILD WITNESS IN FLORIDA

The Missing and Exploited Children Comprehensive Action Program, or M/CAP, has commissioned a number of projects that serve the needs of missing and exploited children in the United States. One facet of the M/CAP concerns the manner in which children are treated in America's courtrooms. Children who have to testify as crime victims are often retraumatized by the truth-finding process of trial. However, a number of states have implemented innovative procedural measures for child witnesses that aim to reduce trauma to the testifying child. The focus of this Florida report is on laws designed to reduce trauma to the missing or exploited child victim who is a witness in any legal proceeding.

Florida is classified as a "progressive" state in terms of the protections it affords child witnesses. Lawmakers there have codified more than thirty trauma reducing procedures over the past ten years. Additionally, Florida's courts have been sympathetic to the child witness in a number of recent appellate court rulings. Legal practitioners within the state receive Continuing Legal Education (CLE) courses on the topic of the child witness as well. The CLE courses provide practitioners with discretionary tools that help to reduce trauma to young witnesses. The combined efforts of these various groups have made Florida a state that other jurisdictions can look to in adopting their own trauma-reducing laws.

OVERVIEW

General

The state of Florida has addressed the unmet needs of children in a number of studies and reports issued during the past year. The governor, legislature, judiciary, and Florida Bar have all written separate reports that indicate that Florida's children are at risk due to a wide variety of societal problems. The reports acknowledge the fact that missing and exploited children often suffer trauma as a result of a legal process that is designed for adults, not children. The diverse reports mentioned above highlight the need to assist the missing/exploited child through all phases of the legal process. A recurrent finding of the reports was that there is no single, yet comprehensive code that practitioners can look to in order to find the tools available to assist them in reducing trauma to the child victim who is a witness. This report is an attempt to provide a first draft compendium of an unofficial code and case law study for use in Florida's communities by professionals who work with child witnesses. In effect, this compilation can serve to reduce the amount of time judges, attorneys, law enforcement officials, clinicians, and others involved with children must spend to find and interpret child witness law in the state. The focus of the compendium is on laws that reduce trauma to the child witness in any legal proceeding.

This study is not limited to practitioners in Florida, however. The fact that people in the state have a profound interest for the child witness has been important in the development of a number of innovative and progressive laws that can serve to protect child victims anywhere. This means that professionals in other states can use Florida's laws as a guide for innovations or changes in their own jurisdictions. Most laws are intended to cover either the missing or exploited child, such as the special oath for young witnesses. Some laws are limited to sexually exploited children though, such as certain exceptions to the hearsay rule. These distinctions are important for communities that have adopted the Missing and Exploited Children Comprehensive Action Program (M/CAP) since not all laws apply to the "missing child witness."

The Research

The Florida research was largely a replication of the child witness study conducted in Connecticut. It was compiled in a two-phase operation. In the first phase, the National Task Force for Children's Constitutional Rights (Task Force) analyzed and assembled all relevant mandatory law existing in Florida during a six-day intensive research swarm. This research included recent U.S. Supreme Court decisions, Florida Statutes, and Florida case law. The research was completed at the Connecticut State Library, which provides access to the most recent laws of every state in the nation.

Phase two was conducted on site in Hillsborough County, Florida. The goal of phase two was to interview as many local practitioners as possible over a seven-day period. Practitioners were carefully selected by Task Force personnel in coordination with the Hillsborough M/CAP chairman and the National Center for Missing and Exploited Children. Among those interviewed by the Task Force were a circuit court criminal judge, a juvenile judge, a family court judge, two former state's attorneys from the sex crime division, the senior attorney from the Department of Health and Rehabilitative Services (HRS), the team coordinator for the Child Protective Team (CPT), a juvenile services guardian ad litem director, pro bono guardians ad litem, a subdistrict administrator at HRS, and a sergeant from the Juvenile Operations Unit at the Hillsborough County Sheriff's Office. An ancillary goal during the on-site visit was to obtain the most up-to-date laws related to child victims in Florida. This was achieved in coordination with the law clerks' office at the circuit court in Hillsborough County. The Task Force had access to the LEXIS research system at that office. This was our first chance to use automated research for the project. The Task Force also used the expertise of the law clerks in obtaining relevant contemporaneous reports issued in Florida, such as recent attorney general opinions, law review weeklies, and pending legislation.

Research Highlights

General. Lawmakers in Florida apparently devote much attention to the child witness. This is manifested in the volume of statutes and case law generated by the legislature and the courts, respectively. The Task Force compiled nearly 30 statutes that serve to protect the interests of child victim witnesses. The courts have not been as sympathetic to the plight of the child witness, however. Cases abound in the state on child witness issues; yet many of the rulings favor not the victim but, rather, the rights of the accused. However, a recent trend has shown that the Florida Supreme Court is willing to uphold laws that tend to reduce trauma to the child, even in cases where the rights of the accused are at stake. See *Glendening v. State*, 536 So.2d 212 (Fla. 1988), *cert. denied*, 109 S.Ct. 3219 (1989).

The courts' rulings on statutes designed to protect child victims are not the only source of concern in the state. It seems that the large volume of statutes also causes problems for attorneys and judges. This translates to problems for the child victim witness. The problem that attorneys and judges have with the large volume of statutes is in knowing which ones are available to them at any given time. The Report of the Study Commission on Child Welfare, *Recommendations*, found that "laws affecting children are now found in many separate chapters in Florida Statutes, which is confusing because some laws are repetitive, others conflicting. A consequence is the fragmented treatment of the problems of children and their families." The Task Force wishes to help treat this malady in our Florida study.

Intermediate Level Appellate Reviews. Florida has five district courts of appeals in the state. Each circuit court falls within the jurisdiction of a district court of appeals. When a new issue has been decided by just one district court of appeals, then that decision controls in all circuit courts in the state. The other district courts of appeals use this decision as persuasive authority when faced with the same issue, but they are not bound by that decision. When one district decrees counter to another district, then circuit courts are bound by the district decree in which they sit. When there are conflicting decrees from district courts, then the Florida Supreme Court will step in to decide the issue for all districts.

The organization of Florida's appellate courts is important for the child witness project. Currently, many district court of appeals rulings hold sway throughout the entire state because only one court has decided the issue or because other districts have agreed with the ruling in a separate case. There are also conflicting rulings that exist in the state that the state's highest court has not yet decided. Two such rulings concern the interpretation of the child hearsay statute. See *Kopko v. State*, 577 So.2d 956 (Fla. 5th DCA 1991) and *State v. Pardo*, 16 FLW D1791 (Fla. 3rd DCA 1991). Certiorari has been granted by the Florida Supreme Court on the issue in conflict. If the supreme court agrees with the cogent argument of the 3rd District Court of Appeals, it will be easier for attorneys to gain admittance of prior consistent hearsay declarations, as reasoned in *Pardo*.

Guardian ad Litem. Florida has an extensive guardian ad litem (GAL) program. Special training courses are set up in the state for GALs, and the frequent use of GALs in criminal proceedings is a phenomenon not encountered too often in other jurisdictions because of the traditional use of GALs in civil matters only. However, there is still a problem of not enough volunteers in a system of ever increasing demands.

Interviews. The practitioners in Hillsborough County indicated that children are interviewed more than is necessary. Despite the circuit court chief judge's rule requiring that a child not be interviewed more than three times during a legal proceeding, attorneys and HRS workers stated that this rule is disregarded frequently. There are interview protocols between law enforcement and CPTs, but these are not always followed either. An awareness of the trauma created by repetitive interviews and an expanded use of videotape or other special procedures can help to reduce this vexation.

Evidence. Florida, unlike Connecticut, has an evidence code. It provides a number of trauma-reducing techniques for the willing attorney. The evidence code is significant in two respects: it is an easy reference for professionals to use, and it encapsules a number of important tools in one concise section of the Florida Code. A newcomer to Connecticut must sift through a number of treatises and cases to gather all of the relevant trauma-reducing methods available in the realm of evidence law. This is not true in Florida.

TRAUMA-REDUCING STATUTES AND RULES

Rules of Criminal Procedure

Rule 3.220, Discovery. This statute requires depositions of children under the age of 16 to be videotaped unless otherwise ordered by the court. The statute states that a defendant "shall not be physically present at a deposition except upon stipulation of the parties or upon court order for good cause shown." See *In re Amendment to Florida Rule Crim. Proc.*, 550 So.2d 1097, 1103 (Fla. 1989). The statute applies to discovery in criminal proceedings only; all child witnesses fall within the purview of this statute.

Juvenile Procedure

Rule 8.590, Guardian ad Litem. This rule states that at any stage of a dependency proceeding "any party may request or the court may appoint a guardian ad litem to represent any child alleged to be dependent." The appointed GAL represents the "best interests" of the child, as opposed to representing the child within the context of counsel-client relationships.

Rule 8.610, General Provisions for Hearings. Children involved in dependency proceedings may be examined by the court outside the presence of other parties (in-camera). The court may exclude all other witnesses if the court finds it necessary to do so; the court must exclude all other witnesses upon request by any party involved in the dependency proceeding. Any party may file a motion to excuse the presence of a child.

Section 39.408, Hearings for Dependency Cases. This statute is akin to Rule 8.610 and similarly allows for an in-camera examination of a child involved in a dependency case. The statute demonstrates the duplicity found in many parts of the Florida Code. The court need not determine that the child would be traumatized to use in-camera exam under this section. See *Castellanos v. Department of Health and Rehabilitative Services*, 545 So.2d 455 (3rd DCA 1989).

Termination of Parental Rights

Section 39.465, Right to Counsel; Guardian ad Litem. "The court shall appoint a guardian ad litem to represent the child in any termination of parental rights proceedings and shall ascertain at each stage of the proceedings whether a guardian ad litem has been appointed."

Dissolution of Marriage

Section 61.001, Purpose of Chapter. This statute requires a liberal construction and application of laws found in Chapter 61 of the Florida Statutes. Obviously, this means that circuit court family judges have wide discretion in custody/dissolution proceedings. Sympathetic judges will interpret this chapter in favor of the child witness. One purpose of the statute is "to mitigate the potential harm to . . . children caused by the process of legal dissolution of marriage."

Section 61.011, Dissolution in Chancery. Simply, this statute provides that divorce proceedings are in chancery or, in other words, in "equity." Judges in equity proceedings are cloaked with the maxim that they will do what is necessary to ensure fairness to all parties concerned. This means that family court judges have great discretion in protecting the child witness and can use many protective measures "sua sponte." See "Discretionary Measures," below.

Evidence

Section 90.5035, Sexual Assault Counselor-Victim Privilege. This statute provides that a communication between a sexual assault counselor and a victim is confidential if it is not intended to be disclosed to third persons other than those persons present to further the victim's interests and/or those persons to whom the disclosure is reasonably necessary to accomplish the purposes for which the sexual assault counselor is consulted. The GAL may claim this privilege for the child.

Section 90.601, General Rule of Competency. Florida has no presumption of competency for child witnesses, unlike some other states (i.e., Connecticut). The general rule of witness competency is that "it is within the sound discretion of the trial judge to decide whether an infant of tender years has sufficient mental capacity and sense of moral obligation to be competent as a witness, and his ruling will not be disturbed unless a manifest abuse of discretion is shown." See *Williams v. State*, 400 So.2d 471 (DCA 1981), aff'd, 406 So.2d 1115 (Fla. 1981). Establishing competency and credibility is discussed in "Discretionary Measures," below. The competency examination must be more than "de minimus," *Griffin v. State*, 526 So.2d 752 (1st DCA 1988).

Section 90.605, Oath or Affirmation of Witness. "In the court's discretion, a child may testify without taking the oath if the court determines the child understands the duty to tell the truth or the duty not to lie."

Section 90.612, Mode and Order of Interrogation and Presentation. Leading questions are generally not allowed on direct or redirect examination of witnesses. Judges have little discretion in Florida concerning leading questions. See *Erp v. Carroll*, 438 So.2d 31 (5th DCA 1983). One exception to this general rule concerns the "reluctant or recalcitrant" witness. The reluctant witness, i.e., potentially the nonverbal child victim, "should always be subject to interrogation by leading question" on direct or redirect examination, *Erp v. Carroll*.

Section 90.614, Prior Statements of Witnesses. This statute does not allow prior inconsistent statements of witnesses into testimony, unless the witness is first afforded the opportunity to explain the inconsistency. While there is no case law on point concerning inconsistent statements of child victims, it seems plausible to infer that an expert should be able to testify as to why certain child victims give inconsistent statements during interviews. Other states recognize such a need (e.g., Connecticut).

Section 90.702, Testimony by Experts. This statute covers a wide array of the admissibility of expert testimony. Two cases are directly on point. The first states that a qualified expert is "entitled to express opinion on [the] issue of whether [a] child has been sexually molested," *Glendening v. State*, 536 So.2d 212 (Fla. 1988) *cert. den'd* 109 S.Ct. 3219. The second case says an expert may testify that a "sexual battery victim demonstrated symptoms indicative of child sexual abuse syndrome," *Calloway v. State*, 520 So.2d 665 (1st DCA 1988).

Section 90.803, Hearsay Exceptions; Availability of Declarant Immaterial. This statute provides a number of relevant hearsay exceptions for the child victim. Spontaneous statements, excited utterances, and statements made for the purposes of medical treatment are among the "traditional" hearsay exceptions located under this statute. The "child hearsay" exception is also treated under this statute, but its application will be discussed under "Relevant Case Law," below, due to the complexities of recent rulings in Florida and at the U.S. Supreme Court on the issue of admissibility.

Section 92.53, Sexual Abuse or Child Abuse Case; Videotaping of Testimony of Victim or Witness Under Age 16. This statute allows the child witness to testify in front of a videotape machine in *lieu* of trial testimony in open court. This procedure is available on motion and a finding that there is a "substantial likelihood that a victim or witness who is under the age of 16 would suffer at least moderate emotional harm if he were required to testify in open court...." The child's GAL may file this motion. This procedure is available in civil and criminal proceedings. The defendant shall be present at the videotaping, unless this right is waived. The trial court may require the defendant to view the videotaping by means of a two-way mirror. Due to the volume of cases delimiting this statute, specific rulings will be dealt with below under "Relevant Case Law, Confrontation."

Section 92.54, Use of Closed-Circuit Television in Proceedings Involving Sexual Offenses Against Victims Under the Age of 16. This statute is nearly identical to Section 92.53, except that it deals exclusively with sexual assault offenses and that it involves contemporaneous viewing. Specific rulings concerning this statute are also treated below under "Relevant Case Law, Confrontation."

Section 92.55, Judicial or Other Proceedings Involving Child Victims or Witnesses Under the Age of 16; Special Protections. This statute is sort of a "catchall" for the courts in protecting child victims. The statute is defined in broad terms, allowing for considerable discretion by the trial court in protecting young victim witnesses. Relevant provisions include allowing motions by any party that relate to protecting the child witness, allowing the court to implement measures as the trial judge deems necessary to protect the child witness, allowing the court to limit the number of interviews of child witnesses, allowing the court to prohibit the deposition of a child, requiring the submission of questions prior to examination of a child, and allowing the court to set the place and time of interviews of the child. An important caveat here is that this statute "requests" the Florida Supreme Court to adopt this statute pursuant to the authority vested in the court by section 2(a), Article V of the state constitution. Essentially, what this means is that the court establishes rules of procedure, including rules of evidence, and the legislature would like the Florida Supreme Court to adopt this statute under the current evidence code. There is, however, no such case law at this time. The effect of the statute is that lower courts may use "special procedures" for child witnesses up until the Florida Supreme Court decides otherwise.

Records

Section 119.07, Inspection and Examination of Records; Exemptions. This statute provides that a public agency's records shall be available for review by the public, except for specific exemptions. One exemption concerns "the identity of the victim of the crime of lewd, lascivious, or indecent assault upon or in the presence of a child. . . ." Another exemption concerns the identity of the victim of the crime of child abuse. . . ."

Witnesses; Criminal Proceedings

Section 914.16, Child Abuse and Sexual Abuse Victims Under Age 16; Limits on Interviews. This statute requires the chief judge of each judicial circuit to limit the number of interviews allowed for each child victim. In Hillsborough County the chief judge has limited the number to three per child victim.

Section 914.17, Appointment of Advocate for Minor Victims or Witnesses. The scope of this statute extends to any minor involved in a criminal proceeding if the minor is a victim of child abuse or neglect, a victim of sexual abuse, or a witness to a sexual offense committed against another minor. The court must appoint a GAL or other advocate under this statute. The GAL is immune from liability in the proceeding.

Criminal Procedure and Corrections

Section 918.0155, Expeditious Disposition of Particular Criminal Cases Involving a Child Under Age 16. The legislature has requested the supreme court to adopt emergency rules for expediting child victim cases. The cogent reasons for the need to have such procedures are outlined in the statute.

Section 918.16, Sex Offenses; Testimony of Person Under Age 16; Courtroom Cleared; Exceptions. This statute closes the courtroom to not too many people actually. For instance, in cases involving sexual assault victims under the age of 16, reporters are permitted to remain in the courtroom during testimony (due to a U.S. Supreme Court ruling). The use of the statute was further circumscribed by a second district ruling in 1990. There the court stated that "application of this section to trial of defendant charged with capital sexual battery violated [the] defendant's constitutional right to [a] public trial, where trial court failed to make any findings to justify closure," *Pritchett v. State*, 566 So.2d 6 (2nd DCA 1990).

Victim Assistance

Section 960.001, Guidelines for Fair Treatment of Victims and Witnesses in the Criminal Justice System. State agencies that provide general services to victims are required to provide informational services to crime victims who use the agency. Such informational services include the availability of crime victim compensation, counseling services available to victims, expectations for the victim in the criminal justice system, the victim's right to be heard, and more. Subparagraph (e) of the statute outlines specific provisions for the minor victim and his or her family and guardian. Subparagraph (i) outlines the right to submit impact statements for the victim.

RELEVANT CASE LAW

General

This section is concerned with federal and state rulings which affect the child witness in Florida. The issues are addressed topically rather than by case because of the sundry cases that may impact each separate issue. For instance, at least five separate cases impact on the Child Hearsay Exception Statute in Florida; at least four impact videotape procedures. Some rulings pertain to the interpretation of Florida Statutes, while other rulings pertain solely to Florida case law (i.e., the common law). Where district courts of appeals cases are given, this is the existing law in Florida, unless otherwise indicated (i.e., in cases where there is a conflict, as between *Kopko* and *Pardo*, supra and infra).

Confrontation

The Sixth Amendment to the U.S. Constitution provides, inter alia, that defendants have a right to face their accusers in *criminal proceedings*. This is the so-called "confrontation clause." The clause has caused problems for child victim advocates in a number of areas because it tends to subvert some of the ameliorative techniques that advocates have attempted to use in reducing trauma to the child witness. As many studies document, avoiding child-to-perpetrator confrontation can be important in reducing trauma to the child. See, generally, D. Whitcomb, *When the Victim Is a Child: Issues for Judges and Prosecutors* (Washington, D.C.: National Institute for Justice, U.S. Department of Justice, 1985). The child hearsay statutes, videotape procedures, and closed-circuit television procedures are just three of the important developments that the confrontation clause has affected.

Child/Residual Hearsay Exception. Florida has adopted a child hearsay exception. See West's F.S.A. Section 90.803(23) (1991). The child hearsay exception is not a firmly rooted or "traditional" hearsay exception, so its application is normally limited to special circumstances (i.e., where a child is nonverbal and the state has a strong interest in prosecuting the case). There are other circumstances where it can be used though. The criterion of the exception that is relevant to the confrontation clause is the "reliability" requirement. That is to say, the child's statement must have certain indicia of reliability before a court will allow it into evidence. The reason that hearsay statements fall under a confrontation clause analysis is due to the fact that the defense cannot effectively cross-examine the statement when it is made. Cross-examination is one aspect of effective confrontation. Courts consider hearsay statements as inherently unreliable, except under special situations. When these special situations are present, courts may allow an exception to the general hearsay rule.

Idaho v.Wright, 110 S.Ct. 3139 (1990). (U.S. Supreme Court endorses the "totality of the circumstances" approach in assessing the reliability of a child's statement offered under the residual or child hearsay exception. However, the Court said that when evaluating the totality of the circumstances, "the relevant circumstances include only those that surround the making of the statement.") When testing the reliability of a residual hearsay statement, the *Wright* ruling essentially eliminates corroborative evidence that does not surround the making of the statement, such as medical or physical evidence of abuse that falls outside the circumstances of the making of the child's statement. In other words, the *Wright* ruling makes it more difficult to admit evidence under the Florida Child Hearsay Statute. The *Wright* ruling overrules the provision in the Florida statute that would allow corroborative evidence to be taken into account, in toto, when determining the reliability of a child declarant's hearsay statement. *Wright* also overrules that aspect of the *Glendening* case, infra, dealing with corroboration. Many have criticized the reasoning of the majority in the *Wright* case, including the dissent of Justice Kennedy, who wrote, "I see no constitutional justification for this decision to prescind corroborating evidence from consideration of the question whether a child's statements are reliable. It is a matter of common sense for most people that one of the best ways to determine whether what someone says is trustworthy is to see if it is corroborated by other evidence or the lack thereof to determine the reliability of hearsay statements not coming within one of the traditional hearsay exceptions," *Wright* at 3153. The Task Force has not uncovered any post *Wright* rulings in Florida concerning the Child Hearsay Statute. There is precedent antedating *Wright* that is still good law in most respects however. See *Glendening, Weatherford,* and *Kopko,* below. Presumptively, the confrontation clause analysis in *Wright* applies to criminal proceedings only. This means that evidence offered under child hearsay statutes in civil proceedings may include "outside" corroborative factors, such as physical abuse. For a good discussion of the residual hearsay statutes, see J. Myers, *Child Witness Law and Practice,* 1991 cumulative supplement (New York: Wiley Law Publications, 1991).

Glendening v. State, 536 So.2d 212 (Fla. 1988). (Florida Child Hearsay Statute ruled constitutional; in order to admit the child's statements, the court was required to find that the "time, content and circumstances of the statement provided sufficiency of guards of reliability.") The court in *Glendening* allowed corroborating medical testimony to be taken into account when determining the reliability of the victim's out-of-court statements. The court in *Wright* declared that this type of corroboration cannot be taken into account when assessing the reliability of a statement that the state has attempted to have admitted under the child hearsay exception. Thus, the *Glendening* ruling should be amended to say, as in *Wright*, that the totality of the circumstances include only those factors surrounding the making of the statement. Factors outside the making of the statement, i.e., evidence of physical abuse not incident to the child's statement, may not be taken into account by the court when assessing reliability. The inference *Wright* presents for *Glendening* is that the child's hearsay statements would not have been allowed in *Glendening* if *Glendening* were a post *Wright* ruling. All other aspects of the *Glendening* ruling, however, remain good law. Thus, time and content of the child's statements may be taken into account when assessing reliability. Corroborative circumstances surrounding the making of the statement may be considered by the trial court as well.

Weatherford v. State, 561 So.2d 629 (Fla. 1st DCA 1990). ("Trial court committed reversible error by not making specific findings of fact on record, setting forth reasons the court determined out-of-court statements of child sexual assault victim to be reliable.") This case is important because it shows the necessity of establishing reliability when attempting to admit hearsay statements under the Child Hearsay Exception Statute. It also shows that some judges do not understand or are unaware of the requirements of this particular hearsay exception. Prosecutors can "appeal-proof" their cases by always establishing the requisite indicia of reliability, as set forth in *Wright* and *Glendening*, when attempting to admit evidence under Section 90.802(23) of the Florida Statutes. Prosecutors should also ensure that this gets into the record so that the issue cannot be raised by the defense with any success on appeal.

Kopko v. State, 577 So.2d 956 (Fla. 5th DCA 1991) and conflict with *State v. Pardo*, 16 FLW D1791 (Fla. 3rd DCA 1991). (Issue in conflict for the Florida Supreme Court: where a child victim's hearsay statements satisfy subsection 90.803[23], Florida Statutes [1989], and the child is able to testify fully at trial, must the hearsay statements be excluded solely because they are prior consistent statements by the child, or is the test for exclusion that found in Section 90.403, Florida Statutes [1989]?) The Child Hearsay Statute may be invoked whether or not the declarant is available. See Section 90.803, Florida Statutes, (1989). The text of this section of the Child Hearsay Statute states this quite lucidly. The court in *Kopko* held otherwise, however. In *Kopko*, the court stated that where a witness testifies at trial, the court may not also admit the prior consistent statements of the witness because this is seen as unfairly bolstering the witness' credibility. The *Pardo* court does not agree. Instead, the 3rd District Court makes a strong argument that prior consistent hearsay statements of a testifying child may be admissible if the statement passes muster under Section 90.403, Florida Statutes (1989). Section 90.403 applies to any inquiry into the admissibility of evidence in Florida. This statute states that a defendant can move for exclusion of evidence "if its probative value is substantially outweighed by the danger of unfair prejudice, confusion of issues, misleading the jury, or needless presentation of cumulative evidence." The 3rd DCA seems to present a more plausible argument for the Child Hearsay Statute since its reasoning rests on the specific language of the statute. The *Kopko* court's reasoning is in conflict with the plain language of the statute. Note, too, that the issue here is not really a confrontation clause analysis because the reliability test is already met. Rather, the issue goes beyond confrontation, into the realm of evidence law in general. The Florida Supreme Court's ruling will affect the Child Hearsay Statute, nevertheless, so it is included in this section.

Videotape and Closed-Circuit Testimony. As Professor Myers of the McGeorge School of Law, University of the Pacific, tells readers, "Some forms of video testimony are the functional equivalent of live, in-court testimony. . . . [S]uch testimony raises few, if any, confrontation problems," *Child Witness Law and Practice* 234, cited above. An example of video testimony that does not raise a confrontation clause problem is where a child testifies via closed-circuit television from a room that is away from the courtroom, but where the defendant and his counsel are also present. This meets all the elements of effective confrontation (cross-examination, oath, an opportunity for the jury to view the witness's demeanor, and face-to-face confrontation between the victim and the accused). Child advocates have met resistance from the courts in situations where the defendant has not been allowed to be present during the child's testimony, or in cases where the defendant has been blocked from the child's view during testimony. See, e.g., *Coy v. Iowa*, 487 U.S. 1012, 108 S.Ct. 2798 (1988). Here the Task Force is concerned with circumstances that have allowed the child to avoid confronting the alleged perpetrator during testimony.

Maryland v. Craig, 110 S.Ct. 3157 (1990). ("A state's interest in the physical and psychological well-being of child abuse victims may be sufficiently important to outweigh, at least in some cases, a defendant's right to face his or her accusers. . . . The requisite finding of necessity must of course be a case specific one: the trial court must hear evidence and determine whether use of the one-way closed-circuit television procedure is necessary to protect the welfare of the particular child witness who seeks to testify.") The court in *Craig* did not outline the factors that constitute a minimum "necessity."

Leggett v. State, 565 So.2d 315 (Fla. 1990). (Child abuse victim was permitted to testify via videotape, where the defendant viewed the child through a two-way mirror so that the child could not see the defendant but the defendant could see the child. For purposes of videotaping a child's testimony, the court must conclude that the child would suffer at least "moderate emotional harm" if required to testify in open court.) The Florida Supreme Court reversed the defendant's conviction in this case, saying that it was reversible error for the trial court to fail to make a specific finding that the child abuse victim would suffer "at least moderate psychological or mental harm if he were required to testify in open court. . . ." The homiletic message of the court here is that prosecutors and judges *must* first establish that the child would suffer at least moderate emotional harm if required to testify in court before dispensing with confrontation and live, in-court testimony. The specific finding of fact must be on the record. The trial court in *Leggett* did not clearly document a specific finding of moderate mental harm, despite the fact that an expert witness set out areas in which the child would suffer at least some harm. The Florida Supreme Court said that this departure from the Florida Videotape Statute was reversible error. The court's reasoning was based on the reasoning espoused in the *Coy* ruling, supra, concerning confrontation.

Fricke v. State, 561 So.2d 597 (Fla. 3rd DCA 1990). ("Absent case specific finding of necessity, allowing a child victim of sexual battery to testify against defendant at trial via closed-circuit television violated defendant's right to confrontation." A "generalized" finding that a child would be protected by testifying via closed-circuit television is not sufficient.) The court in *Fricke* said that this constitutes reversible error in light of the seriousness of the charges against the defendant. The child testified from the judges chambers while the defendant remained in the courtroom in contact with his counsel.

State v. Asfour, 555 So.2d 1280 (Fla. 4th DCA 1990). ("Merely videotaping the out-of-court statement did not transform it into an in-court statement. Frequently, defendants' and witnesses' statements to police officers are audio- or videotaped. Such statements are still hearsay, however, and must therefore fall within some exception to the hearsay rule in order to be admissible.) In this case, law enforcement officials videotaped the child victim's statements during its investigation. The trial court stated that the test to determine whether this evidence was admissible was to be found in the Florida Videotape Statute. However, videotaped testimony is hearsay when there is no confrontation at all, as in this case. Thus, in order to be admitted as evidence, the statement must fall within one of the existing hearsay exceptions. The only possible exception in the instant case would be the child hearsay exception. This brings the videotaped statement under the criterion of *Wright* (court may consider only those circumstances surrounding the making of the statement in assessing reliability). The caveat here is that videotaped interviews conducted during the "investigatory" stage of a case must be treated as hearsay. This procedure is to be distinguished from videotaped testimony in lieu of in-court testimony, which must meet the requirements of the Florida Videotape Statute.

Credibility

In general, a witness' credibility is one for the jury to determine. Problems are created when one witness testifies to the credibility of another witness.

Tingle v. State, 536 So.2d 202 (Fla. 1988). ("It was error for state's expert witness to testify as to truthfulness of victim of sexual assault.") The Florida Supreme Court's ruling in this case is significant because it circumscribes the allowed testimony of an expert witness who testifies to the veracity of a child victim. The expert may aid a jury in assessing credibility "without usurping their exclusive function by generally testifying about a child's ability to separate truth from fantasy, by summarizing the medical evidence and expressing his opinion as to whether it was consistent with the victim's story that she was sexually abused, or perhaps by discussing various patterns of consistency in the stories of child sexual abuse victims and comparing those patterns in the victim's story."

Page v. Zordan, **564 So.2d 500 (Fla. 2nd DCA 1990).** ("Expert witnesses impermissibly intruded into function of jury to determine questions of credibility, even though experts were not directly asked to express opinion as to whether alleged victim of child molestation was being truthful.") This case reaffirms the standard established in *Tingle* and makes clearer what an expert may affirm during his or her testimony concerning the veracity of a child witness. In this case, the plaintiff's experts never stated directly that the child's statements concerning abuse were truthful. The experts did testify to other factors that would lead one to believe that the child was telling the truth. The 2nd District Court said that this invades the province of the jury. It is not necessary for questions to be asked so directly in order to "run afoul of the *Tingle* . . . rule," *id.* at 502. Note that this was a case where a child was attempting to receive money damages for alleged sexual abuse (i.e., a civil liability case). These cases are rarely encountered, but the decisions hold sway in criminal matters as well.

Excited Utterances/Spontaneous Statements

While similar in many respects, there is a difference between an excited utterance and a spontaneous statement. Both are recognized hearsay exceptions under the Florida Evidence Code. See West's F.S.A. Section 90.803(1) and (2) (1991). The difference between the two subsections is in the amount of time that "may lapse between the event and the statement describing the event," C. Ehrhardt, *Florida Evidence* Section 803.2 at 473–474 (2d ed. 1984). Under the excited utterance exception, there is no requirement of contemporaneity between the event and the statement, *id.* at 473.

This means that the excited state can occur after the described event. Time still remains a factor though. Another important consideration for a court is the state of mind of the declarant. The declarant must have made the statements while in a state of "stress or excitement," *id.* at 473. The spontaneous statement, on the other hand, must occur "while the declarant was perceiving the event or . . . immediately thereafter," West's F.S.A. Section 90.803 (1) (1991).

State v. Jano, **524 So.2d 660 (Fla. 1988).** ("The fact that a declarant long after the occurrence of a startling event once again becomes excited in the course of telling about it would not permit the statement to be introduced as an excited utterance. It would be an exceptional case in which a statement made more than several hours after the event could qualify as an excited utterance because it would be unlikely that the declarant would be under the stress of excitement caused by the event.") This case provides a didactic discussion of both the spontaneous statement and the excited utterance. The Florida Supreme Court recognizes the limitations of young child victims in presenting their testimony. However, the court held in favor of the defendant on appeal because the statements were made too long after the occurrence of the startling event. The victim involved in the case was a 2 1/2-year-old girl. The chief worry of the court was that a long period of time between the event and the revelation of the event would provide time for contrivance. The court acknowledges the fact that 2 1/2-year olds have little capacity to contrive; the justices may be more concerned with establishing an unworkable precedent. Bright line rules concerning these hearsay exceptions would prove inadequate because of the arbitrary rulings that could occur as a result. It is important to note that the young girl did not testify in this case. She made the statements to her babysitters and a child protection worker, and each witness testified under the excited utterance exception. There is no record of how long after the startling events had occurred that the child recounted her statements to the babysitters and the child protection worker.

Expert Witnesses

There are relatively few Florida cases concerning expert witness testimony that reduces trauma to the child victim. Commonly, experts can testify in order to bolster the state's case-in-chief, so long as the testimony satisfies the requirements of Section 90.702, Testimony by Experts, Florida Statutes (1990), supra. Frequently, this begins the "battle of the experts" and can increase the length of a trial.

***Ward v. State*, 519 So.2d 1082 (Fla. 1st DCA 1988).** ("The study of child sexual abuse was sufficiently established to permit an expert to state an opinion as to whether the patient's symptoms were consistent with child sexual abuse.") The 1st District Court stated that the trial court has broad discretion in determining the range of subjects on which experts may testify. This is consistent with Section 90.702 , Florida Statutes (1990).

Physical Examination of Child

***State v. Farr* (Fla. 4th DCA 1990).** (On appeal, the 4th District Court held that the trial courts granting of a second gynecological examination of a young sexual assault victim was improper; no "extreme and compelling circumstances" are present that would warrant a second gynecological examination.) The state sought to prohibit the trial court's order granting a second examination of the child. The appeals court prudently quashed the order since the respondents challenged the results of the examination rather than the methodology. In effect, the respondents (the Farrs) challenged the state's witness as a competent medical doctor. Common sense would say that there is no need to put a child through a second exam where the exam would have "little probative value." Quite uniquely, the court made the statement that the examination "is not in the best interest of the child." Such averments are normally used in juvenile proceedings, but the court here has taken an empathetic approach to the plight of the child victim and in so doing has provided a just result for all parties to the proceeding.

DISCRETIONARY MEASURES

General

Judges, prosecutors, attorneys for the child in juvenile proceedings, and guardians ad litem all have a wide range of discretionary measures available to them that can reduce trauma to the missing/ exploited child involved in a court proceeding. Many Florida Statutes specifically state, "This is left to the sound discretion of the trial court." Discretionary measures rarely constitute reversible error on appeal, unless there was some form of abuse in using that discretion and unless its use was prejudicial to the defendant. A judge also has available to him or her the use of certain discretionary tactics that cannot constitute reversible error. Allowing a young child to testify at a time of day convenient to her is one example of this type of discretionary measure.

Prosecutor, attorney for the child, and guardian ad litem discretion is often a matter of common sense. Some of the discretionary procedures available to lawyers working with children require approval from the trial judge; other procedures require nothing more than a sensitivity to the needs of the child. If a certain procedure does require trial judge approval, the attorney must be aware of the standard that must be met prior to requesting its use. The reason is that some judges may grant use of the discretionary tactic where it is not appropriate and where it is prejudicial to the defendant. This is grounds for reversal. A concrete example of how this could happen is clear from the *Weatherford* case, supra.

For a superb discussion of relevant discretionary measures, see B.W. Dziech and C.B. Schudson, *On Trial,* 2d ed. Boston: Beacon Press, 1989.

Judge Discretion

Case Law. There was a paucity of case law on point in Florida on the specific issue of how a judge may reduce trauma to the child witness during testimony. A most persuasive and well-reasoned decision from the Supreme Judicial Court of Massachusetts provides a forcibly convincing analysis on the merits of trauma reducing measures available to a trial court judge however. In *Commonwealth v. Amirault,* 404 Mass. 221, 535 N.E.2d 193 (1989), Massachusetts' highest court wrote, "[A] judge is afforded wide discretion in fashioning procedures and modifying practices to accommodate the special needs of child witnesses. . . . We have recognized the plight of child sexual abuse victims, and the difficulties a particular child may face in trying to testify in a traditional courtroom setting. . . . A judge may require that the environment in which a witness is to give testimony may be made less formal and intimidating," 535 N.E.2d at 207.

The Robe. Criminal court judges are expected to wear their robes in court in Florida. The juvenile court judge whom the Task Force spoke with indicated that he takes his robe off during in-camera interviews with the child. He also stated that he allows the child to wear the robe if he or she desires.

The Small Witness Chair. None of the judges with whom the Task Force spoke in Florida had used a small witness chair during any proceedings.

Time of Day. The Florida judges interviewed by the Task Force routinely allowed child witnesses to testify at a time of day most convenient for the child and the child's daily regimen (i.e., a time of day when the child is most alert and prepared to offer testimony). The responsibility to request a specific time of day for the child's testimony rests with the child's GAL or the state's attorney.

Sitting at Witness Level. One juvenile court judge interviewed by the Task Force indicated that he would often sit on the floor with a child during interviews in dependency proceedings. In court, the judges sat at their benches.

Comfort Aids. Child witnesses in civil proceedings routinely bring a favorite toy or stuffed animal with them during testimony. One Florida circuit court juvenile judge had a ready supply of coloring books and toys for children during in-chamber interviews. The use of comfort aids in criminal trials is less frequent, however. There is no case law in Florida, so far as the Task Force could find, on the use of comfort aids during criminal trial testimony. For persuasive authority, *Commonwealth v. Amirault*, supra, discusses the ramifications of allowing a child witness to bring a toy into the courtroom in a criminal trial. The Supreme Judicial Court ruled that this procedure was valid in Massachusetts, 535 N.E.2d at 207. The only effective objection to such a procedure would be that, in allowing a child to carry a toy to the witness stand, the court has unfairly prejudiced the jury in favor of the state. The Massachusetts court rejected this argument in *Amirault, id.* at 207.

Comfort Person. Trial court judges may use Section 92.55, Special Protections, Florida Statutes (1989) if a support person is necessary during a child's involvement in the proceeding. This statute is broadly written in order to give judges great discretion in protecting the child victim, while simultaneously protecting the defendant's constitutional rights. The Task Force found no case law on the issue of whether a comfort person could be used during criminal proceedings. See, however, *State v. Jones*, 362 S.E.2d 330, 332 (W.Va. 1987), where the West Virginia Supreme Court said that the "defendant was not prejudiced by trial court's decision permitting seven-year-old witness to sit in her foster mother's lap while testifying. Child was extremely anxious. There was no evidence the foster mother prompted the child." In civil proceedings the use of a comfort person raises few concerns.

Age-appropriate Questions. Under Section 92.55 of the Florida Statutes the court may also stipulate that all questions to the child upon direct and cross-examination be appropriate for the child according to the child's level of linguistic and cognitive development. This may mean that both parties submit questions to the court prior to the child's testimony. Additionally, the court may wish to set forth the manner in which objections may be raised and the manner in which attorneys question the child. Attorneys may be required to question the child while sitting, for example.

Attorney Discretion

Background Information. In order to decrease the amount of time a child needs to be on the stand, a prosecutor may use an adult witness known to the child to provide any relevant "background" information that is peripheral but necessary to the child's testimony. This might include such factors as where the child attends school or day care.

Where Child Must Look. There is sufficient case law on record that says that a witness need not look at the alleged perpetrator during testimony. A note of caution here, though, since a jury may interpret this to mean that the child is not telling the truth due to the fact that the child is unwilling to look at the person that the state has accused. There is much to the old maxim, "Look me in the eye and say that." Sensitive jurors, however, will understand why an honest child has trouble in looking at a perpetrator. (That is why jury selection can be so important in these cases.) Attorneys, therefore, ought to let their child witnesses know, if the conditions are right, that they do not have to look at the perpetrator during testimony.

Familiarization. Sensitive prosecutors or GALs familiarize their child witnesses with the courtroom and its procedures prior to the child's appearance in court. This includes meeting a judge, sitting in the judge's chair, sitting in the witness chair, meeting the bailiff and knowing his role as protector, sitting in the jury box, and knowing that the prosecutor selected the jury for the child and that the jury is there to help the child.

Preparation. Education and empowerment of a child victim are important before that child testifies. The prosecutor can get the child used to speaking one-on-one. The prosecutor can let the child know that it is all right to take a break during testimony if the child feels uncomfortable or is tired. The prosecutor can let the child know that it is all right to say "I don't know." One prosecutor from a different jurisdiction indicated that many young witnesses are afraid to say that they do not know the answer to a question. Children want to please their adult interviewers and often believe that they should try to answer any and all questions in order to please the adult. This can be problematic, however, since defense attorneys may ask confusing questions during cross-examination. The child witness should know that he or she can respond "I don't know" or "I don't understand" rather than answer an ambiguous question that may lead to inconsistencies and to questions concerning the child's credibility as a witness.

Special Procedures. The prosecutor or attorney for the child or the GAL has the discretion to request special procedures for the child's testimony. Since some prosecutors may be reluctant to request certain procedures, such as videotaped testimony in lieu of in-court testimony, GALs should be adamant in requesting trauma-reducing procedures when necessary in order to protect the best interests of the child. Special procedures include use of anatomical dolls and pictures, videotape, closed-circuit television, and swearing by an informal oath or no oath at all.

Credibility. Astute prosecutors know the importance of establishing a child's credibility. One effective method of establishing credibility is to ask the child egocentric questions that are unobtrusive. An example would be, "Susan, if I said you were a boy, would that be the truth or a lie?" This shows that a child understands the philosophical concept of truth, but in relatively few words and in a concretized answer (there are probably not too many adults who can readily provide a sufficient answer to the question, "What is truth?"—never mind a child witness). A child might also be asked, "John, what would your teacher do if you told a lie?" The child's answer should establish that the child knows the consequences of telling a lie. This is also an important aspect for the child witness in terms of both the child's credibility to the jury and the court's preliminary competency examination of the victim.

Postpreparation. The attorney can reinforce the child after the child's day in court. A "good job" from the prosecutor or GAL can do wonders for a young witness' morale, especially after a difficult afternoon on the witness stand. The attorney can also speak to the child after the jury has given its verdict. This applies equally to acquittals. It is important to reinforce the child one way or another, said one prosecutor.

Corroboration. The prosecutor has the discretion to call witnesses who corroborate the child's testimony. This can decrease the length of time a child needs to testify. Use of the hearsay exceptions under section 90.803 of the Florida Statutes may be necessary when using corroborating witnesses (i.e., statements made to a medical doctor during the course of a medical examination, etc.).

Interviews. Attorneys can help to reduce the number of interviews of a child in a variety of ways. One approach is to videotape the initial interview with the child so that all parties who need to question the child can view the videotape instead of conducting separate interviews. This is where interview protocols become necessary because the interviewer must ask the right questions in order to provide each agency with the information it needs. Hillsborough County has such a protocol. The videotape can also be used during trial if it falls within one of the hearsay exceptions under Section 90.803 of the Florida Statutes. Another possible way to reduce the number of interviews is to conduct the child's interview using one-way mirrors, where members of the team watch from a position unseen by the child. The interviewer may be linked to the observers via a special listening device if available. One important aspect of the interview is the manner in which it is conducted. Children react better to informal surroundings noted a prosecutor from a jurisdiction outside Hillsborough County. They like to color and to take breaks and to have fun where possible. Prosecutors can make this a part of the interview. Some prosecutors follow special interviewing guidelines, designed to reduce trauma, when speaking with a child witness.

PART II

RESEARCH IN CHILD SEXUAL ABUSE

CHAPTER 8

HIV Transmission by Child Sexual Abuse

Laura T. Gutman   Karen K. St. Claire

Chris Weedy   Marcia E. Herman-Giddens

Barbara A. Lane   Jeanne G. Niemeyer

Ross E. McKinney, Jr.

The authors gratefully acknowledge funding from the National Institutes of Allergy and Infectious Diseases for the Duke Pediatric AIDS Treatment and Evaluation Unit.

Reprinted with permission from the *American Journal of Diseases of Children* (1991) *145*: 137–41.

INTRODUCTION

The Duke Pediatric AIDS team began accepting child patients in 1987 and by December 1989 had a census of 96 patients who were HIV antibody positive and were known to the AIDS team social worker. These children were at all stages of HIV-related illness and ranged in age from newborn to 17 years. All children received integrated multidisciplinary services which delivered optimal therapy and management of the complex problems which characterize children with AIDS.

During this period, 14 children from the AIDS team population were confirmed to have been sexually abused. The medical and social conditions of the lives of the abused children were reviewed for known risk factors for the acquisition of HIV and for the known risk factors for child sexual abuse (CSA). This study describes the results of the evaluation of the sexually abused children, the circumstances surrounding the abusive experiences, the perpetrators, and the data regarding the means by which the children had acquired HIV.

METHODS

Evaluation Process

All children seen by the AIDS team who presented with or developed indications of possible abuse or neglect were referred to the child protection team for evaluation. Data for this study were collected at the time of the assessment of each child and represent cumulative information regarding the child's environment from the families, child, child protection team, AIDS team, local social service agencies, schools, and, often, charitable agencies. Child sexual abuse was defined in 1977 as the involvement of dependent developmentally immature children and adolescents in sexual activities that they do not fully comprehend, to which they are unable to give informed consent, or that violate the social taboos of family roles.[1] CSA includes rape, pedophilia, child prostitution, child pornography, child sex rings, and incest.

Multiple issues often led to the referral to the child protection team. The instigating events included: (a) the child or a caretaker volunteered the suspicion of or disclosure of CSA (2 children); (b) routine medical examination had revealed abnormal genital findings (5); (c) suspected physical abuse or neglect, or a chaotic family environment (3); (d) medical or behavioral histories indicative of CSA (5); (e) children older than six years at onset of HIV disease, or with no known risk factor for HIV (3); and (f) the child was an HIV (+) sib of a sexually abused child (1). All of the children were known to be HIV (+) prior to the diagnosis of CSA.

Evaluation for CSA

The evaluation of a child for CSA began with a family interview regarding the family constellation, patterns of care for the child, interactions of family members, behavioral characteristics of the child, and concerns or knowledge the caretaker may have had regarding possibly abusive events. Five groups of data needed for adequate evaluation of possible CSA were then obtained: (a) a review of the behavioral history of the child; (b) a review of the medical history of the child; (c) diagnostic interview(s) with the child; (d) the physical examination, and (e) assessment for other sexually transmitted diseases.[2,3,4]

The diagnostic interviews followed a standard format. Drawings and anatomically correct dolls were available for use when appropriate.[5] In the present study, "disclosure" refers to the disclosure by the child or witness of a specific sexually abusive act. Perpetrators were "identified" if the child or a caretaker had specifically identified the person as an assailant. Perpetrators were considered "suspected" if the interview or historical information indicated sexually inappropriate interactions with the study child or another child and unsupervised access to the study child.

Each child received a complete physical examination and external genital examination using standard techniques.[6,7] For the girls, genital examinations included identification of hymenal type and contour, measurement of the horizontal diameter of the hymenal opening, and anal examination.[8,9] Samples of vaginal secretions were examined for indicators of bacterial vaginosis and trichomonas. Cultures of the introitus or vaginal canal of girls and of the anus of boys for *Neisseria gonorrheae* and *Chlamydia trachomatis* were taken unless the child was receiving antimicrobial therapy. Cultures of other sites and assessments for other infectious diseases were made when indicated.

Sexual abuse was confirmed if: there was a detailed account from the child or a witness; a sexually transmitted disease in addition to HIV was found; the genital examination was abnormal with findings clearly indicative of abuse as defined at the 1985 National Child Sexual Abuse Summit meeting[10] and subsequently updated[2,11,12]; serial genital examinations showed significant changes; or there was acknowledgement by the perpetrator.

Mode of Acquisition of HIV by Study Children

The five possible routes of transmission of HIV which were separately assessed for each child were: (a) vertical transmission, (b) transfusion, (c) clotting factor concentrates, (d) intravenous drugs, and (e) sexual abuse (including child prostitution).

Data regarding vertical transmission included date(s) and result(s) of maternal HIV serology relative to the birth of the child or HIV-related illness of the child. Data regarding transfusion-transmitted HIV disease included dates of transfusion to the child and the results of retrospective blood-bank HIV surveillance. None of the study children had received clotting factor concentrate therapy or had engaged in IV drug abuse. Data regarding transmission by sexual abuse included available information on the HIV status of the perpetrator(s), and the type of abuse.

Since many of the abused children had multiple possible modes of acquisition of HIV, the influence of each on the development of the HIV infection was stratified into categories of "proven", "possible", "disproven", and "unknown".

The following criteria were used to define the categories for vertical transmission. "Proven"—the mother was HIV (+) prior to or within six months of the birth, or the child's mother was first shown to be HIV (+) six or more months after delivery and the child had an opportunistic infection or lymphocytic interstitial pneumonia by the age of two years. "Possible"—the mother was first known to be HIV (+) at six or more months after delivery. "Disproven"—the mother was HIV (-) six or more months after delivery. "Unknown"—the mother's HIV seroreactivity was unknown.

Criteria to define the categories for transmission by transfusion were: "Proven"—the mother was HIV (-) at or after delivery and the child was known to have received an HIV contaminated transfusion. "Possible"—the mother was first known to be HIV (+) six or more months after delivery and the child received an HIV (+) transfusion. "Disproven"—the child either received no transfusion, or it was HIV (-). "Unknown"—the child received a transfusion and retrospective surveillance was not able to trace the unit.

The criteria to define the categories for transmission of HIV through CSA were: "Proven"—either (a) all other risk factors were disproven, or (b) the child was older than 12 years of age when HIV was first diagnosed, sexual contact had been high-risk for HIV, and no other factor had been "proven". "Possible"—the perpetrator was either HIV (+) or unknown, and no other risk factor was "proven". "Disproven"—identified perpetrator(s) was HIV (-). "Unknown"—

additional risk factor was "proven". Inclusion in this report required that sexual abuse of the child had been confirmed. A conservative definition of "proven" transmission of HIV by CSA gave priority to other known modes of transmission.

Sociological Setting

The social settings of the subjects were evaluated for five socio-logical risk factors for CSA identified from the 1987 National Survey of Children.[13] In that study, a significantly greater incidence of CSA was experienced by girls who: (a) had lived apart from their biological parents before age 16 years; (b) had been raised in poverty; (c) had an emotional, physical or mental handicap; (d) had family members who were alcoholic; or (e) had family members who were drug abusers.

Other aspects of the social setting which were recorded in the present study included prostitution by adults in the home; the presence of multiple, unrelated, and frequently changing live-in visitors to the household; significant personality disorder of a caretaker; and AIDS encephalopathy or other AIDS-related disability of a caretaker.

RESULTS

Fourteen HIV (+) children were confirmed to have been sexually abused. The children included three males and 11 females (78% female) whose ages at the time of the diagnosis of CSA ranged from 3.5 to 13 years and whose mean age was 6.2 years. Thirteen of the 14 children were CDC class P-2 at the time they were diagnosed to be HIV (+). Eleven children were black, two were white, and one was Native American.

Diagnosis of CSA

Each of the 14 children with confirmed CSA had either disclosed sexual abuse, had genital or anal findings strongly indicative of CSA, or both. All of the 11 girls had abnormal examinations of the introital area and/or hymen. Two of the three boys had abnormal anal examinations. The genital findings indicative of abuse were: scars or healed lesions of the posterior fourchette, (4); scars, tears, notches or significant distortions of the hymen (5); persistent vaginal discharge and odor or vaginal bleeding, (6); hymenal opening size ≥ 8 mm in a prepubertal child, or a significant change in the genital examination on serial evaluations, (8); perianal scars, (2); significant and rapid anal dilation, (4); and perianal lesions (1). Neither *Neisseria gonorrheae* nor *Chlamydia trachomatis* were isolated from the vagina, throat, or rectum of any study child. Three children had a sexually associated disease other than HIV; two had bacterial vaginosis[14] and one had condylomata acuminatum.[15]

Eight children were able to disclose their abuse. Two made partial disclosure and four were unable to disclose. Four of the disclosing children were aided in their descriptions by the use of art, and six children were assisted by the use of anatomically correct dolls. The forms of sexual abuse described by the eight children who were able to disclose are listed in Table 8–1.

All identified or suspected perpetrators were male. The number of known or suspected assailants and their relationship to the child when information was available are shown in Table 8–2. For four children the number and identity of perpetrator(s) was unknown. A single perpetrator was identified for three children, and for three children multiple perpetrators were identified. For two children a single perpetrator was suspected. For one child, one perpetrator was identified and additional perpetrators were also suspected. For another child, one perpetrator was suspected while the multiple perpetrators known to have abused the child were unidentified.

Acquisition of HIV

Using the criteria stated in methods, an assessment was made of the mode of transmission of HIV when all data were considered. The results are shown in Table 8–3. For four of the 14 children (28%), CSA was the only means of transmission of HIV to the child. A brief synopsis of the histories of these children follows. In order to protect the identities of the children, gender identification is not provided.

Case 1. The child was an emotionally abused, physically well child who lived in fear of the stepfather. At age 13, the child ran away from home and lived as a child prostitute for three months, during which time sexual practices included unprotected anal-receptive intercourse with multiple high-risk adult clients. Intrave-

TABLE 8–1
FORMS OF CHILD SEXUAL ABUSE
(EIGHT DISCLOSING CHILDREN)

	Female Children <u>(n=7)</u>	*Male Children* <u>(n=1)</u>
Genital vaginal	–7	Not applicable
Digital vaginal	–2	Not applicable
Genital rectal	–4	–1
Genital oral	–3	–0
Unknown	–4	–2

nous drugs were never used. The child had never had a transfusion and was not hemophiliac. The mother was not tested but had no risk factors for HIV. At age 15, the child requested an HIV assay because of the high-risk history. The test was positive by ELISA and Western blot, and the child was CDC class P-1 subclass B. It was concluded that the child had acquired HIV while a child prostitute.

Case 2. At age 3–9/12 years this child was HIV ELISA (+) and Western blot (+) and the child was CDC class P-2 subclass A. The child's mother was HIV (-). The child had not received a transfusion or blood products and was not hemophiliac. Genital examination was abnormal and included *condyloma acuminatum* which had first been noted at age 3–3/12 years. After partial disclosure it was concluded that the abuse had occurred during a chaotic family episode when numerous caretakers had had access to the child, and that the child had acquired HIV during the abuse.

TABLE 8–2
RELATION OF IDENTIFIED AND SUSPECTED
PERPETRATOR(S) TO AN ASSAULTED CHILD

	Number	
	Identified	*Suspected*
Brother	1*	—
Father	1	3
Uncle	2	1*
Grandfather	2*	—
Foster father	1*	—
Foster brother	1*	—
Non-related assailants of child prostitute	7*	—

*One of multiple identified or suspected assailants of a single child.

TABLE 8–3
ASSESSED MODE OF ACQUISITION OF HIV
IN SEXUALLY ABUSED CHILDREN
(n=14)

	Proven	*Possible*	*Disproven*	*Unknown*	*Total*
Child Sexual Abuse	4	6	—	4	14
Vertical-transmission	3	5	5	1	14
Transfusion	2	—	12	—	14

Note: Acquisition of HIV by clotting factor concentrate and by intravenous drug use was disproven for each of the 14 children.

Case 3. This child was age 2–2/12 years when diagnosed to be HIV (+) by ELISA confirmed by Western blot, and the disease was CDC class P-2 subclass F. The mother was HIV (-) by ELISA, Western blot and HIV culture. Although the child had received a transfusion, the donor was HIV (-). The child was not hemophiliac. Genital examination was positive for traumatic abuse. Although verbal disclosure was obtained, identification of the assailant was not made, and a suspected assailant refused HIV testing. Because of the disclosure and the fact that another child had been sexually abused in the same home, the child was removed from the household and restricted from contact with the suspected perpetrator. Re-abuse was subsequently documented by the development of new physical signs and symptoms, but specific identification of the perpetrator again could not be made. It was concluded that the child had acquired HIV during abuse by multiple perpetrators.

Case 4. This child was diagnosed at 6–2/12 years to be HIV (+) by ELISA and Western blot when at CDC class P-2 subclass C. At the time of the diagnosis, the mother was HIV (-), the child had never had a transfusion, and the child was not hemophiliac. The genital examination revealed definitive evidence of traumatic abuse, as did the medical history. Two assailants were identified, one of whom was known to be HIV (+). It was concluded that the child had acquired HIV infection during child sexual abuse by an HIV (+) assailant.

TABLE 8–4
SOCIAL CONDITIONS IN HOMES OF SEXUALLY
ABUSED CHILDREN WITH AIDS
(n=14)

Descriptors	**Number (%)**
Lived apart from both biological parents*	6/14 (43%)
Raised in poverty*	10/14 (71%)
Child was handicapped*+	9/14 (63%)
Alcoholic family member*	7/14 (50%)
Drug abusing family member*	10/14 (71%)
Prostitution in home	4/14 (29%)
Transient adults living in home	8/14 (57%)
Mental illness of caretaker	5/14 (36%)
AIDS-related disability of caretaker	2/14 (14%)

* Risk factors for CSA identified by Moore.[13]
+Handicap was apparent at a time that probably preceded onset of CSA.

Knowledge by the Assailant of the Possibility of HIV Transmission To or From the Child

Three of the assailants who were identified or suspected were HIV (+) and knew of their HIV status at the time they assaulted the child. There was no indication from the child that "safe sex" precautions had been taken.

Eight identified or suspected assailants were aware that the child was HIV (+) at the time of the assault. Five of these eight were themselves either HIV (-) or HIV unknown at the time that the child was assaulted. Again, there was no indication from the child that "safe sex" precautions had been taken.

Outcomes of Diagnosis of CSA for Child and for Assailant(s)

In Table 8–5 are presented the outcomes of the diagnosis of CSA for the 14 children and for the 22 identified or suspected assailants. Members of both the AIDS team and child protection team advocated for the needs of the child patients for therapy and for a safe environment. All cases were reported to the Department of Social Services. The environments of seven children remained unchanged following the diagnosis of CSA. Only four children received counseling or therapy for abuse, only one identified assailant was restricted from

TABLE 8–5
OUTCOMES OF DIAGNOSIS OF CSA

For the 14 Children	n	For 22 Identified or Suspected Assailants*	n
In therapy	4	Charged with offense	2
Removed from home	6	Barred from home	1
No change	7	No repercussion	20*

*Includes seven clients of child prostitute

contact with the child, and only two assailants are known to have been charged with an offense. Six children were themselves removed from their homes for their protection.

DISCUSSION

In a recent review of the data from the 1987 National Survey of Children, social settings were identified which increased the risk of CSA.[13] All but one child in the present study had two or more of these risk factors, and the proportion of children who had a given risk factor ranged from 43% to 71% (Table 8–4). In the National Survey of Children study, 6% of girls with no risk factor, 9% of girls with one risk factor, 26% of girls with two risk factors, and 68% of girls with three or more risk factors had been sexually abused as children. In the present study, five of these identified factors were assessed, and 11 of 14 (78%) children each had three or more of these risk factors, demonstrating that the living circumstances of the abused children in the present study included previously described indicators for increased risk of sexual abuse.

Many of the circumstances surrounding the sexual abuse of these children are also previously identified risk factors for adult HIV transmission. First, promiscuous sexual activity with multiple partners is a well defined risk factor for adult HIV.[16] In the present series, seven of 14 (50%) children were known or suspected to have been assaulted by multiple perpetrators, eight (57%) children lived in homes in which casual adult acquaintances frequently slept in the home, thereby creating opportunities to abuse a vulnerable child, and four of these eight homes were also the sites for prostitution by adult caretakers. One of the study children had turned to child prostitution, itself a form of CSA.[17] A second risk factor for adult HIV is sexual contact which is physically traumatic or involves impaired mucosal barriers. Both anal-receptive and oral-receptive sex have been associated with increased rates of transmission of HIV in adults, and are acts which these children described.[18-20] Furthermore, the study children had an unusually high incidence of physical signs of genital injury compared with usual groups of sexually abused children. A third risk factor for adult HIV is sexual intercourse without barrier protection. Assailants of children in this study practiced high-risk and unprotected sex even when the assailant knew himself to be HIV-infected or when he knew the child to be HIV-infected. A fourth risk factor for adult HIV, which was also found in most study children, is genital mucosal lesions, as evidenced by vaginal bleeding, discharge, infections and scars, and perianal infections, lesions, scars, and other sexually transmitted diseases.[21] Finally, the adult population with whom many children lived were at increased risk of HIV from the use of illicit drugs. Use by caretakers of drugs and alcohol may also have diminished their ability to protect the child and lowered their threshold for sexual aggression.[22,23] Consequently, these children were subjected to forms of sexual intercourse which were known from adult studies to be especially hazardous regarding transmission of HIV, and the children lived in family and social settings in which many adults who were their caretakers were at increased risk of being HIV infected.

In spite of the multiple risk factors for CSA which characterize the lives of many children with HIV, acquisition of HIV by children through abusive sexual assault has been infrequently considered or reported in previous medical literature. Although individual case reports have provided evidence that this route of transmission should be examined for children with HIV,[24,25] few medical reviews of the routes of transmission of HIV or of unsolved epidemiologic problems with HIV allude to transmission through CSA.[2,26-29] The lack of data and the need for policies on the testing of abused children for HIV has been the subject of a recent review.[30] The present study indicates that, at a minimum, four of 96 (4.2%) children with HIV, and four of 14 (28%) sexually abused children with HIV, acquired the infection through CSA. These represent the minimal percentages of pediatric HIV disease which can be attributed to CSA since the abused children were identified during standard, non-directed pediatric interactions rather than by specific screening for abuse. In addition, children who also had other "possible" modes of transmission, such as maternal HIV, could not be proven to have acquired their disease through CSA. It was notable that four of the five children for whom vertical transmission of HIV was assessed to have been "possible" because the mother was HIV (+) were older than three years of age when AIDS-like illness first began. This would be a long incubation period for perinatally transmitted HIV,[31] and some of these children may instead have acquired their disease through CSA. This likelihood is exemplified by one of the study cases in which the HIV (+) male who was identified as the perpetrator of a child's abuse was also the source of the mother's HIV infection.

The diagnosis of CSA in children who have AIDS or who are in a high risk environment is of particular importance because some immediate and delayed behavioral sequelae of CSA put the adolescent and adult survivor at increased risk of exposure to HIV or transmission of HIV to others if they are infected. First, high-risk sexual behaviors which may characterize female CSA survivors include early entry into sexual activities, sexual promiscuity and a particular vulnerability to further abuse and sexual exploitation, including prostitution and unintended pregnancy at an early age. [32-40] Male victims of CSA may develop a cycle of sexual behavior in which the child victim becomes a sexual aggressor of other children, either immediately or in adulthood.[41] Multiple victims may be involved.[42] The consequences of the intersection of child sexual abuse with immediate and late risk factors for acquisition of HIV are dramatically highlighted in New York "street" children.[43] Many of these children had been sexually abused in earlier childhood, presumably providing their motivation for leaving their homes at a highly vulnerable, adolescent age.

In conclusion, this study has demonstrated that child sexual abuse was the proven mode of transmission in at least 4% of all study children with HIV followed by the pediatric AIDS team, and may have been the mode of transmission for a considerably larger proportion of cases. The abused children lived in circumstances which were high-risk for both CSA and HIV, and these risk factors often overlapped. Assailants were known to have abused children in spite of knowing themselves to be HIV (+) or of knowing the child to be HIV (+). Prevention of HIV transmission in populations of children and adolescents cannot be successful without the development of policies and resources to identify and eliminate the underlying sexual abuse to which these children are exposed. Sexual abuse and its consequences provide a major mechanism for the introduction of HIV to children and adolescents.

REFERENCES

1. Kempe, H.C. (1978). Sexual abuse, another hidden pediatric problem: the 1977 C. Anderson Aldrich Lecture. *Pediat* 62:382–389.

2. Herbert, C.P. (1987). Expert medical assessment in determining probability of alleged child sexual abuse. *Child Abuse Neg* 11:213–221.

3. Sargent, D.A. et al. (Panel member). (1985). AMA diagnostic and treatment guidelines concerning child abuse and neglect. *J Amer Med Assn* 254:796–800

4. Berson, N., & Herman-Giddens, M., eds. (1986). *Duke University Medical Center Child Protection Team Manual 1990*. Published by the Child Protection Team. Duke U. Medical Center.

5. Berkowitz, C.D. (1987). Sexual abuse of children and adolescents. *Adv Pediat* 34:275–312.

6. Finkel, M.A. (1988). "The medical evaluation of child sexual abuse," in D. Schetky and A. Green (eds.), *Child Sexual Abuse*. New York: Brunner-Mazel.

7. McCann, J.; Voris, J.; Simon, M.; et al. (1990). Comparison of genital examination techniques in prepubertal girls. *Pediat* 85:182–187.

8. Goff, C.W.; Burke, K.R.; Rickenback, C.; et al. (1989). Vaginal opening measurement in prepubertal girls. *Amer J Dis Child* 143:1366–1368

9. Herman-Giddens, M.E., & Frothingham, T.E. (1987). Prepubertal female genitalia: examination for evidence of sexual abuse. *Pediat* 80:203–208.

10. Tipton, A.C. (1989). Child sexual abuse: physical examination techniques and interpretation of findings. *Adolesc Pediat Gynecol* 12:10–25

11. Emans, S.J.; Woods, E.; Flagg, M.; et al. (1987). Genital findings in sexually abused symptomatic and asymptomatic girls. *Pediat* 79:778–785

12. White, S.T.; Ingram, D.L.; & Lyner, P.R. (1989). Vaginal introital diameter in the evaluation of sexual abuse. *Child Abuse Neg* 13:217–224

13. Moore, K.A.; Nord, C.W.; & Peterson, J.L. (1989). Nonvoluntary sexual activity among adolescents. *Family Planning Persp* 21:110–114

14. Hammerschlag, M.R.; Cummings, M.; Doraiswamy, B.; et al. (1985). Nonspecific vaginitis following sexual abuse in children. *Pediat* 75:1028–1031.

15. Herman-Giddens, M.E.; Gutman, L.T.; & Berson, N.L. (1988). Duke Child Protection Team. Association of coexisting sexually transmitted diseases and multiple abusers in female children with genital warts. *Sex Transm Dis* 15:63–67.

16. Pape, J.W.; Liautaud, B.; Thomas, F.; et al. (1985). The acquired immunodeficiency syndrome in Haiti. *Ann Int Med* 103:674–678.

17. Cohen, M.I. (1988). Effective low enforcement strategies for handling juvenile prostitution. *Nat Sheriff* 40:49–52.

18. Fischl, M.A.; Dickinson, G.M.; Scott, G.B.; et al. (1987). Evaluation of heterosexual partners, children, and household contacts of adults with AIDS. *J Amer Med Assn* 257:640–644.

19. Padian, N.; Marquis, L.; Francis, D.P.; et al. (1987). Male-to-female transmission of human immunodeficiency virus. *J Amer Med Assn* 258:788–790.

20. Frederick, W.; Olopoenia, L.; Delapenha, R.; et al. (1989). Sexual practices associated with HIV transmission among female sexual partners of HIV seropositive men. Presented at the 29th International Conference on Antimicrobial Agents Chemotherapy, Houston, Texas, Sept. 17–20.

21. Greenblatt, R.M.; Lukehart, S.A.; Plummer, F.A.; et al. (1988). Genital ulceration as a risk factor for human immunodeficiency virus infection. *AIDS* 2:47–50.

22. Browning, D.H., & Boatman, B. (977). Incest: Children at risk. *Amer J Psych* 1134:69–72.

23. Famularo, R.; Stone, K.; Barnum, R.; et al. (1986). Alcoholism and severe child mistreatment. *Amer J Ortho Psych* 56:481–485.

24. Leiderman, I.Z., & Grimm, K.T. (1986). A child with HIV infection. *J Amer Med Assn* 256:3094.

25. Gellert, G.A., & Durfee, M.J. (1989). HIV infection and child abuse. *New Eng J Med* 321:685.

26. Gellert, G.A., & Mascola, L. (1989). Rape and AIDS. *Pediat* 83:Suppl. 644–645.

27. Fuller, A.K., & Bartucci, R.J. (1988). HIV transmission and childhood sexual abuse. *J Amer Med Assn* 259:2235–2236.

28. Osterholm, M.T., & MacDonald, K.L. (1987). Facing the complex issues of pediatric AIDS: a public health perspective. *J Amer Med Assn* 258:2736–2737.

29. Novick, B.E., & Rubinstein, A. (1987). AIDS—the paediatric perspective. *AIDS* 1:3–7.

30. Gellert, G.A.; Durfee, M.J.; & Berkowitz, C.D. (1990). Developing guidelines for HIV antibody testing among victims of pediatric sexual abuse. *Child Abuse Neg* 14:9–17.

31. Johnson, J.P.; Nair, P.; Hines, S.E.; et al. (1989). Natural history and serologic diagnosis of infants born to human immunodeficiency virus-infected women. *Amer J Dis Child* 143:1147–1153.

32. Browne, A., & Finkelhor, D. (1986). Impact of child sexual abuse: A review of the research. *Psychol Bull* 99:66–77.

33. Briere, J., & Runtz, M. (1987). Post sexual abuse trauma: Data and implications for clinical practice. *J Interpersonal Viol* 2:367–379.

34. Miller, J.; Moeller, D.; Kaufman, A.; et al. (1978). Recidivism among sexual assault victims. *Amer J Psych* 135:1103–1104.

35. Sedney, M.A., & Brooks, B. (1984). Factors associated with a history of childhood sexual experience in a nonclinical female population. *J Amer Acad Clinic Psych* 23:215–218.

36. Finkelhor, D., & Browne, A. (1985). The traumatic impact of child sexual abuse: a conceptualization. *Amer J Ortho Psych* 55:530–541.

37. Bagley, C., & McDonald, M. (1984). Adult mental health sequels of child sexual abuse, physical abuse and neglect in maternally separated children. *Canad J Comm Mental Health* 3:15–26.

38. Silbert, M.H., & Pines, A.M. (1981). Sexual child abuse as an antecedent to prostitution. *Child Abuse Neg* 5:407–411.

39. James, J., & Meyerding, J. (1977). Early sexual experience and prostitution. *Amer J Psych* 134:1381–1385.

40. Gershenson, H.P.; Musick, J.S.; Ruch-Ross, H.S.; et al. (1989). The prevalence of coercive sexual experience among teenage mothers. *J Interpersonal Violence* 4:204–219.

41. Longo, R. (1982). Sexual learning and experience among adolescent sexual offenders. *Int J Offender Therapy Comp Criminol* 26:235–241.

42. Abel, G.G.; Becker, J.V.; Mittelman, M.; et al. (1987). Self-reported sex crimes of nonincarcerated paraphiliacs. *J Interpersonal Viol* 2:3–25.

43. Stricof, R.; Novick, L.F.; Kennedy, J.; et al. (1988). HIV seroprevalence of adolescents at covenant house/under 21, New York City. Presented at American Public Health Association Conference, Boston, Mass., Nov.

CHAPTER
9

Sexually Exploited Children: Assessing Competency to Testify

Christine A. Grant

INTRODUCTION

This chapter presents a child competency tool for clinicians who interview children suspected of sexual exploitation. Fifty videotaped interviews were analyzed by the process of content analysis. Through the use of coding instructions the content of each videotaped interview was coded according to four competency categories: personal, interpersonal, academic, and truthfulness competency. Content that indicated sexual exploitation was coded according to a separate category for abuse. The content was analyzed using predetermined categories developed from the competency requirements of the Federal Rules of Evidence. The tool proved reliable among trained coders and experts in the area of child sexual exploitation.

When parents or professionals suspect child sexual exploitation, a myriad of interventions from public and private agencies and services are set into motion. Parents seek information from the child directly, from the alleged perpetrator, or from an outside source to either confirm or deny the possibilities of abuse. When suspected abuse is raised by the professional, then the parents are questioned as to symptomatology and a range of behaviors that have been correlated with sexual abuse. The professional seeks information to confirm their findings. When substantial clinical material or parental information is gathered then legal proceedings are initiated. Numerous interviews with child protective services, law enforcement agencies and district attorneys are conducted. The majority of the public agencies are concerned with the disclosure of the exploitation. The child's statement in particular is paramount for legal intervention including prosecution. The verbal hearsay statements of the child are critical, and the records and reports by professionals that reflect these statements are very important (Myers, Bays, Becker, et al., 1989). Statements by the child are frequently the most telling and the most useful evidence indicating abuse. The child's statement must be clear, truthful and competent.

Victim advocates have proposed that a child's testimony will be assisted if the child is not required to face the defendant in court (Whitcomb, Shapiro, & Stellwagen, 1985). Closed-circuit television had been introduced as one technique to spare children potential psychological injury as a result of testifying in court and was confirmed constitutionally in Nebraska, Kentucky and Pennsylvania (Dziech & Schudson, 1989). But the United States Supreme Court has declared its use unconstitutional because of the defendant's right to confront his or her accuser (*Coy v. Iowa*, 1988). Justice Antonin Scalia explained that "face-to-face presence may, unfortunately, upset the truthful rape victim or abused child; but by the same token it may confound and undo the false accuser or reveal the child coached by a malevolent adult." The frustration that professionals in the field of sexual abuse experienced over the decision is reduced because four justices took the opportunity in *Coy* to express their beliefs that techniques such as the one-way screen are constitutional and truly needed to serve "the compelling state interest of protecting child witnesses" (Dziech & Schudson, 1989).

Even in the shadow of the Supreme Court's decision the videotaping of a child's disclosure should be considered, for such methods enable the professional to search for the truth. Videotaping a formal statement or complaint is not new to the criminal justice system, and despite the Court's ruling has application to child victims. Initial disclosure statements to law enforcement personnel, protective service workers, and medical professionals preserved on videotape may have the following benefits: (1) children's memory may fade over time; (2) family members may pressure a child to retract statements as a case progresses; (3) videotaping may reduce the number of interviews children are required to endure; (4) a videotape may be permitted as hearsay evidence; and (5) a videotaped interview may prompt a guilty plea when viewed by the defendant (Whitcomb, Shapiro & Stellwagen, 1985).

This study examined 50 videotaped interviews of children by experts in the field of child sexual abuse. The children were all suspected victims of child sexual exploitation and the interviews were conducted in order for the professional to validate if the exploitation had occurred. An instrument to assess a child's ability to testify was developed from the videotaped content and is presented for clinicians in the discussion that follows.

Incidence of Child Sexual Exploitation

Identification and reporting of sexual exploitation of children increased dramatically in the 1980s as child abuse legislation and public awareness has increased. Accurate statistics for the incidence of child sexual victimization are difficult to obtain. The National Incidence Study (NCCAN, 1981) collected data from 600 child protective agencies during a one-year period (May 1979 to April 1980) and concluded that of the estimated 351,000 children abused annually, 44,700 or 13% were sexually exploited. Woodling and Kossoris (1981) estimate that one girl out of every four in the United States will be sexually abused in some form before she reaches the age of 18. In a review of 19% studies of the prevalence of child sexual abuse, rates varied from 6% to 62% for females and from 3% to 31% for males (Finkelhor, 1986). Both researchers and clinicians in the child abuse field agree that the majority of child sexual abuse cases remain undetected (Russell, 1983). No one knows precisely how many children are sexually abused each year, but professionals concur that the figure is appallingly high (Myers, 1990). The American Humane Association estimated that in 1986 there were 132,000 substantiated cases of child sexual abuse in the United States. Yet the majority of child sexual abuse cases are not reported, and the number is clearly higher (Peters, Wyatt & Finkelhor, 1986).

Institutional Response: Legal, Social, and Medical

Institutional responses to child sexual victimization and their impact on the child have not been addressed in the research literature on child sexual abuse. The quality and extent to which the legal, social, and medical professions intervene and interact with the child who has been sexually abused has not been studied. Minimizing system-induced trauma is an important issue for medical, legal, mental health, and social service professionals (Conte, 1984). Insensitive interactions, poor interviewing techniques, and mismanagement of cases by these groups may result in further trauma to the victim, plus contribute to delays in prosecution and therapeutic intervention for the child (de Chesney, 1984; Whitcomb, Shapiro, & Stellwagen, 1985).

Typically six months or more can elapse from the time of the assault, or report of the assault, to the child's appearance in court (Goodman, 1984). This raises concerns regarding the child's ability to recall events over time, the effects of repeated questioning by law enforcement personnel and others, and the effects of reliving the event. The legal response to the child victim who has experienced sexual victimization is often burdened by protocol and procedure. Burgess and Holmstrom (1978) described court processes such as recapitulation of the molestation, preparation of the child by the district attorney, and facing the defendant as factors that could increase stress. The child, already psychologically vulnerable, is faced coping with a legal system that at times induces more anxiety in the child and is insensitive to the child's needs (Schudson, 1987; Weiss, 1982).

Professionals are drawing attention to the need for reform in the prosecution of offenses against children. Numerous innovations are being tried across the United States to spare children the potential trauma of the legal system. Collaborative efforts are needed among legal, social, and medical professionals, and the use of videotaped interviews of children may prove advantageous if properly applied. Constitutional as well as practical objections have been raised regarding using children's videotaped testimony. The defendant's right to face-to-face confrontation and cross-examination are issues that will require continued judicial scrutiny.

A properly conducted videotaped interview may have the potential to spare children future interviews. The professional who combines therapeutic and investigative interviewing must have extensive skills and experience. Conducting videotaped interviews in accordance with the competency requirements of the rules of evidence may demonstrate the child's ability to be a valuable witness. The child competency tool developed during this study may help guide clinicians during the interviewing process.

As a traumatic event, sexual victimization has the potential to precipitate not only immediate, but long-range difficulties for the victim (Burgess & Grant, 1988). The initial emotional and behavioral reactions demonstrated by the child can be prolonged or intensified when legal proceedings are involved (Berliner, 1985, 1988). The literature is replete with case documentations by clinicians, prosecutors, and experts in child sexual abuse that children suffer additional psychological harm by insensitive legal procedures (Berliner & Stevens, 1980; Bulkley, 1981; Conte & Berliner, 1987; De Francis, 1969; MacFarlane, 1978; Russell, 1983; Sgroi, 1978).

English Common Law allowed children as young as 7 years of age to testify in court (Wigmore, 1976) but with an understanding that the child first demonstrate that he or she could comprehend the nature of an oath. English Common Law established in the landmark case of *Rex v. Brasier* (1779) that there be no minimum age requirement for allowing children to testify. Although most of the old rules have been abolished, children can still be judged competent or incompetent on the basis of arbitrary rules (Collins & Bond, 1953; Whitcomb, Shapiro & Stellwagen, 1985).

Today a child is usually asked to demonstrate, for the court, an ability to distinguish the truth from a lie and know that it is wrong to tell a lie. The legal trend is to adopt Rule 601 of the Federal Rules of Evidence, which eliminates all grounds for incompetence, including age (Bulkley, 1982; Melton, Bulkley, & Wulkan, 1983; Whitcomb, Shapiro, & Stellwagen, 1985). Competency examinations are being removed in many jurisdictions, but the obstacle that remains is that children 4 years of age and younger are seldom called as witnesses. Their poor communication skills and inability to withstand cross-examination prevent calling them to testify.

VIDEOTAPING

A child's testimony may be key in the prosecution of an offender, but this testimony need not necessarily be given in court. Some jurisdictions allow grand jury indictments on the basis of the child's out-of-court deposition and in some cases even through the use of videotaped testimony (Berliner & Barbieri, 1984). Bulkley (1982) reports the use of videotaped testimony in the case of sexual assault as being appropriate if the defendant is also present at these depositions. Yet the presence of the offender may negate the reasons for encouraging videotaping.

Videotaping interviews with children who have disclosed their sexual victimization could reduce the numerous grueling interviews, repeated continuances, and painful questioning in the courtroom. The link for professionals to the legal system is a basic understanding of the rules of evidence, including hearsay, and the application of such knowledge to their videotaped interviews.

Memory and Recall

A child as a witness to sexual victimization raises two immediate concerns for the courts: (1) the accuracy and completeness of the child's reports and (2) the credibility of the child as a witness. Therefore, more important than simply capturing every session with a child on videotape is the understanding of memory and its development in children.

For children there are three principal factors that account for the relative instability of their memories. First, children lack an organized and differentiated cognitive structure. This prevents retention of events in a relevant, stable conceptual foci (Ausubel, Sullivan, & Ives, 1980). Second, memory also depends on the potential meaningfulness of the material that is to be related (Ausubel, 1968; Brown, 1975), and, finally, in the absence of an adequate vocabulary much early experience remains unspecifiable (Mandler, 1967).

There is little evidence to support the notion that a child's lower recall equates with a defect in the memory itself. Children may be at a disadvantage because they do not have the amounts of acquired knowledge as they would as adults, and, further, they have not had opportunities to establish such strategic skills as establishing cognitive relations between events (Johnson & Foley, 1984). When the child can produce and use spontaneous rehearsal strategies, then recalling events is more accurate (Flavell & Wellman, 1977; Yussen & Paquatte, 1978). A study by Dent (1982) revealed that any form of prompting impaired the accuracy of children's verbal recall. Free reporting produced a more accurate, though less complete, recall than did answers to general or specific questions. The results revealed that narrative information was more robust and even enhanced when minimal prompting was involved. These are important factors to consider when conducting interviews with children.

The implication for testimony of children is that they will perform better from directive questioning. What a child remembers often indicates what he or she can retrieve under the specific form of testing used rather than what may actually be stored in memory (Fivush, Gray, & Fromhoff, 1987; Goodman & Reed, 1986). It is important to note that even though children may recall less than what adults do, their recall may be very accurate. It is important to recognize the impact that leading questions might have on young witnesses. Children who are allowed to recount their own events in their own way at their own pace with their own emphasis recall more details (Pynoos & Eth, 1984; Saywitz, Goodman, & Myers, 1990).

The interest level for an event, the ability to understand the event, the encoding process, delay intervals, and the child's language level may all be influencing factors. The interviewer and the techniques employed may be counterproductive. Highly suggestive phrasing and preconceived impressions of the event may interfere with the accuracy of the children's reports. Children may be more susceptible to pressure from the interviewer because of their greater dependency relationship with authorities. The interviewer's preconceptions can bias the questions asked and lead to misinterpretation of the child's report (Goodman & Helgeson, 1985). A highly trained, neutral interviewer would seem to be the best possible person for dealing with a child who has been sexually abused, yet the ability to form a trusting relationship with such a person may be difficult for a child. Videotaping these interviews and having them accessible to prosecuting attorneys, law enforcement personnel, and clinicians could allow the content to be evaluated for the type of questioning used, the demeanor of the child, and the credibility of the child's testimony. Clinicians who use videotapes have an obligation to understand the law and how it applies to the tapes and an obligation to conduct the interviews in a most judicious style. Interviewing style needs to be addressed so that questions and statements are not leading in nature, are not overly influential, and do not mirror the therapist's preconceptions of the case.

SAMPLE STUDY

Methods

The sample consisted of 50 videotaped interviews of 50 children. The limitations placed on the recruitment of videotapes included the following: (1) the child was 12 years of age or under, which omitted adolescent victims because of the additional problems that may accompany the adolescent; (2) the child was able to understand and speak English; and (3) the interviewer in the videotape was a nurse clinician, social worker, psychologist, or physician. For the study 30 videotaped interviews were obtained from district attorney's offices and 20 videotapes from therapists in private practice.

The range of the ages was from 2 years to 10 years, the mean age was 4.5 years. Forty-eight (96%) of the subjects were Caucasian, one (2%) was black, and one (2%) was of Spanish descent. The 68% of the children in the videotapes were in preschool.

Instrument

The child competency instrument was developed by the author so that the videotapes could be readily coded in the four predetermined areas of child competence: personal, interpersonal, academic, and truthfulness. The competency categories for this study were derived from the well-established procedure known as the voir dire examination, which is held outside the presence of a jury (Federal Rules of Evidence, 1975). The standards for competency set forth by the Federal Rules of Evidence (1975) are as follows: (1) present understanding of or intelligence to understand, on instruction, an obligation to speak the truth; (2) mental capacity at the time of the occurrence in question truly to observe and to register such occurrence; (3) memory sufficient to retain an independent recollection of the observations made; and (4) capacity truly to translate into words the memory of such observation. The videotapes were analyzed by coding the content under the competency categories. The predetermined categories, derived from the literature on child development and the competency standards for legal proceedings, were established to represent the conditions necessary in order for the child to be considered competent to testify in a court of law.

Content validity was established through a review of the literature and by having the tool examined by an assistant district attorney in charge of child sexual assault cases in a large metropolitan city and by two legal experts in the field of child sexual abuse.

The coding procedure involved the use of the coding instructions on the entire videotaped interview. The coding procedure was examined for content validity by an expert in the area of evidence and child sexual assault. Each videotape was viewed with a written transcription. Following the identification of each competency item, the manner in which the information was elicited from the child, the manner of nonverbal interaction, and the verbal interaction from the therapist was coded.

The videotapes were obtained through letters of request to the district attorneys' offices and through personal contact with the private therapists. Consent was obtained from the contacts who agreed to allow the videotapes to be included in the study. The investigator then completed the child competency instrument for each individual videotape.

RESULTS OF THE STUDY

The videotapes were analyzed through content analysis. Content analysis is a technique that allows replicable and valid contextual inferences to be made from data.

Each videotaped interview was transcribed by hand to paper by the investigator for ease of coding. The transcriptions contained verbatim responses from all individuals in the videotape. Instructions were written to describe how the videotapes were to be coded. Personal, interpersonal, academic, and truthfulness competence were defined. In addition, instructions were written to define how to analyze the questions and responses of the interviewer. The coding instrument contained 278 individual items and each was recorded independently.

Percentage of agreement was the method of choice for the reliability estimation as the data were categorical or nominal. The percentage of agreement was determined across all raters. Agreement was considered to occur only when all raters recorded the same response. Only the agreed-upon items were compared to the total number of items to determine the percentage of agreement. Agreement above 70% was needed before the coding instructions could be used on the remainder of the videotaped interviews. An overall percentage of agreement was calculated at .94.

CHILD COMPETENCY EXAMINATION CHECKLIST

The checklist was developed for the study and is suggested for others to follow or to use as a model. (See the appendix at the end of this chapter).

Personal Competence

The personal competence category included items relating to the individual child. Content coded from the videotape included children's knowledge of their first, middle, and last names; age; birthday; address; phone number; grade in school; name and location of school; rank in school, names of present and past teachers; activities at school; ability to dress themselves, feed themselves, and tie their own shoes. Competency in these areas would assist the legal system in determining if the child had sufficient memory and mental capacity. Of the 17 items determined by the legal experts and the investigator to comprise the personal competency category, the following 12 were coded from the videotapes: first and last name; age; birth date; address; grade in school; name and location of school; present and past teacher; school activity; and, dressing self.

The most frequently coded item in the personal competency category was to determine the child's knowledge of his or her age. Nearly half (46%) were asked their age during the interview. Identification of a school activity was the second most frequently coded item. This item was identified in 42% of the videotapes. Coding for past teacher was completed for 34% of the cases, and knowledge of present teacher was established in 14% of the tapes. Interviewers asked children to identify their first names and their birth dates in 24% of the tapes, while knowledge of last names was coded in only 10% of the videotaped sessions. The item establishing if the child knew the name of the school was coded in 14% of the tapes. The interviewers asked the children their grade in school in 8% of the videotapes. School location, child's address, and the child's ability to dress self was coded in 2% of the tapes. Rank in school, home telephone number, the child's middle name, and whether the child could feed self and tie shoes were the three items not present on the tapes and therefore not coded.

During the establishment of reliability the coders expressed concern that all 17 personal competency items should remain in the coding tool even though 5 of the items did not appear during that phase. The concern was that these items were important for competency and that they might appear in future taped interviews. Completion of coding revealed that these items were never coded.

Interpersonal Competence

The six item interpersonal competence category included coding children's identification of members of their household; neighbors; friends; activities with friends; chores; and family activities. Identification of chores was the only item not coded from the videotapes for this category. Interpersonal competency was established as a separate category to determine information pertinent to the child's life external to the individual. Competency in this area would assist the legal community to assess memory and the ability to translate into words the memory of observations and events. The item most frequently coded was the child identifying activities with friends. The second most frequently coded item was the child identifying a friend by name.

Intellectual Competency

The academic competency category determined the cognitive capabilities of the child. Items in this category included counting, adding, reading, writing, identifying colors, time elements (weekdays, months), body parts, feelings, relational concepts, and the order in which clothing is put on and removed. The most frequently asked item was to identify the child's body parts. This item was coded in 60% of the videotaped interviews.

Moral Competency Category

These items were important to determine if the child could demonstrate an ability to translate into words events and observations that were experienced and the veracity of these statements. The category was devised to code whether a child could identify a "story," something make-believe, a lie, a truth, consequences to either a lie or a truth, and whether the child could identify qualities in a person that were bad and/or good. The item most frequently coded was the child identifying qualities in a person that were bad. Yet this item was only present in 22% of the videotapes. Coding items that revealed a child understood the nature of a truth was only present in 6% of the tapes, and coding for a lie was present in 10% of the tapes.

Abuse Information

Additional analysis of the videotapes in the sample study included coding for allegations of sexual abuse. The coding for the videotapes preceded any court trial, thus prevented access to the legal outcomes of the cases. Conclusive statements could not be made concerning whether or not the child had been a victim of sexual abuse. The method for determining the coding of abuse was identical to the method developed for the competency categories. The coding of abuse occurred in 17, or 34%, of the videotaped interviews. The items coded for the abuse information included an ability to relate the abuse event, emotionality of the relating of the abuse, amount of details, and ordering of events. Of the tapes that were coded for sexual abuse information, only 20% were coded for detailed information.

DISCUSSION

The purpose of the study was to develop methodology to analyze responses of children, suspected to have been sexually victimized, from videotaped interviews to determine if the content could be applied to the competency requirements of the basic rules of evidence. The literature suggests that children should not be forced to testify in the courtroom proceedings as these experiences may be traumatic. To alleviate the courtroom trauma, many professionals endorse the use of videotaped interviews. The study analyzed the content of

50 videotaped interviews with children and determined that these tapes did not adhere to the basic rules of evidence establishing competency. The Federal Rules of Evidence and the competency requirements for a witness provided the framework from which the four competency categories were developed. Normal cognitive and social development of a child determined the items within each competency categories. The literature on memory further directed the study as the items selected within each category were from everyday events and "known" to the child.

The coding instrument to analyze the videotapes proved reliable among legal experts in the area of child sexual abuse. The competency categories were shown to assess the child's mental capacity and ability to communicate facts while also assessing the memory of the child. Coding the content into categories assessed the child's memory by examining the child's capacity to recall events, separate fact from fantasy, and maintain the memories independently.

The limitations of the study included that fact that the clinician who interviewed the child on videotape was not accessible to this investigator for questioning. The clinician may have had prior knowledge about the individual child's case and may have guided the interview session based on this knowledge. This information may have allowed the interview to progress logically for the clinician but when coded for the competency categories it appeared fragmented and leading.

Another limitation was that the developed competency categories were not consistently coded and some items were never used. Statements could not be made concerning the overall competency of a child, or the overall competency of the sample of videotapes. The competency categories that were used may restrict content that would otherwise be useful to the legal system.

Recommendations for further study include training clinicians in terms of the forensic use of tapes and then analyzing the videotaped content and looking at the effects of children's testimony on jurors. Analysis of the actual testimony of children admitted into court proceedings and the reliability of competency examinations are issues that also need to be addressed.

REFERENCES

Ausubel, D.P. (1968). *Educational Psychology: A Cognitive View.* New York: Holt, Rinehart & Winston.

Ausubel, D.P.; Sullivan, E.V.; & Ives, S.W. (1980). *Theory and Problems of Child Development.* (3rd ed.) New York: Grune & Stratton.

Berliner, L. (1985). The child and the criminal justice system. In A.W. Burgess (ed.), *Rape and Sexual Assault.* Pp. 199–208. New York: Garland.

Berliner, L. (1988). Deciding whether a child has been sexually abused. In J. Bulkley (ed.), *Sexual Abuse Allegations in Custody and Visitation Cases.* Washington, D.C.: American Bar Association, National Legal Resource Center for Child Advocacy and Protection.

Berliner, L., & Barbieri, M.K. (1984). The testimony of the child victim of sexual assault. *Journal of Social Issues* 40(2): 125–137.

Berliner, L., & Stevens, D. (1980). Advocating for sexually abused children in the criminal justice system. In J. Bulkley (ed.), *Sexual Abuse of Children.* Washington, D.C.: American Bar Association.

Berliner, L., & Stevens, D. (1982). Clinical issues in child sexual abuse. In J.R. Conte & D.A. Share (eds.), *Social Work and Child Sexual Abuse.* New York: Haworth Press.

Brown, A.L. (1975). The development of memory: knowing, knowing about knowing, and knowing how to know. In H.W. Reese (ed.), *Advances in Child Development and Behavior.* Vol. 10. New York: Academic Press.

Bulkley, J. (1981). *Innovations in Prosecution of Child Sexual Abuse Cases.* Washington, D.C.: American Bar Association.

Bulkley, J. (1982). *Intrafamily Child Sexual Abuse Cases.* Washington, D.C.: American Bar Association.

Burgess, A.W., & Grant, C.A. (1988). *Children Traumatized in Sex Rings.* Arlington, Va.: National Center for Missing and Exploited Children.

Burgess, A.W., & Holmstrom, L.L. (1978). The child and family during the court process. In A.W. Burgess, A.N. Groth, L.L. Holmstrom, & S.M. Sgroi (eds.), *Sexual Assault of Children and Adolescents.* Pp. 205–230. Lexington, Mass.: Lexington Books.

Collins, G.B., & Bond, E.C. (1953). Youth as a bar to testimonial competence. *Arkansas Law Review* 8: 100–107.

Conte, J. (1984). Progress in treating the sexual abuse of children. *Social Work* (May–June): 258–263.

Conte, J. R., & Berliner, L. (1987). The impact of sexual abuse on children: the empirical findings. In L. Waler (ed.), *Handbook on Sexual Abuse of Children: Assessment and Treatment Issues*. New York: Springer.

Coy v. Iowa. No. 86-6757, United States Supreme Court, June 29, 1988.

de Chesney, M. (1984). Father-daughter incest. *Journal of Psychosocial Nursing, 22*(9), 9–16.

deFrancis, V. (1969). *Protecting the Child Victim of Sex Crimes Committed by Adults*. Denver, Col.: American Humane Association.

Dent, H.R. (1982). The effects of interviewing strategies on the results of interviews with child witnesses. In A. Trankell (ed.), *Reconstructing the Past*. Pp. 279–298. Deventer, Netherlands: Kluwer.

Dziech, B.W., & Schudson, C.B.(1989). *On Trial: Sexually Abused Children in America's Courts*. Boston: Beacon Press.

Federal Rules of Evidence for United States Courts and Magistrates (1975).

Finkelhor, D. (ed.). (1986). *A Sourcebook on Child Sexual Abuse*. Newbury Park, Calif.: Sage.

Fivush, R.; Gray, J.; & Fromhoff, F.A. (1987). Two year olds talk about the past. *Cognitive Development* 2:393–409.

Flavell, J.H., & Wellman, J.H. (1977). Metamemory. In R.V. Kail & J.W. Hagen (eds.), *Perspectives on the Development of Memory and Cognition*. Hillsdale, N.J.: Erlbaum.

Goodman, G.S. (1984). Children's testimony in historical perspective. *Journal of Social Issues* 40(2): 9–31.

Goodman, G.S., & Helgeson, V.S. (1985). Child sexual assault: children's memory and the law. In J. Bulkley, (ed.), *Papers from a National Policy Conference on Legal Reforms in Child Sexual Abuse Cases*. Washington, D.C.: American Bar Association.

Goodman, G.S., & Reed, R.S. (1986). Age differences in eyewitness testimony. *Law and Human Behavior* 10: 317–332.

Johnson, M.K., & Foley, M.A. (1984). Differentiating fact from fantasy: the reliability of children's memory. *Journal of Social Issues* 40(2): 33–50.

MacFarlane, K. (1978). Sexual abuse of children. In J. Chapman & M. Gates (eds.), *The Victimization of Women*. Newbury Park, Calif.: Sage.

Mandler, G. (1967). Verbal learning. In E. Galanter, G. Mandler, R. Brown, & E.H. Hess (eds.), *New Directions in Psychology III*. New York: Holt, Rinehart and Winston.

Melton, G.; Bulkley, J.; & Wulkan, D. (1983). Competency of children as witnesses. In J. Bulkely (ed.), *Child Sexual Abuse and the Law*. Washington, D.C.: American Bar Association.

Myers, J.E.B. (1990). The child sexual abuse literature: a call for greater objectivity. *Michigan Law Review* 88 (6): 1709–1733.

Myers, J.E.B.; Bays, J.; Becker, J.; et al. (1989). Expert testimony in child sexual abuse litigation. *Nebraska Law Review* 68 (1 & 2).

National Center on Child Abuse and Neglect (NCCAN) (1981). National study of incidence and severity of child abuse and neglect. Washington, D.C.: NCCAN.

Peters, S.D.; Wyatt, G.E.; & Finkelhor, D. (1986). Prevalence. In D. Finkelhor (ed.) *A Sourcebook on Child Sexual Abuse*. Newbury Park, Calif.: Sage.

Pynoos, R.S., & Eth, S. (1984). The child as witness to homicide. *Journal of Social Issues* 40 (2): 87–108.

Rex v. Brasier 1779, 1 Leach 199, 168 Eng. Rep 202.

Russell, D.E.H. (1983). The incidence and prevalence of intrafamilial and extrafamilial sexual abuse of female children. *Child Abuse and Neglect* 7: 133–146.

Saywitz, K.J.; Goodman, G.S.; & Myers, J.E.B. (1990). Can children provide accurate eyewitness reports? *Violence Update* (September).

Schudson, C.B. (1987). Making courts safe for children. *Journal of Interpersonal Violence* 2 (1): 120–122.

Sgroi, S.M. (1978). Child sexual assault: some guidelines for intervention and assessment. In A.W. Burgess, A. N. Groth, L.L. Holmstrom, & S.M. Sgroi (eds.), *Sexual Assault of Children and Adolescents*. Pp. 129–142. Lexington, Mass.: Lexington Books.

Weiss, E., & Berg, R. (1982). Child victims of sexual assault: impact of court procedures. *Journal of Child Psychiatry* 21 (5): 513–518.

Whitcomb, D.; Shapiro, E.R.; & Stellwagen, I.D. (1985). When the victim is a child: issues for judges and prosecutors. Washington, D.C.: National Institute of Justice.

Wigmore, J.H. (1976). *Evidence in Trials at Common Law*. Rev. by J. Chadborn. Vol. 6. Boston: Little, Brown.

Woodling, B., & Kossoris, P. (1981). Sexual misuse: rape, molestation and incest. *Pediatric Clinics of North America* 28 (2): 481–499.

Yussen, S.R., & Paquatte, N.S. (1978). Developmental changes in predicting recognition memory for semantically related and unrelated sentences. *Developmental Psychology* 14: 107–113.

APPENDIX—COMPETENCY CHECKLIST

Section# (__________)

Defendant (__________________)
Case identifier (______________________)
Child identifier (____________________)

Please check one: ___ Separate competency
hearing (voir dire)
___ Competency questions
after child is sworn

Child Competency Examination Checklist
Personal Competency

Item	Asked?		Response Used to Disqualify Witness?		If disqualified, please explain
	No	Yes	No	Yes	
Child's first name	__	__	__	__	___________________
Child's middle name	__	__	__	__	___________________
Child's last name	__	__	__	__	___________________
Child's age	__	__	__	__	___________________
Child's birthday	__	__	__	__	___________________
Child's address	__	__	__	__	___________________
Telephone	__	__	__	__	___________________
Grade in school	__	__	__	__	___________________
Name of school	__	__	__	__	___________________
Rank in school	__	__	__	__	___________________
Name of present teacher	__	__	__	__	___________________
Name of past teacher	__	__	__	__	___________________
Identifies a school activity	__	__	__	__	___________________
Ability to dress self	__	__	__	__	___________________

Interpersonal Competency

Item	Asked?		Response Used to Disqualify Witness?		If disqualified, please explain
Identifies people in home	__	__	__	__	___________________
Identifies neighbors	__	__	__	__	___________________
Identifies friends	__	__	__	__	___________________
Identifies an activity with a friend	__	__	__	__	___________________
Identifies chore	__	__	__	__	___________________
Identifies a family activity	__	__	__	__	___________________
Other: ____________			__	__	___________________
Other: ____________			__	__	___________________
Other: ____________			__	__	___________________
Other: ____________			__	__	___________________
Other: ____________			__	__	___________________

Intellectual Competency

Item	Asked?		Response Used to Disqualify Witness?		If disqualified, please explain
	No	Yes	No	Yes	
Can count	—	—	—	—	__________________
Can add	—	—	—	—	__________________
Knows colors	—	—	—	—	__________________
Can read	—	—	—	—	__________________
Can write	—	—	—	—	__________________
Identifies body parts	—	—	—	—	__________________
Identifies a favorite food	—	—	—	—	__________________
Identifies clothing	—	—	—	—	__________________
Identifies relationship	—	—	—	—	__________________
Identifies a feeling	—	—	—	—	__________________
Identifies a relational concept	—	—	—	—	__________________
Identifies a time concept	—	—	—	—	__________________
Other: __________			—	—	__________________
Other: __________			—	—	__________________
Other: __________			—	—	__________________
Other: __________			—	—	__________________
Other: __________			—	—	__________________

Moral Competency Category

Item	Asked?		Response Used to Disqualify Witness?		If disqualified, please explain
	No	Yes	No	Yes	
Identifies something as make believe	—	—	—	—	__________________
Identifies a truth	—	—	—	—	__________________
Identifies a lie	—	—	—	—	__________________
Identifies the consequences of telling a lie	—	—	—	—	__________________
Identifies good qualities in a person	—	—	—	—	__________________
Identifies bad qualities in a person	—	—	—	—	__________________
Identifies an event as right	—	—	—	—	__________________
Identifies an event as wrong	—	—	—	—	__________________
Other: __________			—	—	__________________
Other: __________			—	—	__________________
Other: __________			—	—	__________________
Other: __________			—	—	__________________
Other: __________			—	—	__________________

<u>Questioning Style Toward Witness</u>

Prosecutor
___1) Appropriate for child witness   ___2) More appropriate for adult witness

Defense attorney
___1) Appropriate for child witness   ___2) More appropriate for adult witness

Judge
___1) Appropriate for child witness   ___2) More appropriate for adult witness

<u>Manner Toward the Witness</u>

Prosecutor
___1) Businesslike   ___2) Supportive
___3) Condescending/descending   ___4) Intimidating
Defense attorney
___1) Businesslike   ___2) Supportive
___3) Condescending/descending   ___4) Intimidating
Judge
___1) Businesslike   ___2) Supportive
___3) Condescending/descending   ___4) Intimidating

<u>Location of Witness While Testifying</u>

___1)Sitting at a table   ___2)Standing
___3)Sitting in a witness box   ___3)In judge's chambers
5)Other: ___________________

10

Stress Responses of Children and Parents to Sexual Abuse and Ritualistic Abuse in Day Care Centers

Susan J. Kelley

Sections of this chapter were reprinted, with permission, from *Journal of Interpersonal Violence* 4 (4): 502–513 and *Nursing Research* 39 (1): 25–29.

INTRODUCTION

The sexual abuse of a child constitutes a major crisis for child victims and their parents. While the existing empirical evidence indicates that sexually abused children are negatively impacted by the experience (Anderson, Bach, & Griffith, 1981; Conte & Schuerman, 1987; Friedrich, Urquiza, & Beilke, 1986; Gomes-Schwartz, Horowitz, & Sauzier, 1984; Tong, Oates, & McDowell, 1987) to date there has been no systematic examination of parental responses to sexual victimization. What appears in the literature is largely anecdotal, based on clinical observations, and lacking standardized instruments to measure parental reactions.

IMPACT OF SEXUAL ABUSE ON CHILD VICTIMS AND PARENTS

Existing research suggests that sexually abused children display a variety of disturbed behaviors immediately following disclosure of

231

the abuse. Initial effects of sexual abuse reported in the research literature include fear (Conte & Schuerman, 1987; Gomes-Schwartz, Horowitz, & Sauzier, 1984), anger and hostility (Gomes-Schwartz, Horowitz, & Sauzier, 1985), and guilt and shame (DeFrancis, 1969). In addition, sexually abused children often demonstrate inappropriate sexual behaviors (Friedrich, Beilke, & Urquiza, 1988; Friedrich, Urquiza, & Beilke, 1986; Gomes-Schwartz, Horowitz, & Sauzier, 1985; Tong, Oates, & McDowell, 1987). Sexual victimization and the resulting disclosure are stressful events that alter the homeostatic balance of the family, interfering with previously effective coping abilities (Sesan, Freeark, & Murphy, 1986). The few studies that have attempted to examine the reaction of parents to sexual abuse have primarily involved cases of intrafamilial sexual abuse (Anderson, Bach & Griffith, et al., 1981; deYoung, 1982; Gomes-Schwartz, Horowitz, & Sauzier, 1984; Herman, 1981). This poses a serious methodological problem since it is difficult to separate the effect of sexual abuse from membership in a dysfunctional incestuous family.

It is a generally held belief that sexually abused children incorporate their parents' reactions to the abuse (De Vine, 1980; Esquilin, 1987; MacFarlane & Waterman, 1986). Anderson, Bach & Griffith (1981) found increased behavioral symptomatology in children who had encountered negative reactions from their parents, such as blaming the child, compared to victims whose parents were responsive to their needs. Gomes-Schwartz, Horowitz, and Sauzier (1984) report that when mothers react to disclosure of sexual abuse with anger and punishment, children manifest more behavioral disturbances. Friedrich and Reams (1987) suggest that the symptoms seen in sexually abused children reflect not only the trauma they have experienced directly, but also their family environment, the amount of support the child feels, and the level of disruption that follows the disclosure of abuse. Thus, based on the available data, it appears that the reactions of parents to their child's victimization critically influence the child's reaction.

SEXUAL ABUSE IN DAY CARE CENTERS

In recent years there has been a sharp rise in the number of reported cases of sexual abuse in day care centers. Finkelhor, Williams, and Burns (1988) identified 270 day care centers where sexual abuse occurred involving a total of 1,639 victims during a three-year period. Based on their national survey, they estimate the incidence rate of sexual abuse in day care to be 5.5 per 10,000 children compared to 8.9 cases of intrafamilial abuse per 10,000 children under 6 years of age. Although a disturbing number of children are sexually abused in day care, the researchers concluded that these large numbers do not indicate a particularly high risk to children in day care, but rather reflect the large number of children in day care and the risk of sexual abuse to children in all settings.

RITUALISTIC ABUSE

A particularly disturbing type of child maltreatment that has recently come to the attention of professionals is ritualistic abuse. Ritualistic abuse refers to repetitive and systematic sexual, physical, and psychological abuse of children by adults as part of cult or satanic worship (Kelley, 1988). Reports of ritualistic abuse are often characterized by forced ingestion of human excrement, semen, or blood; ceremonial killing of animals; threats of harm from supernatural powers; ingestion of drugs or "magic potions"; and use of satanic songs, chants, or symbols (Gould, 1987; Kaye & Klein, 1987; Kelley, 1988). Sexual abuse occurs within the context of group rituals or ceremonies and is a means of inducing a religious experience for adult perpetrators.

Reliable estimates of the extent of this problem are not yet available for several reasons. Many professionals are unaware of the nature of ritualistic abuse and fail to recognize indicators of ritualistic abuse. Even when cases are identified, child protective agencies do not categorize them according to ritualistic involvement. Another major obstacle to determining the extent of ritualistic abuse is the skepticism with which allegations of ritualistic abuse are met. The more horrible and bizarre the child's allegation, the less likely that he or she will be believed. In the national study of sexual abuse of children in day care centers (Finkelhor, Williams, & Burns, 1988) 13% of the cases involved ritualistic abuse, suggesting that this is not a rare phenomenon.

The purpose of this study was to examine the stress responses of young children and their parents to sexual victimization in day care. Specifically, it was predicted that children who were sexually abused in day care would demonstrate more behavioral disturbances than a carefully matched group of nonabused children. It was also predicted that parents of children abused in day care would demonstrate more psychological distress than the comparison group of parents of nonabused children. Furthermore, because of the severe nature of ritualistic abuse, it was hypothesized that children who were subjected to ritualistic abuse and their parents would manifest the most severe psychological difficulties.

METHOD

Subjects

The 134 families in the study were divided into three groups. Group I consisted of 32 children and their parents. Half of the children were male, aged 4 to 8 years, who were sexually abused in day care centers. Their age at the time the abuse began ranged from 1 to 4 years, with a mean of 2.38 years. The time elapsed between the end of the abuse and data collection ranged from 8 to 36 months, with a mean of 26 months.

The parents in Group I included 32 mothers and 25 fathers. The mean age of the mothers was 33.5 years (range = 26–42) and of the fathers, 36 years (range = 30–45). The majority of families were of middle to high socioeconomic status, with 82% falling into social classes I and II on the Hollingshead Index of Social Status (Hollingshead, 1974); 44% were college graduates; and 72% earned more than $26,000 a year.

Group II included 35 children who were ritually abused in day care centers and their parents. Of the children in this group, 40% were male and 60% were female. Their age at time of data collection ranged from aged 4 to 11 years. The ages of the children at the onset of the abuse ranged from 1 to 7 years, with a mean age of 3.2 years. The time elapsed between the end of the abuse and data collection ranged from 6 to 47 months, with a mean of 29 months.

The parents in this group included 33 mothers and 21 fathers, representing all 35 children. The mean age of the mothers was 34.6 years (range = 28–43); of the fathers, 37 years (range = 26–55). The majority of the families were of middle to upper socioeconomic status, with 75% scoring within social classes I and II of the Hollingshead Index of Social Status (Hollingshead, 1975); 59% were college graduates; and 91.2% earned more than $26,000 per year.

Subjects were assigned to Group II if the children reported involvement in satanic rituals. The satanic rituals involved worship of the devil; participation in ceremonial acts that involved adults wearing costumes or robes and using occult symbols; and threats of harm from supernatural powers. Other important differences between the types of abuse experienced by children in Groups I and II will be described in the Results section.

Group III, the comparison group, was comprised of 67 nonabused children and their parents. The subjects in the comparison group were matched to the children in Groups I and II on the following variables: age, gender, socioeconomic status, and length of attendance at a day care center. The children's age ranged from 4 to 11 years, with a mean age of 6.6 years.

The parents of children in Group III included 66 mothers and 53 fathers representing families of all 67 nonabused children. The Hollingshead Index of Social Status was employed to match abused subjects on socioeconomic status. In this group 63% were college graduates, and 90% of the families earned over $26,000 annually.

The subjects in Groups I and II were recruited nationally through the criminal justice system, a parent organization, and mental health agencies. With the permission of the potential subjects, the cooperating agencies provided the researcher with the names of 81 parents whose children had been sexually abused in day care centers. Questionnaires were mailed to the 81 parents; 67 were returned, resulting in a response rate of 83%. The subjects represented 16 day care centers in 12 different states where sexual abuse occurred. The researcher did not have access to all children who alleged abuse in each of the day care center cases, since access was limited only to those subjects involved with the cooperating agencies.

Allegations of sexual abuse were substantiated by the child protective agency in the jurisdiction responsible for investigating charges of sexual abuse for all cases involved in this study. The types of abuse reported in this study are based on statements made by the children to parents or their therapists. Criminal charges were brought against the abusers in 92% of cases. When criminal charges were filed, 80% resulted in convictions of one or more offenders at the day care center. Of the remaining cases, 5% resulted in innocent verdicts, 7% had charges dismissed, and 7% had trials in progress.

The comparison subjects (Group III) were recruited through three day care centers and two public school systems in the Northeast. Questionnaires were mailed to 250 potential subjects for the comparison group. Of these, 189 were returned, resulting in a response rate of 76%. The first 67 nonabused subjects who matched subjects in Groups I and II on age, gender, SES, and history of having attended day care were selected for the comparison group. The Hollingshead (1975) two-factor index of social status was used to match families according to the five categories of social strata.

Measures

The parents of the child victims completed three standardized instruments, the Child Behavior Checklist (Achenbach & Edelbrock, 1983), the Symptom Checklist-90-R (Derogatis, 1977), and the Impact of Event Scale (Horowitz, Wilner, & Alvarez, 1979). In addition, parents completed a questionnaire on the child's case history and demographic data.

Child Behavior Checklist

The Child Behavior Checklist (CBCL) developed by Achenbach and Edelbrock (1983) measures children's behavioral functioning. Scales on the CBCL include the Total Behavior Scale, Internalizing Scale, Externalizing Scale, Social Competency Scale, and the following subscales: somatic complaints, schizoid, uncommunicative, immature, obsessive compulsive, hostile, withdrawn, delinquent, aggressive, sex problems, and hyperactive. Norms are available for each of the eight gender/age groups (males and females, 2 to 3, 4 to 5, 6 to 11, and 12 to 16 years). Normalized T scores are available for each age/gender group.

The psychometric properties of the CBCL have been extensively evaluated. Reliability has been established for 2 to 16 year olds. Intraclass correlation coefficients of .838 have been obtained on the 118 behavior problem items and .978 on the 20 social competency items. Interparent agreement reliability is .985 on the behavior problem items and .978 on the social competence items. The correlations on a one-week test-retest reliability of each of the different scales range from .78 to .96 with a median correlation of .89. A Chronbach alpha reliability coefficient of .97 was obtained to establish internal consistency on the 118 items of the Total Behavior Problem Score for this sample.

Several studies have supported the construct and content validity of the CBCL. Tests of criterion-related validity using clinical status as the criterion support ($p < .001$) support its validity.

The Child Behavior Checklist was initially scored with a software program that transforms raw scores into normalized T scores. The utilization of T scores allows for comparisons of scores when there are age and gender differences. T scores were obtained for Internalizing, Externalizing, Social Competence, Total Behavior Problem scales and the five subscales appropriate for the four age/gender groups included in the sample. The Delinquent, Hyperactive, Schizoid, Depressed, and Withdrawal scales exist for the four age/gender groups included in this sample. Since, according to Achenbach and Edelbrock (1983), the Aggressive and Somatic Complaint scales are reasonably similar among the age/gender groups and suitable for comparisons among the age/gender groups, they were analyzed as well. One additional scale, Sex Problems, was derived as previously described by Friedrich, Beilke, and Urquiza (1988). The scale was based on the total raw score of the six CBCL items pertaining to sexual behavior.

Symptom Checklist-90-R

The Symptom Checklist-90-R (Derogatis, 1977), a 90-item multidimensional self-report symptom inventory, was used to measure symptomatic psychological distress in the parents. The Symptom Checklist-90-R (SCL-90-R) reflects psychopathology in terms of nine primary symptom dimensions (somatization, obsessive-compulsive, interpersonal sensitivity, depression, anxiety, hostility, phobic anxiety, paranoid ideation, and psychoticism) and three global indices of distress (General Severity Index, Positive Symptom Total, and Positive Symptom Distress Index). The General Severity Index (GSI) combines information on numbers of symptoms and intensity of distress, and is considered to be the best single indicator of distress in subjects. Therefore, it was chosen as the summary measure of psychological distress for parents in this study. Each item of the SCL-90-R represents distress in terms of a discrete 5-point scale ranging from "not at all" (0) to "extremely" (4). The SCL-90-R scores reported in this study are normalized T scores for adult nonpatient normals, which have a mean score of 50 and a standard deviation of 10.

The SCL-90-R has shown high levels of both internal consistency and test-retest reliability. Derogatis (1977) reports coefficient alphas between .77 and .90 for the nine primary symptom dimensions, and test-retest coefficients between .78 and .90. Cronbach's alpha was computed on the responses of subjects in this sample and resulted in a reliability coefficient of .98.

Validity of the SCL-90-R has been well established. A very high convergent and discriminate validity between the SCL-90-R and the MMPI has been established. The SCL-90-R has been shown to be highly sensitive to stress-related changes.

Impact of Event Scale

The Impact of Event Scale (IES) is a 15-item instrument that focuses on the quality of conscious experiences during a recent period with a stressful life event specific to the individual written on the form as the referent for response to the list of experiences. For the purposes of this study "the event" is the sexual abuse of the subject's child in a day care center.

The Impact of Event Scale was developed by Horowitz, Wilner, Kaltreider, and Alvarez (1980) through sequential refinement of items and studies of reliability and validity of the instrument. Subscales of coherent items were found to be both logically and empirically consistent and yielded intrusion and avoidance subscales. The split half reliability of the total scale is .86. The internal consistency of these subscales, using Cronbach's alpha, was .78 and .82, respectively. The test-retest reliability for the total stress score is .87—.80 for the intrusion subscale and .79 for the avoidance subscale. Cronbach's alpha was computed for internal consistency of items on the IES for this sample. The reliability coefficient obtained on mothers was .93 and for fathers rwas .94.

The two subscales of avoidance and intrusion index symptoms on the two dimensions that characterize the DSM-III diagnosis of posttraumatic stress disorder. These two dimensions are (1) intrusion into consciousness of unbidden ideas, feelings, and images and (2) consciously recognized denial or avoidance of stress related themes and emotional responses (Horowitz, Wilner, & Alvarez, 1979).

Procedures/Data Collection

The researcher collected the data through mailed questionnaires. Subjects in Groups I and II completed the three self-administered standardized instruments described above as well as a questionnaire developed by the researcher to collect information related to the sexual abuse, a brief inventory of 12 stressful life events, and demographic data. Comparison subjects completed the Child Behavior Checklist (Achenbach & Edelbrock, 1983), the Symptom Checklist-90-R, and the questionnaire on demographic data and stressful life events. A letter for informed consent was included with the instruments; anonymity and confidentiality of responses were assured.

Results

Data analysis was performed utilizing the SPSS-X program on an IBM mainframe computer. Initial analyses were performed to examine potential sources of confounding by demographic, stressful life events, and abuse-related variables. Analysis of variance (ANOVA) and planned comparisons were conducted to compare the mean scores of the three groups on CBCL, SCL-90-R, and IES scale scores and interval-level demographic and abuse-related variables. Chi square analyses were performed to test for significant differences among groups on demographic and abuse-related variables. There were no significant differences between the three groups on socioeconomic status, income, marital status, race, number of children in the family, and length of time the child attended day care.

Demographic Data

There were no significant differences among groups on parental marital status, race, subjects' gender, number of siblings in the family, length of attendance at day care, SES as measured by the Hollingshead Index of Social Status (1975), or total number of stressful life events. Of the subjects, 82% fell within the two highest social classes on the Hollingshead. The parents in the study were generally well educated: 96% were high school graduates and 58% were college graduates. Over $26,000 per year was earned by 84% of the families.

There are several variables on which significant differences among groups were found. The mean number of hours of day care attendance per week was significantly greater for children in Group II (mean =

26.09) than in Group I (mean = 14.72; t = 3.54, p < .01). Children in Group II were significantly older than children in Group I (t = 4.01, p < .01). It is important to note that there were no significant correlations between hours of attendance in day care or age of subject and scores on the dependent measures; therefore, the differences on these two variables would not appear to explain any differences found among groups.

Variables Related to the Abuse

The mean number of child victims per day care center case was 38.4 children, with a range of 2 to 100 victims per day care center case. The child victims were sexually abused by an average of 3.4 different offenders, with a range from 1 to 17 different offenders per child. Ritualistic abuse was associated with significantly more victims per day care center (t = 2.03, p < .05) and significantly more offenders per child (t = 5.01, p < .0001). When the number of times the children were abused was divided into the categories of less than 20 times and more than 20 times, children in the ritualistic abuse group experienced proportionately more abuse than the children who were sexually abused without ritualistic abuse (X2 = 4.32, df = 1, p < .05). There were no significant differences between the two abuse groups on the duration of the abuse or months elapsed since the abuse ended. The majority of children in both abuse groups received therapy, with 90.4% of children in Group I and 94.3% of children in Group II receiving therapy. There were no significant differences between the groups in length of therapy or time elapsed since therapy ended.

Types of Abuse

Victimization in day care was associated not only with extensive sexual abuse, but with serious physical and psychological abuse as well (Table 10–1). The data reported in Table 10–1 were provided by the subjects' parents and are based on the children's disclosure to their parents, therapists, and law enforcement officials.

Sexual Abuse

The types of sexual abuse ranged from fondling of the genitals to vaginal and rectal intercourse. Only female subjects were included in the items on vaginal intercourse and vaginal penetration with a

TABLE 10–1

COMPARISON OF SEXUAL AND RITUALISTIC ABUSE GROUPS ON
SEXUAL, PHYSICAL, AND PSYCHOLOGICAL ABUSE

	Group 1 Sexual Abuse (n = 32)	Group 2 Ritualistic Abuse (n = 35)	p
Type of Sexual Abuse			
Fondling of breasts/chest	21.9%	54.2%	.0065
Fondling of genitals	93.8%	91.4%	NS
Digital penetration	71.9%	88.6%	NS
Oral genital sex	59.4%	88.6%	.0061
Vaginal intercourse	31.3%	71.4%	.0151
Rectal intercourse	28.1%	66.7%	.0019
Object in vagina	56.3%	60.9%	NS
Object in rectum	56.3%	80.0%	.0363
Pornographic pictures taken	59.4%	88.6%	.0061
Satanic rituals	0.0%	100.0%	.0001
Sexual activity with other children	43.8%	94.3%	.0001
Mean number of different types of abuse per child	4.81	8.34	.0001
Type of Physical Abuse			
Child physically abused	81.3%	97.1%	.0371
Given drugs	28.1%	74.3%	.0002
Deprived of meals	18.8%	31.4%	NS
Hit by abuser(s)	68.8%	68.6%	NS
Consumption of excrement	25.0%	51.4%	.0266
Physically restrained	37.5%	71.4%	.0053
Psychological Abuse/Threat			
Child threatened with harm	96.9%	100.0%	NS
Child would be killed	56.3%	85.7%	.0075
Parents would be killed	75.0%	94.1%	.0304
Sibling would be killed	31.3%	31.4%	NS
Dismemberment	15.6%	37.1%	.0472
Loss of parents love	28.1%	8.6%	.037
Ritualist Abuse			
Threatened with supernatural powers	39.3%	100.0%	.0001
Chants/songs used	7.1%	86.2%	.0001

foreign object. Of particular concern is the severity of the sexual abuse experienced by subjects in both groups with the majority of subjects reporting one or more forms of penetration. The children each experienced a mean of 6.6 different types of sexual abuse.

Children in the ritualistic abuse group experienced significantly more (mean = 8.34, t = 5.67, p < .0001) types of sexual abuse than children in the sexual abuse group (mean = 4.81). The results presented in Table 10–1 indicate that children involved in ritualistic abuse experienced significantly more forms of penetration (vaginal, rectal, and oral) than children abused without rituals. In addition, children abused with rituals were more likely to report having pornographic pictures taken, being forced into sexual acts with other children, and having their breasts fondled.

Physical Abuse

Eight-nine percent of the child victims were physically abused by the offenders. The majority of the children were hit by their abusers. Seventy-four percent of children abused in rituals and 28% of those abused without rituals were forced to drink a substance or drug that made them drowsy, perhaps in an effort to make them less resistant to abusive acts and less likely to accurately recall details of the traumatic events. Over 50% of the children reported being physically restrained during the abuse. The consumption of human excrement, including urine, feces, and semen, was described by 38% of the children, with significantly more children in the ritualistic group reporting this type of abuse. These findings indicate that children who are sexually abused in day care experience extensive physical abuse at the hands of their abusers, with those in the ritualistic group recounting the most severe physical abuse.

Psychological Abuse

Severe intimidation was used to prevent victims from disclosing their abuse. The perpetrators threatened some form of physical harm to 98% of the abused children, with death threats being the most prevalent type of threat—71% were told they would be killed, 85% were threatened that their parents would be killed, and 31% were told a sibling would be killed if the abuse were ever disclosed. The threats used were often very specific, such as "I'll kill your mommy while she's sleeping" or "A UPS truck will come to your house and run you over if you ever tell." Offenders often convinced their victims that they had magical powers. For instance, some children were told that the offender would "come through the walls in their home and take them away." Over one-fourth of the children were threatened with a form of dismemberment, ranging from "Jesus will cut your arms off" to demonstrations of animal mutilation accompanied by the promise "This is what will happen to you if you ever tell."

Parents in 95% of the cases reported that their child was extremely frightened by the threats made by the offenders. Despite the fact that a mean of 2.2 years had elapsed since the abuse, 80% of the parents reported that their children had persistent fears related to the abuse. A significantly greater proportion (X2 = 4.13, df = 1, p < .05) of children abused with rituals (88.6%) continued to experience fears related to the abuse compared to the sexual abuse group (71.9%).

Ritualistic Abuse

Children in Group II all reported participation in satanic rituals and threats with supernatural powers. The satanic rituals described often involved wearing robes or costumes and use of paraphernalia, including candles, drugs or "magic potions," and satanic symbols, such as inverted crucifixes and pentagrams. In the ritualistic abuse group 86% of the children described the use of chants and songs to invoke the power of Satan during the ceremonial abuse. The threats with supernatural powers were most often related to Satan, evil spirits, or demons, and included warnings such as, "Satan always knows where you are and what you are doing".

Child Stress Responses to Sexual Victimization

The results of the planned comparisons on the CBCL reported in Table 10–2 indicate that children sexually abused in day care (Groups I and II) demonstrated significantly more behavioral disturbances than nonabused children (Group III). The mean scores on the total behavior problem scale were significantly greater (t = 16.38, p < .0001) for the children abused in day care (mean = 66.74) than for the comparison subjects (mean = 43.19). Scores ≥ 70 on the behavior problem total score are at the 98th percentile and are considered to be in the clinical range (Achenbach & Edelbrock, 1983). Of the

TABLE 10–2
CHILD BEHAVIOR CHECKLIST MEAN SCORES

	Group 1 Sexual Abuse (n = 32)	Group 2 Ritualistic Abuse (n = 35)	Group 3 Comparison (n = 67)
Behavior problem total score[a]			
M	64.78	68.69	43.19
SD	9.84	8.72	7.17
Internalizing score[a]			
M	64.84	69.26	44.19
SD	8.88	7.46	6.68
Externalizing score[b]			
M	.03	63.89	44.80
SD	10.08	9.31	7.07
Social competency score[c]			
M	43.33	45.17	51.33
SD	10.80	11.41	10.64
CBCL Subscales			
Depressed[b]			
M	66.69	69.54	55.43
SD	8.96	8.76	1.47
Aggressive[b]			
M	64.59	66.14	55.36
SD	8.99	9.86	1.81
Schizoid[b]			
M	65.40	67.11	55.63
SD	7.84	7.85	1.80
Social withdrawal[b]			
M	64.31	67.83	55.52
SD	7.25	7.72	1.59
Somatic complaints[b]			
M	64.63	67.54	55.78
SD	8.64	8.64	2.05
Sex problems (raw score)[b]			
M	1.27	1.59	.16
SD	1.51	1.94	.51

[a]Group 1 and Group 2 > Group 3, p < .0001; Group 2 > Group 1, p < .05.
[b]Group 1 and Group 2 > Group 3, p < .0001.
[c]Group 3 > Group 1 and Group 2, p < .0001.

abused subjects, 40% scored in the clinical range (scores ≥ 70), whereas only 2% of the general population would be expected to fall into this range, indicating far greater behavior problems in this sample than in a normative group.

The internalizing dimension mean score was significantly greater ($t = 17.64$, $p < .0001$) for the abused subjects (mean = 67.05) than for the comparison subjects (mean = 44.19). Almost half (47%) of the abused subjects scored in the clinical range (scores ≥ 70) on the internalizing dimension. In addition, the externalizing dimension mean score for the abused subjects (mean = 62.46) was significantly greater ($t = 12.013$, $p < .0001$) than the mean for the comparison subjects (mean = 44.80). On the externalizing dimension 25% of the abused subjects scored in the clinical range (scores ≥ 70). Sexually abused children scored significantly lower on social competence than nonabused children ($t = 3.69$, $p < .0001$), indicating that sexual abuse had a negative impact on their social functioning. There was 11% of the abused subjects who scored in the clinical range (scores ≤ 30) on social competence.

Sexually abused subjects (Groups I and II) scored significantly higher than nonabused children on all six subscales (Table 10–2): sex problems ($t = 5.622$, $p < .0001$), depression ($t = 11.543$, $p < .0001$), social withdrawal ($t = 11.276$, $p < .0001$), somatic complaints ($t = 9.49$, $p < .0001$), schizoid $t = 10.00$, $p < .0001$), and aggression ($t = 8.538$, $p < .0001$).

Child Stress Responses to Ritualistic Abuse

Children in the ritual abuse group demonstrated significantly more behavior problems than children in the sexual abuse group ($t = 1.73$, $p < .05$). In the ritualistic abuse group 48% of the children scored in the clinical range on the total behavior problem scale as compared to 32% of children in the 20 sexual abuse group. Children in this group had significantly higher mean scores on the internalizing dimension of the Child Behavior Checklist ($t = 2.19$, $p < .05$): 57% scored in the clinical range on the internalizing dimension as compared to 38% of the sexual abuse group.

Parental Stress Response

Results of the ANOVA and planned comparisons of mean T scores of parents on the General Severity Index (GSI) and the nine subscales of the Symptom Checklist-90-R are presented in Table 10–3 (mothers) and Table 10–4 (fathers). As hypothesized, parents of sexually abused children (Groups I and II) reported greater psychological distress than parents of nonabused children as indicated by their significantly higher mean T scores on the GSI (mothers, t = –9.32, p < .0001; fathers, t = –8.86, p < .0001). Fifty-two percent of parents of abused children had GSI T scores ≥ 63, which are at the 90th percentile and considered in the clinical range (Derogatis, 1977).

Parents of abused children (Groups I and II) scored significantly higher on each the nine subscales of the SCL-90-R than parents of nonabused children. Both mothers and fathers of abused children had the highest elevations in same five primary dimensions: depression, interpersonal sensitivity, hostility, paranoia, and anxiety.

The next research question examined whether parents of ritually abused children would report more psychological distress than parents of children abused without rituals, due to the extreme nature of ritualistic abuse. As predicted, parents of ritually abused children reported the most psychological distress, with significantly higher mean GSI T scores than parents of children abused without rituals (mothers, t = 1.79, p < .05; fathers, t = 2.08, p < .05): 65% of parents whose children were abused with rituals scored in the clinical range as compared to 40% of parents whose children were abused without rituals.

Next, paired t-tests were conducted to compare the mean scores of mothers and fathers in Groups I and II on the GSI and the nine primary dimensions of the SCL-90-R. The mean GSI T score of fathers (mean = 63.53, SD = 10.47) was significantly greater (t = –2.52, p < .05) than the mean score of mothers (mean = 59.64, SD = 11.49), indicating that two years post disclosure fathers were experiencing greater psychological distress than mothers. The only subscale in which there was a significant difference between mothers and fathers was the depression subscale, in which the mean score of fathers (mean = 63.44, SD = 10.97) was significantly greater (t = –3.15, p < .05) than the mean score of mothers (mean = 58.84, SD = 10.82).

Mean scores obtained on the Impact of Event Scale (IES) indicate that although an average of 2.2 years had elapsed since the sexual

TABLE 10–3

SCL-90-R SCORES OF MOTHERS

SCL-90-R Dimension	Group 1 Ritualistic Abuse (n = 32)	Group 2 Comparison Abuse (n = 33)	Group 3 (n = 67)
General Severity Index (GSI)[a]			
M	58.16	62.64	44.69
SD	10.85	9.26	9.25
Depression[b]			
M	58.25	61.30	47.24
SD	10.71	8.26	8.90
Interpersonal sensitivity[b]			
M	60.09	61.76	49.68
SD	10.92	10.89	8.10
Hostility[b]			
M	61.09	59.79	49.55
SD	9.86	11.23	7.30
Paranoid[b]			
M	59.29	62.33	46.39
SD	10.79	9.66	6.77
Anxiety[a]			
M	56.81	62.76	45.19
SD	10.99	8.39	8.10
Obsessive-compulsive[b]			
M	57.06	60.88	46.06
SD	10.83	9.55	8.18
Psychoticism			
M	58.56	60.24	48.27
SD	9.93	9.97	6.56
Somatization[b]			
M	50.56	55.12	43.94
SD	9.11	10.06	7.48
Phobic[b]			
M	54.48	56.85	45.49
SD	9.87	10.59	4.06

[a]Groups 1 and 2 > Group 3, p < .0001; and Group 2 > Group 1, p < .05.
[b]Groups 1 and 2 > Group 3, p < .0001.

abuse of their child, parents continued to experience intrusive thoughts and images as well as conscious avoidance of ideas and emotions related to their child's abuse. Paired t-tests revealed that mothers (mean = 19.52, SD = 12.78) scored significantly higher than fathers (mean = 15.41, SD = 12.21) on the intrusion subscale (t = 2.36, p < .05). No significant difference was found on the avoidance subscale (mothers, mean = 13.60, SD = 10.21; fathers, mean = 13.00, SD = 10.77). A comparison of Groups I and II revealed no significant difference in mean scores on the IES.

Pearson's correlation was used to test for significant relationships between parental stress scores and variables related to the abuse (Table 10–5). Parental stress as measured by the General Severity Index (GSI) was strongly correlated with the IES intrusion subscale (r = .74, p < .001) and moderately correlated with the IES avoidance subscale (r = .53, p < .001). GSI T scores were moderately correlated with child behavior problems (r = .30, p < .01) as measured by the Child Behavior Checklist (Achenbach & Edelbrock, 1983). There was a weak but significant inverse relationship between GSI scores and time elapsed since the sexual abuse (r = –.22, p < .05) indicating that parental stress decreases with distancing in time from their child's sexual victimization.

The next analyses sought to determine whether parents who had themselves been sexually abused during childhood experienced increased psychological distress. Twenty-two percent of mothers (n = 15) and 9% of fathers (n = 6) reported having been victimized as children. The t test for independent samples was used to compare the GSI T scores of abused and nonabused parents. The mean GSI T score of mothers who had been abused during childhood (mean = 64.2, SD = 10.21) was significantly higher (t = –1.66, p <. 05) than the mean GSI T scores of mothers without a childhood history of victimization (mean = 59.3, SD = 10.08). There was no significant difference between GSI T scores of fathers who had been abused and those who had not been abused.

The relationship between child behavior problem scores and parental history of victimization was explored next. The mean behavior problem score as measured by the Child Behavior Checklist for children whose mothers had been abused (mean = 71.07, SD = 8.75) was significantly higher (t = –2.03, p < .05) than the behavior

TABLE 10–4

SCL-90-R SCORES OF FATHERS

SCL-90-R Dimension	Group 1 Sexual Abuse (n = 25)	Group 2 Ritualistic Abuse (n = 21)	Group 3 Comparison (n = 53)
General Severity Index (GSI)[a]			
M	60.68	66.71	47.91
SD	11.05	8.64	7.52
Depression[a]			
M	61.36	65.76	49.00
SD	11.34	9.96	8.68
Interpersonal sensitivity[b]			
M	60.64	65.48	50.06
SD	9.38	7.45	7.36
Hostility[b]			
M	62.52	63.81	48.09
SD	11.15	9.84	7.44
Paranoid[a]			
M	59.16	65.91	46.91
SD	11.19	10.31	7.85
Anxiety[a]			
M	57.84	65.81	48.81
SD	11.31	8.70	7.91
Obsessive-compulsive[b]			
M	58.92	63.67	49.30
SD	12.03	8.44	8.19
Psychoticism[a]			
M	55.52	62.29	47.55
SD	9.5	8.67	5.69
Somatization[a]			
M	52.96	60.86	47.32
SD	11.67	8.74	9.05
Phobic[b]			
M	54.48	58.05	48.09
SD	9.70	9.30	4.16

[a]Groups 1 and 2 > Group 3, p < .0001; and Group 2 > Group 1 p < .05.
[b]Groups 1 and 2 > Group 3, p < .0001.

TABLE 10–5

CORRELATION MATRIX OF PARENTAL GENERAL SEVERITY INDEX AND
VARIABLES RELATED TO SEXUAL ABUSE

	1	2	3	4	5
1. GSI[a]					
2. Intrusion	.74***				
2. Avoidance	.53***	.79***			
4. Time elapsed	–.22*	–.17	–.07		
5. CBC total problems[b]	.30**	.26*	.19	.14	
6. Stressful life events	.15	.15	.30**	.26*	–.09

[a]General Severity Index, Symptom Checklist-90-R
[b]Behavior problem total score, Child Behavior Checklist
*p < .05
**p < .01
***p < .001

problem scores of children whose mothers did not have a childhood history of abuse (mean = 65.60, SD = 9.31). However, paternal history of sexual abuse did not appear to be related to child behavior problem scores.

DISCUSSION

The findings from this study support and extend earlier reports (Conte & Schuerman, 1987; Friedrich & Reams, 1987; Gomes-Schwartz, Horowitz, & Sauzier, 1985; Tong, Oates, & McDowell, 1987) that children are negatively affected by sexual abuse. Although the follow-up period was relatively short (2.2 years), this study does suggest that this group of children has persisting behavioral disturbances. Consistent with findings reported in earlier studies (Friedrich, Beilke, & Urquiza, 1988; Gomes-Schwartz, Horowitz, & Sauzier, 1985), the sexually abused children in this study displayed more sexual problems than the nonabused subjects.

It is generally agreed that the degree of emotional impact of sexual abuse varies by the closeness of the relationship between the child and offender, with sexual abuse by a close relative, such as a father or father figure, having the most serious impact (Conte & Schuerman, 1987; Friedrich, Urquiza, & Beilke, 1986). The severity of impact of sexual abuse by nonfamily members found in this study suggests that the relative-nonrelative distinction is not always an accurate predictor of the impact.

The extreme forms of physical, sexual, and psychological abuse experienced by the majority of subjects in this study is alarming. The offenders deliberately and systematically terrified their young victims in order to ensure their silence. Given the severity of the abuse, it is understandable that the majority of children still experienced fears related to the abuse although two years had elapsed since removal from the abusive environment. These continued fears may in part explain the children's persistent symptomatology. Therapists who treat children abused in day care centers not only must focus on issues related to sexual abuse, but also must address issues related to the wide range of abusive behaviors children often experience.

The increased impact of ritualistic abuse found in this study is consistent with what has been reported by Finkelhor, Williams, and Burns (1988) and is most likely attributable to the extreme physical, sexual, and psychological abuse associated with ritualistic abuse. Survivors of ritualistic abuse are considered at risk for severe psychiatric problems, especially dissociative disorders such as multiple personality disorder (Gould, 1987; Kaye & Klein, 1987). As there is currently a dearth of scholarly literature on ritualistic abuse, research on the nature, incidence, and mental health consequences of ritualistic abuse is needed to counteract both the skepticism and sensationalism surrounding reports of ritualistic abuse.

The increased psychological distress found in parents of sexually abused children in this study empirically validates the clinical literature that asserts that sexual victimization is a major stressor for nonoffending parents (DeJong, 1986; Esquilin, 1987; Sesan, Freeark, & Murphy, 1986). The parents of children abused in day care centers were found to be highly symptomatic and present strong evidence of experiencing posttraumatic stress disorder. According to Horowitz, Wilner, Kaltreider, and Alvarez (1980), posttraumatic stress disorder occurs in reaction to a major traumatic event and is characterized by intrusive ideas and feelings, ideational denial, and emotional numbing as well as recurrent or prolonged episodes of depression, anxiety, guilt, shame, and hostility. Parents of sexually abused children reported clinical indicators of intrusion and avoidance as measured by the Impact of Event Scale, as well as elevated scores on the depression, anxiety, interpersonal sensitivity, and hostility dimensions of the Symptom Checklist-90-R.

The findings of this study support and extend the findings of earlier studies that identified relationships between parent and child responses to sexual victimization (Finkelhor, Williams, & Burns, 1988; Gomes-Schwartz, Horowitz, & Sauzier, 1984). When parents are overwhelmed by the discovery that their child has been abused, the child may be deprived of needed emotional support. In addition, the behavioral disturbances commonly manifested by sexually abused children are difficult for parents to manage. Most notably, parents have difficulty dealing with their child's sexual acting-out behaviors, developmental regressions, and extreme fears and anxieties (Kelley, 1986). Thus, the stress responses of parents and children to sexual victimization appear mutually to influence each other.

The stress response of parents to their child's sexual victimization identified in this study have important implications for clinicians and researchers. In order to intervene effectively, professionals need to recognize sexual victimization as both an acute and a chronic stressor for parents. During the acute phase parents are dealing with feelings of shock, anger, denial, and guilt (DeJong, 1986; DeVine, 1980; Finkelhor, 1986; MacFarlane & Waterman, 1986) as well as entanglement in the complex legal, mental health, and social service systems. Sexual abuse is also experienced by parents as a chronic stressor due to the long-term impact on the child, the need for extended therapy, and, in many instances, lengthy legal proceedings, which may prevent the family from achieving closure on the event. Even when a guilty verdict is rendered, most verdicts end up in a lengthy appeal process, which further prolongs the stress reaction. Although, on average, two years had elapsed since the discovery of their child's sexual abuse, 52% of parents in the study had psychological distress scores in the clinical range. This persistent symptomatology suggests a chronic form of posttraumatic stress disorder. It is important to note that the psychological distress levels found in parents in this study are comparable to those found in parents two years after their child had died from cancer (Moore, Gilliss, & Martinson, 1988).

Despite the fact that two-thirds of the parents in the study received therapy, the majority continued to display persistent psychological distress. Most parents received less than six months of therapy, which suggests that more extended therapy is needed for successful resolution of this traumatic event. The question must be raised as to whether effective treatment is currently available to parents in cases of extrafamilial abuse. Studies which examine the efficacy of various intervention strategies for parents in cases of extrafamilial abuse are needed.

The higher distress levels found in fathers in this study is in contrast to the findings of other studies that compared the stress responses of mothers and fathers. Moore, Gilliss, and Martinson (1988) found greater psychological distress in mothers than fathers after the death of their child from cancer. Likewise, Klein and Nimorwicz (1982) found greater psychological distress in mothers than fathers of hemophiliac children. Possibly, the fathers were experiencing a delayed stress response, since fathers have been reported as having increased difficulty discussing thoughts and feelings related to their child's victimization (Zimmerman, Wolbert, Burgess, & Hartman, 1987).

The finding that parental stress levels decreased over time is clinically relevant in that it underscores the importance of reassuring parents that the intense psychological distress they initially experience will decrease with time and therapeutic intervention. However, it has yet to be determined how long symptoms persist after the discovery that one's child has been sexually abused. A longitudinal study of parental responses beginning immediately after discovery of the abuse with periodic evaluations of psychological distress levels would provide valuable insight into how parents process this stressful event over time. Such knowledge is fundamental to developing effective interventions to facilitate parental adaptation.

The increased psychological distress found in mothers with childhood histories of victimization is of important clinical significance. For mothers victimized as children, the sexual abuse of their child precipitates a twofold crisis in which they must deal simultaneously with their own unresolved trauma as well as the knowledge that their child has been sexually abused, resulting in a compounded stress reaction. It is therefore imperative for professionals to elicit parental histories of childhood sexual abuse when assessing families of child victims and to provide appropriate support to adult survivors of sexual abuse.

Parents of ritually abused children experienced the greatest psychological distress. This finding could be related to several factors, including parental knowledge of the severe forms of abuse their child suffered, increased impact associated with ritualistic abuse (Finkelhor, Williams, & Burns, 1988), lack of information currently available to parents and professionals on ritualistic abuse, and the skepticism with which some reports of ritualistic abuse are met (Kelley, 1988).

There are several limitations to the study that make generalizations beyond the sample difficult. First, a sample of convenience was utilized. The fact that all of the children in the sample were abused in day care centers also presents limitations since child and parental response to sexual abuse in a day care center may be quite different from child and parental reaction to intrafamilial abuse. Further research is necessary utilizing a longitudinal design, with a larger sample of families, including those whose children have been involved in intrafamilial and extrafamilial sexual abuse.

In conclusion, the sexual victimization of a child in day care is a traumatic event for children and parents often resulting in post-traumatic stress disorder, possibly of a chronic nature. Since resolution of the victimization experience by the child can be facilitated or hindered by parental response, professional intervention is imperative for parents, as well as children. Unfortunately, attention in the past has focused almost exclusively on the treatment needs of incestuous families, while overlooking the needs of families who experience extrafamilial abuse. More extensive research needs to be conducted on the effects of extrafamilial abuse on all family members, including nonabused siblings. Factors that may mediate reactions to sexual abuse, such as coping style, family dynamics that predate the abuse, cultural and religious influences, and social supports need to be carefully examined.

REFERENCES

Achenbach, T. M., & Edelbrock, C.S. (1983). *The Child Behavior Checklist Manual*. Burlington: University of Vermont.

Anderson, S.C.; Bach, C.M.; & Griffith, S. (1981). Psychosocial sequelae in intrafamilial victims of sexual assault and abuse. Paper presented at the Third International Conference on Child Abuse and Neglect, Amsterdam, the Netherlands.

Conte, J., & Schuerman, J. (1987). Factors associated with an increased impact of child sexual abuse. *Child Abuse and Neglect* 11: 201–211.

DeFrancis, V. (1969). *Protecting the Child Victim of Sex Crimes Committed by Adults*. Denver: American Humane Association.

DeJong, A.R. (1986). Childhood sexual abuse precipitating maternal hospitalization. *Child Abuse and Neglect* 10: 551–553.

Derogatis, L.R. (1983). *The SCL-90-R: Administration, Scoring, and Procedures Manual II*. Baltimore: Clinical Psychometrics Research.

DeVine, R.A. (1980). The sexually abused child in the emergency room. In *Sexual Abuse of Children: Selected Readings*. Washington, D.C.: U.S. Department of Health and Human Services.

de Young, M. (1982). *The Sexual Victimization of Children*. Jefferson, N.C.: McFarland.

Esquilin, S.C. (1987). Family response to the identification of extra-familial child sexual abuse. *Psychotherapy in Private Practice* 5 (1): 105–113.

Finkelhor, D. (1986). *A Sourcebook on Child Sexual Abuse*. Newbury Park, Calif.: Sage.

Finkelhor, D.; Williams, L.; & Burns, N. (1988). *Nursery Crimes: Sexual Abuse in Day Care*. Newbury Park, Calif.: Sage.

Friedrich, W.N.; Beilke, R.L.; & Urquiza, A.J. (1988). Behavior problems in young sexually abused boys. *Journal of Interpersonal Violence* 3 (1): 21–28.

Friedrich, W.N., & Reams, R.A. (1987). Course of psychological symptoms in sexually abused children. *Psychotherapy* 24 (2): 160–170.

Friedrich, W.N.; Urquiza, A.J.; & Beilke, R. (1986). Behavioral problems in sexually abused young children. *Journal of Pediatric Psychology* 11: 47–57.

Gomes-Schwartz, B.; Horowitz, J.M.; & Sauzier, M. (1985). Severity of emotional distress among sexually abused preschool, school-age, and adolescent children. *Hospital and Community Psychiatry* 36 (5): 503–508.

Gomes-Schwartz, B.; Horowitz, J.M.; & Sauzier, M. (1984). Sexually exploited children: service and research project. Final report for the Office of Juvenile Justice and Delinquency Prevention. Washington, D.C.: U.S. Department of Justice.

Gould, C. (1987). Satanic ritual abuse: child victims, adult survivors, system response. *California Psychologist* 22 (3): 1.

Herman, J.L. (1981). *Father-Daughter Incest.* Cambridge: Harvard University Press.

Hollingshead, A.B. (1975). Four-factor index of social status. Working paper. New Haven: Yale University Department of Sociology.

Horowitz, M.; Wilner, N.; & Alvarez, W. (1979). Impact of event scale: a measure of subjective stress. *Psychosomatic Medicine* 41 (3): 209–218.

Horowitz, M.; Wilner, N.; Kaltreider,N.; & Alvarez, W. (1980). Signs and symptoms of posttraumatic stress disorder. *Archives of General Psychiatry* 37 (1): 85-92.

Kaye, M., & Klein, L. (November 1987). Clinical indicators of Satanic cult victimization. Paper presented at the Fourth International Conference for the Study of Multiple Personality Disorder, Chicago.

Kelley, S.J. (1986). Learned helplessness in the sexually abused child. *Issues in Comprehensive Pediatric Nursing* 9: 193–207.

Kelley, S.J. (1990). Parental stress response to sexual abuse and ritualistic abuse of children in day care centers. *Nursing Research* 25 (1): 25–29.

Kelley, S.J. (1988). Ritualistic abuse of children: dynamics and impact. *Cultic Studies Journal* 5 (2): 228–236.

Kelley, S.J. (1989). Stress responses of children to sexual abuse and ritualistic abuse in day care centers. *Journal of Interpersonal Violence* 4 (4): 502–513.

Klein, R.H., & Nimorwicz, P. (1982). The relationship between psychological distress and knowledge of disease among hemophilia patients and their families: a pilot study. *Journal of Psychosomatic Research* 26 (4): 387–391.

MacFarlane, K., & Waterman, J. (1986). *Sexual Abuse of Young Children.* New York: Guilford Press.

Moore, I.M.; Gilliss, C.L.; & Martinson, I. (1988). Psychosomatic symptoms in parents two years after the death of a child with cancer. *Nursing Research* 37 (2): 104–107.

Sesan, R.; Freeark, K.; & Murphy, S. (1986). The support network: crisis intervention for extrafamilial child sexual abuse. *Professional Psychology, Research, and Practice* 17 (2): 138–146.

Tong, L.; Oates, K.; & McDowell, M. (1987). Personality development following sexual abuse. *Child Abuse and Neglect* 11 (3): 371–383.

Zimmerman, M.L.; Wolbert, W.A.; Burgess, A.W.; & Hartman, C.R. (1987). Art and group work: interventions for multiple victims of child molestation. *Archives of Psychiatric Nursing* 1 (1): 40–46.

CHAPTER
11

Parental Response to Child Sexual Abuse Trials Involving Day Care Settings

Ann Wolbert Burgess, Carol R. Hartman, Susan J. Kelley, Christine A. Grant, Ellen B. Gray

This study was funded, in part, by the following:
National Center on Child Abuse and Neglect
Grant 90-CA-1273; Department of Justice Office
for Victims of Crime Grant 88-VR-GX-K001; and
a Sigma Theta Tau grant to Susan J. Kelley.
Reprinted with permission from the *Journal of
Traumatic Stress* 3 (3): 395–405, 1990.

Advances have been made in the 1980s through judicial reform for minimizing trauma to the child witnesses (Arthur, 1986; Berliner, 1985; Bulkley, 1985). However, while much has been written and speculated upon regarding whether young children should testify (Yates, 1987), innovative approaches at trial (Whitcomb, 1986), children's memory and credibility (Benedek & Schetky, 1987; Landwirth, 1987), and the impact of court procedures (Goodman, 1984; Weiss & Berg, 1982), little has been written about the psychological impact that the court experience has on parents of the child witness.

The literature on parental response to stressful life events encountered by their children has been primarily in the area of illness (Leahey & Wright, 1987) and general posttraumatic stress disorder (Figley, 1988). There is little empirical evidence as to the response patterns of parents whose children have been criminally victimized except in the area of homicide (Masters, Friedman, & Getzel, 1988;

Rinear, 1988). The literature on the court process for the child and the family suggests that testifying as a witness can be as much of a crisis as the actual sexual abuse. Victims and their families develop a multitude of intense reactions in going through the court process. Several general psychological responses are magnified. First, time becomes suspended. The energies needed to prepare and go to court interrupt schooling and family life. Second, the sexual abuse is resurfaced. The court process recapitulates, in a psychological manner, the original assault situation. The child must relive the assault mentally and verbally in a public setting and be cross-examined by defense counsel. Third, victims become aware that people are skeptical about their story and a feeling of silent suspicion is felt. Few people, except in the courtroom, may be so blatant as to tell the child they do not believe him or her, but this suspicion is communicated in subtle ways. And fourth, the child and family may feel betrayed by people previously considered supportive (Burgess et al., 1978).

This chapter seeks to add to the empirical literature by comparing parental response to child sexual abuse by whether or not their child testified in a trial.

CONCEPTUAL FRAMEWORK

The conceptual framework for this study is predicated on human response to stressful life events (Hill, 1949) and posttraumatic stress disorder (Eth & Pynoos, 1985; Horowitz, 1976; van der Kolk, 1984). A major assumption is that parents experience posttraumatic stress associated with the victimization of their child. The parent, as well as the child, psychologically has to process the perceptions, meanings, and ideations engendered by knowledge of the child's abuse. This processing has been previously conceptualized in a phase-specific model of information processing of trauma, from which posttraumatic behaviors emerge (Burgess et al., 1987; Hartman & Burgess, 1988). This processing model helps explain how a child victim attempts to modify the sensory, perceptual, and cognitive alterations that occurred during abuse, whether it was physical, sexual, or psychological in nature. It hypothesizes how these behavioral adaptations, at these three levels, emerge in overt behavioral patterns specifically reflective of the abuse itself and how the memory constructs, over time, are influenced by the psychological survival mechanisms. These behaviors, reflecting how the event is stored and processed, are referred to as "trauma learned." This framework focuses on how individuals organize their thinking and memories or reconstructions of a critical event.

METHOD

Sample

This study involved a convenience sample of parents of 67 children who were sexually abused in 16 different child care settings within 12 states. Subjects were recruited nationally through therapists, law enforcement officials, and a parent advocacy group. Of 81 parents who received a questionnaire, 83% returned them.

A parent population of the 67 children, comprised of 65 mothers and 46 fathers, participated in the study. The mean age of mothers was 34.05 years (range = 26–43) and for fathers was 36.5 years (range = 30–45). Families were of middle to high socioeconomic status, with over three-quarters of the parent population dividing into social classes I and II on the Hollingshead Index of Social Status (Hollingshead, 1974). College graduates comprised 61% of the subjects, and 81.6 percent earned more than $26,000 a year.

The mean age of the subjects' children at the time they were sexually abused in day care was 2.8 years (range = 1–7). The mean duration of the abuse was 14.95 months. The time elapsed between the disclosure of the abuse and data collection ranged from 6 to 47 months, with a mean of 27.5 months. Of the children, 55% were female and 45% male. The types of sexual abuse the children experienced ranged from fondling of the genitals to vaginal and rectal intercourse, with the majority of children experiencing one or more forms of penetration.

The sexual abuse of each of the child subjects was substantiated by the agency responsible for investigating the allegation of sexual abuse in the respective jurisdiction. Criminal charges were brought against the abusers in 92% of the cases. When criminal charges were filed, 80% resulted in criminal conviction of one or more offenders. Of the remaining cases, 5% resulted in acquittals, 7% had charges dismissed, and 7% of the cases had trials in progress (Kelley, 1989). Of this 67-child sample, 17 children testified in a court proceeding and 50 did not testify.

Data Collection and Procedures

Data collected on parental response to their child's sexual abuse was completed through mailed questionnaires. This study reports on parent completion of two standardized instruments: the Symptom Checklist-90-R (Derogatis, 1977) and the Impact of Event Scale (Horowitz, Wilner, & Alvarez, 1979). A questionnaire asking whether the parent and/or the child received therapy after disclosure of abuse, whether the mother or father was abused as a child, the types of sexual abuse experienced by the child, marital status, family income, stressful life events since disclosure, and reactions to court involvement was also completed. The Symptom Checklist-90-R (SCL-90-R), a 90-item multidimensional self-report symptom inventory, was used to measure symptomatic distress in parents. The General Severity Index (GSI) of the SCL-90-R combines information on numbers of symptoms and intensity of distress. The SCL-90-R has shown high levels of both internal consistency and test-retest reliability. Derogatis (1977) reports coefficient alphas between .77 and .90. A high convergent and discriminate validity between the SCL-90-R and the MMPI has been established (Derogatis, 1977).

The Impact of Event Scale (IES) is a 15 item instrument that focuses on the quality of conscious experiences during a recent period with a stressful life event specific to the individual written on the form as the referent for response to the list of experiences. For the purposes of this study "the event" is the sexual abuse of the subject's child. The two IES subscales, avoidance and intrusion, are index symptoms of the two dimensions that characterize posttraumatic stress disorder. The two dimensions are (1) intrusion into consciousness of unbidden ideas, feelings, and images and (2) consciously recognized denial or avoidance of stress-related themes and emotional responses. The internal consistency of the two scales are .79 and .82, respectively.

RESULTS

Data analysis was performed utilizing a SPSS-X program. Planned comparisons were conducted to compare mean scores on the SCL-90-R and IES and mean scores of interval level demographic data. Chi square analysis was used to compare nominal level demographic data as well as variables related to parental distress.

Parental Response

The General Severity Index T (GSIT) score of the SCL-90-R was used as the singular measure of stress. GSIT scores of mothers of children who testified were significantly greater (mean = 64.94) than mothers of children who did not testify (mean = 58.83, t = 2.17). These scores were significant at the p = .02 level. Of the mothers of children who did testify, 58.8% scored in the clinical range compared to 45.8% of mothers whose children did not testify. A GSIT score greater than or equal to 63 is considered in the clinical range (Derogatis, 1983).

Mothers of children who testified scored higher in the avoidance scale of the Impact of Events Scale (mean = 18.24) than mothers of children who did not testify (mean = 12.30). This finding was significant at the p = .01 level. Mothers of children who testified also scored higher on the intrusion subscale (mean = 24.06) than mothers of children who did not testify (mean = 17.43). This finding was significant at the p = .03 level, t = 1.96.

The fathers of children who testified scored significantly higher on the GSIT (mean = 71.3) compared to fathers of children who did not testify (mean = 61.25). This finding was highly significant at the p = .003 level of significance, t = 2.93. Of the fathers whose children testified, 90% scored in the clinical range compared to 44.4% of fathers whose children did not testify.

The mean score on the avoidance subscale of the IES of fathers whose children testified (mean = 23.0) was significantly greater than fathers of children who did not testify (mean = 9.62, t = 3.91). This finding was highly significant at the p = .000 level of significance. Fathers whose children testified also scored significantly higher (mean = 26.9) on the intrusion subscale compared to fathers of children who did not testify (mean = 12.49). This finding was highly significant at the p = .000 level.

Sample Characteristics of Testifying and Nontestifying Groups

Of the characteristics summarized in Table 11–1, two are significantly different: the child's gender and the marital status of the parents. Of the children testifying, more females testified (76.5%) than males (23.5%), significant at p = .04. In the testifying group, only 70.6% of the parents were married compared to 90% of the nontestifying group, significant at p = .05.

Other Stress Factors Associated with Symptom Distress

Table 11–2 summarizes comparison of the groups on stressful life events. There is a significant difference in the total number of negative life events reported by parents in the testifying group (2.58 vs. 1.56, p = .01). Of the events themselves, three are significantly different for the testifying group: partner separation occurred in 23.5% vs. 2% (p = .003); death in the family was 41.1% vs. 18% (p = .05); and a reported decrease in income was 52.9% vs. 12% (p = .0005).

DISCUSSION

The major finding of this preliminary descriptive study is that parents of testifying children are highly symptomatic and present strong evidence of experiencing chronic posttraumatic stress disorder. In addition, the reported stress is higher in fathers than mothers with regard to symptoms, intrusive thinking, and avoidant behaviors. These findings are higher than parents' distress by type of abuse (Kelley, 1990). Also, the parents of testifying children have more stressful life events following disclosure of the abuse and the court experience suggesting that cumulative stress could serve to heighten anxiety.

TABLE 11–1

SAMPLE CHARACTERISTICS OF TESTIFYING AND
NONTESTIFYING GROUPS

	Group 1 Testifying (n = 17)	Group 2 Nontestifying (n = 50)	p
Child received therapy	100.0%	90.0%	0.1753
Parent received therapy	82.3	61.2	0.1113
Child ritually abused	47.1	54.0	0.6206
Mother abused as child	11.8	26.0	0.2238
Father abused as child	5.9	10.0	0.6075
No. types of sexual abuse experienced per child			
Mean	7.29	6.44	0.283
SD	2.62	3.23	
Child's gender			
Female	76.5%	48.0%	
Male	23.5	52.0	0.0414
Hollingshead Group			
I	23.5%	55.0%	
II	47.1	28.6	
III	12.0	6.0	
IV	17.6	10.0	0.1660
Parental marital status			
Married	70.6%	90.0%	
Not married	29.4	10.0	0.0523

The findings suggest that for parents of sexually abused children, entry into the judicial system not only resurrects the trauma that surfaced at time of disclosure to the knowledge of their child's abuse, but now introduces the parent to a process that raises more anxiety rather than bringing closure to a stressful situation.

What can be the factors that account for this strong response in parents over time? First, the length of time that knowledge of their child's abuse is consciously operant may be one factor influencing the chronic stress. The mean age of the child when the abuse began was 2.7 for the nontestifying group and 3.0 for the testifying group; the average length of duration of the abuse was 15 months. The mean age at time of testifying was 6.8. The length of time between the disclosure of the abuse and final court action is particularly difficult for those parents whose child is involved in testifying, for they are subjected to the review of the case and other activities that constantly resurrect in their mind the whole event and perhaps periods of time when their child was overtly distressed. During this length of time the parent has to deal with his or her own distress, the symptoms of the child (Kelley, 1990), and attempt to return to a precrisis level of activity.

To gain a greater appreciation of the nature of the parents' response to their child testifying, responses were tallied to the following questions, "Before the trial, what did you fear most about your child testifying? Did this happen?" Parents' thoughts that noted their fears did not happen were as follows:

TABLE 11–2

COMPARISON OF GROUPS ON STRESSFUL LIFE EVENTS

	Group 1 Testifying (n = 17)	Group 2 Nontestifying (n = 50)	p
Divorce	5.8%	2.0%	0.4165
Separation	23.5	2.0	0.0035
Death in family	41.4	18.0	0.0528
Unwanted pregnancy	0.0	0.0	NS
Decrease in income	52.9	12.0	0.0005
Alcohol or drug problem	17.6	8.0	0.2613
Death of close friend	0.0	8.0	0.2291
Moved to new location	17.6	28.0	0.3968
Changed schools	23.5	24.5	0.9365
Changed jobs	47.1	26.0	0.1059
Difficulty with boss	17.6	16.0	0.8742
Serious illness or injury	11.8	12.0	0.9794
Total number of stressful events			
M	2.58	1.56	0.011
SD	1.37	1.163	

> *"I thought that my daughter would go back to the way she was after the school was closed."*

> *"I thought that she would just cry and wouldn't talk."*

> *"I thought that the controversy created would filter down to her and that she would fall apart."*

> *"I thought that she would be bullied by the defense attorney and made to feel stupid and inadequate."*

> *"I was afraid that seeing those people again, confronting them, and talking about what happened would start her worrying about the threats coming true."*

> *"I thought that he would feel more guilty about what happened."*

> *"I thought that the defense attorney would harass and frighten her."*

> *"I thought she wouldn't be able to say anything at all. I thought she might have a seizure."*

> *"I thought that there might be acts of violence or vengeance against our family."*

The fears of the parents can be classified into two groups: (1) fears that focus on the child being frightened, disqualified, or pressured in some manner that could precipitate acute symptoms and behaviors and (2) concerns focused on the community response to the family, in particular that there would be a type of retaliation or revenge.

Statements made by parents that they reported did happen follow.

> *"I thought that he would be badgered by the prosecutor."*

> *"I thought that she would cry and not answer the questions asked by the defense lawyer; that the defense lawyer would try to confuse her."*

> *"I thought facing the defendants would make her regress."*

These examples indicated that several parents experienced their worst fears after their child testified. Such an experience challenges the parents as to their decision to permit their child to testify and requires that they cope with their doubts on their decision and of the retraumatizing trial experience. That parents were able to identify their fears about their child testifying suggest that this anticipatory anxiety can be a self-reinforcing process that sustains high levels of symptomatology. It may be that this same anticipatory anxiety is operant in the nontestifying parents but has not been compounded by the additional experience of the trial. Further research will be needed to explore and sort out this hypothesis.

What motivates parents to permit their child to testify? In 4 of the 17 cases, the parents stated they left the decision up to the child. In the majority of cases, however, the decision was made by the parents in conjunction with consultation with the prosecutor or the child's therapist. The analysis of motivation revealed parents primary motive was to create safety for their child; 80% of the parents whose child testified emphasized safety for their child as well as for other children. Safety was defined in terms of the child feeling safe, to know the perpetrator was "locked up" and that the child would be believed and protected during testifying.

Would parents do it over again? The question was asked: "Looking back, do you think the decision to have your child testify was the right one?" The majority of parents (n=12) indicated that they thought they made the right decision.

The fact that parents whose children testified reported more stressful life events than those whose child did not testify raises the question of source of psychological distress. Is the reporting of more stressful life events a function of the stress response itself; that is, parents are more sensitive to life events and recollect them as more stressful because they are presently under stress, or is this a visitation of more noxious life events? The prior interpretation may be warranted when noting that parents in both groups manifested psychological distress and further that fathers were significantly more distressed than mothers. This suggests that the trauma has not been resolved and that for parents that agree to testify there is every indication that the process activates and prolongs the traumatic recognition of their child's abuse in two ways. First, the trial demands a sorting and recounting of details of the child's abuse and, second, the trial itself, even with verdicts of guilty, is inconclusive (Montan, Burgess, Grant, & Hartman, 1988).

The alternate interpretation of cumulative negative life events suggests that parental distress over child sexual abuse may be mediated by interim stress due to death in the family, separation, and reduction in income. These three factors certainly have to be taken into account when examining response of parents to their child testifying. The decrease of family income was associated in the descriptive data with mothers withdrawing from the work role for a period of time until safe child care was secured. This withdrawal from the work role, the trauma of the sexual abuse, the burden of their child testifying further interact with marital harmony and become a stressor that may, in fact, explain separation.

This study reveals the impact on parents who decided to permit their child to testify, and it uncovers the high distress level of the fathers. The fathers are confronted with trying to manage the mother-child dyad, sustain the economic stability of the family, and manage their own response to the sexual abuse. The nature of the symptoms and reactions and the high intrusive imagery scales suggest that there is a strong visual component to how these men process information regarding the abuse of their child and their child in the justice system. This suggests a self-traumatizing mechanism operative in the fathers as well as the mothers. We have no consistent information on the structure of ideation in the fathers and its association to past trauma in their life, anticipated trauma, or, for that matter, fearful identification with sexually aggressive acts in themselves. Since these children were abused in day care settings where some of the perpetrators were females, there is little information on how parents deal with the realization that sexual and ritualistic abuse was initiated as well as condoned by female as well as male perpetrators.

The need of trauma-specific interventions for parents for their own adjustment to their child's trauma is strongly suggested in these findings. The therapeutic issues of how men process and deal with sexual abuse has only been eluded to in the clinical literature with regard to spouses and boyfriends of rape victims (Holmstrom

& Burgess, 1979; Silverman et al, 1978). There have been minimal efforts to provide support groups for males whose spouse or girlfriend has been raped. One finding in child trauma work is that fathers are not involved in the therapy of their children (Zimmerman, Wolbert, Burgess, & Hartman, 1987).

Parents whose child testifies are carrying the double burden of resolving their own stress surrounding the abuse of their child as well as the stressful aspects of a court trial. This dilemma involves complex decision making to permit their child to testify as well as the monitoring of behaviors regarding stress and anxiety prior to trial, during trial, and after trial. At the same time, parents must pursue what efforts they have established to assist their child in resolving the impact of the abuse.

This awareness of the complex dimensions of parenting deserves attention in the overall framework of the justice system. That more parents of testifying children received counseling than nontestifying parents (82.3% vs. 61.2%) and still had high distress levels suggests the need to study further the nature of trauma therapy and the consideration of additional life events.

REFERENCES

Arthur, L.G. (1986). Child sexual abuse: improving the system's response. *Juvenile and Family Court Journal* 37 (2): 1–75.

Benedek, E.P., & Schetky, D.H. (1987). Problems in validating allegations of sexual abuse. Part I: Factors affecting perception and recall of events. *Journal of the American Academy of Child and Adolescent Psychiatry* 26 (6): 912–915.

Berliner, L. (1985). The child witness: the progress and emerging limitations. Papers from a National Policy Conference on Legal Reforms in Child Sexual Abuse Cases. Pp. 93–107. National Legal Resource Center for Child Advocacy and Protection, American Bar Association. Washington, D.C.

Bulkley, J. (1985). Evidentiary and procedural trends in state legislation and other emerging issues in child sexual abuse cases. *Dickinson Law Review* 89 (3): 645–668.

Burgess, A.W.; Groth, A.N.; Holmstrom, L.L.; & Sgroi, S.M. (1978). *Sexual Assault of Children and Adolescents.* Lexington, Mass.: Lexington Books.

Burgess, A.W.; Hartman, C.R.; Wolbert, W.A.; & Grant, C.A. (1987). Child molestation: assessing impact in multiple victims. *Archives of Psychiatric Nursing* 1 (1): 33–39.

Derogatis, L.R. (1977). *The SCL-90-R: Administration, Scoring, and Procedures Manual I*. Baltimore: Clinical Psychometrics Research.

Eth, S., & Pynoos R.S. (1985). *Post-Traumatic Stress Disorder in Children*. Washington, D.C.: American Psychiatric Press.

Figley, C.R. (1988). A five-phase treatment of post–traumatic stress disorder. *Journal of Traumatic Stress* 1 (1): 127–141.

Goodman, G.S. (1984). The child witness: conclusion and future directions for research and legal practice. *Journal of Social Issues* 40 (2): 157–175.

Hartman, C.R., & Burgess, A.W. (1988). Information processing of trauma: application of a model. *Journal of Interpersonal Violence* 3 (4): 443–457.

Hill, R. (1949). *Families Under Stress*. New York: Harper & Row.

Hollinshead, A.B. (1975). Four-factor index of social status. Working paper. New Haven: Yale University Department of Sociology.

Holmstrom, L.L., & Burgess, A.W. (1979). Rape: the husband's and boyfriend's initial reactions. *Family Coordinator* 28 (3): 321–330.

Horowitz, M. (1976). *Stress Response Syndromes*. New York: Aronson.

Horowitz, M.; Wilner, N.; & Alvarez, W. (1979). Impact of event scale: a measure of subjective stress. *Psychosomatic Medicine* 41 (3): 209–218.

Kelley, S.J. (1990). Parental stress response to sexual abuse and ritualistic abuse of children in day care settings. *Nursing Research* 37 (2): 104–107.

Kelley, S.J. (1989). Stress responses of children to sexual abuse and ritualistic abuse in day care settings. *Journal of Interpersonal Violence* 4 (4): 501–512.

Landwirth, J. (1987). Children as witnesses in child sexual abuse trials. *Pediatrics* 80 (4): 585–589.

Leahey, M.L., & Wright, L.M. (1987). *Families and Life-Threatening Illness*. Springhouse, Penn.: Springhouse Corporation.

Masters, R.; Friedman, L.N.; & Getzel, G. (1988). Helping families of homicide victims: a multidimensional approach. *Journal of Traumatic Stress* 1 (1): 109–126.

Montan, C.; Burgess, A.W.; Grant, C.A.; & Hartman, C.R. (1989). The case of two trials: father-son incest. *Journal of Family Violence* 4 (1): 95–103.

Rinear, E.E.; (1988). Psychosocial aspects of parental response patterns to the death of a child by homicide. *Journal of Traumatic Stress* 1 (3): 305–322.

Silverman, D., et al. (1978). Sharing the crisis of rape—counseling the mates and families of the victim. *American Journal of Orthopsychiatry* 48: 166–73.

van der Kolk, B.A. (1984). *Post-Traumatic Stress Disorder: Psychological and Biological Sequelae*. Washington, D.C.: American Psychiatric Press.

Weiss, E.H., & Berg, R.F. (1982). Child victims of sexual assault: impact of court procedures. *Journal of the American Academy of Child Psychiatry* 21 (5): 513–518.

Whitcomb, D. (1986). Prosecution of child sexual abuse—new approaches. *National Institute of Justice Reports* 197: 2–6.

Yates, A. (1987). Should young children testify in cases of sexual abuse? *American Journal of Psychiatry* 144 (4): 476–480.

Zimmerman, M.L.; Wolbert, W.A.; Burgess, A.W.; & Hartman, C.R. (1987) Art and group work: interventions for multiple victims of child molestation. *Archives of Psychiatric Nursing* 1 (1): 40–46.

PART III

TREATMENT INTERVENTIONS AND PREVENTION PROGRAMS

Resilient Peer Training: Systematic Investigation of a Treatment to Improve the Social Effectiveness of Child Victims of Maltreatment

John W. Fantuzzo

Anne Holland

Many families in the United States, particularly disadvantaged families in large cities, are facing horrendous social stressors. This sadly is reflected in the incidence of child abuse and neglect. In 1986 there were over 1 million substantiated cases of children suffering harm as a result of maltreatment and 1,100 deaths (U.S. Department of Health, 1988). Since the early 1960s extensive professional efforts have produced hundreds of articles and many specialized journals documenting professional responses to this social problem. However, despite heightened awareness and professional activity, scientifically validated treatment of child victims is nearly nonexistent (Walker, Bonner, & Kaufman, 1988). Extensive reviews of the child physical abuse and neglect treatment literature have identified only a handful of studies that assessed the relative effectiveness of interventions for child victims, met minimal standards of experimental design (i.e., random assignment of subjects to multiple groups) and included dependent variables derived from the child maltreatment research literature (Fantuzzo, 1990).

The lack of an adequately researched treatment technology for child victims is directly related to the urgency and complexity of this problem. Growing public awareness of the nature and extent of child maltreatment has pressured mental health professionals to implement treatment strategies without careful assessment of the problem or research data to support their interventions. Additionally, unique characteristics of this population make it extremely difficult for investigators to conduct rigorous psychotherapy outcome research. Fantuzzo and Twentyman (1986) have identified a number of issues that complicate research in this area. For example, we do not have data-based definitions of child maltreatment that operationalize the type, extent, and severity of maltreatment. Without valid and reliable definitions we are unable to identify precisely the relationship between treatment components and various aspects of maltreatment. Additionally, since abusive families are typically required to participate in many agencies (e.g., protective services, the judicial system, and various treatment agencies), there are many potential confounds that could affect the integrity of treatment outcome research. Redundant assessment procedures across agencies could affect the quality of data used to evaluate the effectiveness of a treatment strategy. Also, different agencies may be using strategies that are antagonistic and produce results that distort research evaluations. What we desperately need to develop is a strategic research plan that adequately reflects our current data base in child abuse and neglect and takes into consideration the needs of child victims and the realities of conducting research with this population.

The purpose of this chapter is threefold. First, we will outline the major components of our research strategy. Second, we will share the results from a series of three studies investigating a proposed intervention, Resilient Peer Training (RPT), which illustrate our strategy. Finally, we will discuss possible next steps in this line of research.

BASIC COMPONENTS OF TREATMENT STRATEGY

Our overarching strategy involves two major components: (1) identification of strategic treatment targets and (2) assessment and cultivation of available resources for treatment.

Treatment Targets

The first component involves establishing a data-based rationale for (1) targeting the most vulnerable child and family populations for treatment and (2) identifying the areas of child development that have been found to be the most adversely affected by maltreatment.

Official national reporting statistics and empirical investigations of psychological factors associated with child abuse and neglect identify targets for a comprehensive treatment strategy. Review of the most recent national reporting data indicate that there were over 2.1 million reports of maltreatment in 1986—a 212% increase in reports from 1976 (American Humane Association, 1988). These reports reveal an overrepresentation of younger child victims. Of the child victims, 43% were in the age group 0–5 years. This is particularly true for the most severe forms of physical maltreatment. Even though the average age of all child victims was 7.27 years, the average age for fatalities and victims of major physical injury was 2.8 and 5.54 years, respectively.

Since over 80% of the perpetrators have been found to be the child victim's primary caregiver, consideration of family factors is an essential component of treatment planning. Family data from these official reports indicate a disproportionate number of poor, disadvantaged minority families experiencing multiple stressors. A large percentage of these families (33%) have a single female as the head of the household. Of the reported families, 49% are on public assistance as compared to about 12% of all U.S. families. Additionally, reports indicate a strong association between child maltreatment and stress factors associated with poverty and disadvantage (Pelton, 1981). Cohn and Daro (1987) reviewed 19 demonstration projects from 1978 to 1982 targeting about 1,000 families associated with relatively severe cases of maltreatment and found the following distribution of problems: 80% suffered financial difficulties, 36% had employment problems, 74% evidenced marital conflict, 67% were socially isolated, 54% were involved with substance abuse, and 42% evidenced spouse abuse.

Since the late 1970s there has been a growing number of studies that have investigated various aspects of the psychological functioning of child victims. Investigations of the social domain of child functioning provide the most consistent findings of deviancy associated with maltreatment (Conaway & Hansen, 1989). In comparison with nonmaltreated children, maltreated children have been reported as significantly more aggressive, resistant, and avoidant with both adults and peers (Cicchetti & Carlson, 1989). Cross-sectional studies of maltreated preschool children have revealed that a very important preschool developmental task—the ability to be a full participant in other children's play activities and to be socially accepted by them—is adversely affected by maltreatment. Peer relations of preschool and early school-aged maltreated children also have been found to be marked by aggression, avoidance, and insensitivity during play activities. In addition to poor peer relationships, maltreated early school-aged children display low self-esteem and very poor adaptation to school. This is a serious problem. To fail in play with other children is the strongest indicator of social maladjustment in childhood, and it is the best predictor of later social maladjustment and psychopathology in adulthood (Cowen, Pedersen, Babigian, et al., 1973; Roff & Ricks, 1970).

The design, implementation, and evaluation of a strategic treatment plan for maltreated children should be guided by two major findings from the empirical knowledge base. First, treatment outcome investigations should attend carefully to developmental considerations and place a high priority on improving the social effectiveness of young victims. Second, researchers should recognize the multiple problems and minimal resources of the most vulnerable group of child victims (children coming from low-income, single-parent, minority households) and consider the need for practical and acceptable service delivery systems.

Treatment Resources

The reality of highly stressful environments and minimal resources should compel treatment planners to optimize the potential of existing resources. Instead of creating an artificial treatment context or sending parents and child victims to treatment facilities that are outside of their community, a planner's task is to develop and investigate specific treatment interventions in the context of culturally sensitive, community-based facilities that are already successfully providing services to abusive families.

One promising service delivery system for child victims and their families is the community-based preschool program. These programs, which are generally government funded (like Headstart), typically provide a comprehensive set of services (e.g., nutritional, health/medical, educational, social, and psychological services) and require active parent involvement. The preschool environment provides child victims and parents with many opportunities to be part of a supportive social network. Preschool settings have great untapped potential for using indigenous, high-functioning parents and peers to assist in providing treatment services to maltreated families. Parents could be systematically exposed to many nonthreatening situations where they could observe parents successfully interact with their children. Children also could benefit from their experience with resilient peers who display a high level of prosocial behavior despite their family and neighborhood conditions.

Program evaluations have indicated that child victims participating in these types of comprehensive preschool programs have evidenced general improvements on standardized developmental tests (Culp, Heide, & Richardson, 1987; Culp, Richardson, & Heide, 1987). Howes and Espinosa (1985), for example, demonstrated beneficial effects of consistent involvement of this type of program for maltreated preschoolers. After a period of time of regular involvement in preschool, maltreated children were similar to a group of normal children and displayed more adaptive and skillful interactions than maltreated children in the newly formed peer groups.

This type of treatment context also provides a foundation from which researchers and clinicians can investigate systematically the merits of specific interventions. Because this type of context involves a safety network of day-treatment personnel monitoring children and families on a daily basis, evaluators can randomly assign participants to multiple comparison groups (including no-treatment control conditions) to evaluate interventions without putting the participants in any jeopardy.

It is essential that researchers and clinicians carefully consider the complex needs and environmental stressors of abusive family when they develop and test treatment strategies. Specific treatment of skill deficiencies should be developed in the context of providing comprehensive family services in a culturally sensitive manner. Failure to attend to these realities will lessen or completely nullify the effects of promising treatment technology.

RESILIENT PEER TRAINING (RPT)

RPT is an intervention strategy developed by Fantuzzo and his associates. This research team has conducted a series of three studies evaluating the effectiveness of RPT for child victims of maltreatment (Fantuzzo et al., 1987, 1988, 1989). Because these studies were guided by the above mentioned strategic treatment components, they share the following characteristics. First, subjects were drawn from the most vulnerable population of maltreated children. Participants were economically disadvantaged, maltreated preschool children evidencing social dysfunction. Second, interventions targeted the social effectiveness of this vulnerable group of maltreated preschool children. Third, treatments were carried out in an environment easily accessible to the target children and their families and sensitive to the multiple needs and minimal resources of these individuals. Subjects were all enrolled in community-based preschool programs that provided comprehensive services to economically disadvantaged preschoolers and their families (i.e., nutritional, health/medical, educational, psychological, and social services), and interventions were carried out in these settings during regular preschool hours. Fourth, primary treatment agents were individuals natural to the target children's preschool environment or community. High-functioning peers, teachers' aides, or community volunteers carried out the interventions. The following provides a description and rationale for this sequence of studies.

The first step in the process of developing and evaluating RPT treatment strategies was a careful review of the preschool treatment literature. Although several intervention strategies had been proposed to treat socially withdrawn preschool children, peer social initiation interventions had the best documented success rate (Strain, Guralnick, & Walker, 1986). Basically, these strategies, developed by Strain and his colleagues, involve training higher functioning peers to make social overtures to withdrawn children. During play sessions adults directly prompt trauned peers to initiate specific prosocial behaviors and provide these peers with contingent rewards for social initiations.

The RPT intervention was based on a modified version of Strain's peer initiation strategy. Changes in this strategy were made to capitalize further on the natural potency of using peers as treatment agents and utilizing play as a context for enhancing preschoolers' social effectiveness. The first set of modifications involved identifying and training resilient peers from the target children's natural preschool environment to serve as treatment agents. Resilient peers are children who function exceptionally well even though they face the same set of environmental stressors as the target children. Researchers have found that these resilient children are socially at ease and productive (Anthony & Cohler, 1987). In the midst of their stressful life situations, they appear to be able to create play oases—play activities that they can master.

The second set of modifications was based on the recognition that the motive force in preschool play interactions is not adult prompting or reinforcement but the dynamic and vigorous sociodramas that the children create and sustain themselves. In the play literature the richness and durability of social interactions are a function of the potency of the sociodrama and the tactics children use to maintain the play and keep all players actively involved (Corasaro, 1981). From this perspective, individual competency is related to a player's ability to enter (or create) the drama, assume roles, follow the plot and play direction, and transact cooperatively with the other players. Therefore, dramas coming from competent players must be flexible and allow the players freedom to adjust the drama to fit their skills and motivation. For these reasons, efforts were made to identify the productive sociodramas of the resilient children and to set up play environments that encouraged resilient peers to include target children in ongoing play dramas. This strategy involves less emphasis on direct adult control and interruption of the play activity (delivering prompts and rewards) and more emphasis on supporting and facilitating the target child's inclusion.

The first in a series of three studies was a small-scale pilot study designed to assess the effectiveness of the RPT strategy for socially withdrawn, maltreated preschoolers (Fantuzzo, Stovall, Schactel, et al., 1987). Four withdrawn preschool children who were victims of child neglect served as subjects, and two maltreated children who displayed high levels of prosocial behavior were trained to carry out the RPT intervention. Play sessions were conducted in a playroom containing toys and materials identical to those in the children's regular preschool classrooms. The social behavior of the withdrawn children was recorded during play sessions and during free-play time in the children's classrooms. The specific experimental design was a single-case, reversal design within subjects superimposed on a multiple-baseline design across subjects (Barlow & Hersen, 1984). After a stable baseline was obtained, the RPT treatment was implemented for a period of time, then withdrawn, and then re-instituted (reversal design). Across subjects the time at which the intervention was implemented was staggered (multiple baseline).

Figure 12–1 reveals, that the RPT intervention resulted in increases in positive social behavior directly associated with the introduction of the intervention in treatment (playroom) and generalization (classroom) settings. Reports from classroom teachers validated the treatment gains achieved. Posttreatment, teachers reported that the subjects (as well as the resilient peers) were displaying more positive social behavior in the classroom during unstructured play activities and structured learning activities.

The second study (Fantuzzo, Jurecic, Stovall, et al., 1988) was designed to replicate the previous pilot study on a larger scale using more rigorous experimental procedures and to assess the relative effects of using a resilient peer or a familiar adult as a treatment agent. For this study, 36 withdrawn, maltreated preschoolers were randomly assigned to one of three experimental groups: peer-treatment (RPT), adult-treatment, or control conditions. The peer-treatment condition was identical to that used in the first study. High-functioning, maltreated peers were trained to involve the subjects in their play activity. The adult-treatment condition followed similar procedures, except that a familiar adult, specifically a teacher's aide, made the play overtures to the subjects. To control for the number of overtures made, adults were yoked to resilient peers (the adults were instructed to make the same number play overtures as the peers). The control condition was a placebo control condition. Subjects in this group were exposed to identical situations as the children in the other conditions, except that no play overtures were made by an adult or peer during the play sessions. Data were collected to ensure the treatment was implemented accurately, and pre- and posttreatment assessments of the subjects' social behavior were conducted in both treatment (playroom) and generalization (class-room) settings. Moreover, standardized teacher ratings of the subjects' adjustment and development were collected prior to and following treatment.

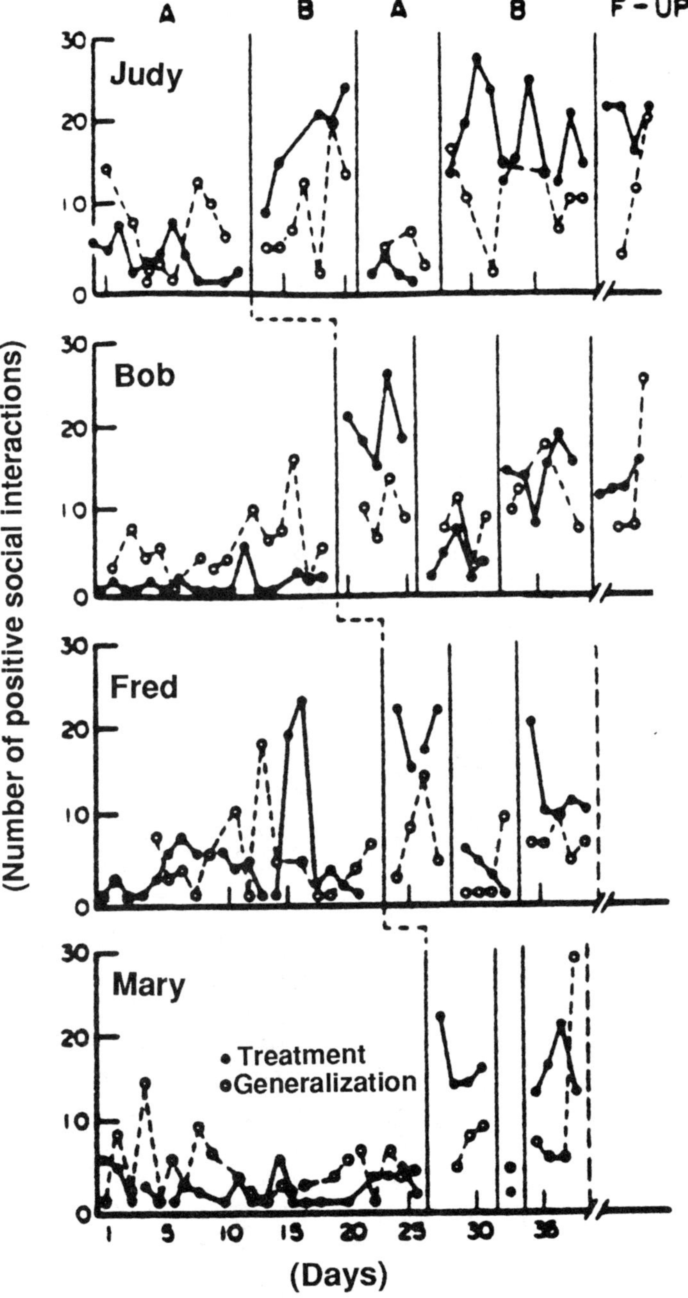

Figure 12–1
Daily number of positive social interactions in treatment (solid circle) and generalization (open circle) settings across experimental phases. Figure taken from published first study (Fantuzzo, Stovall, Schachtel, et al., 1987).

Findings indicate that children in the peer-treatment condition evidenced significant increases in positive social behaviors in treatment and generalization settings, while children in the adult-treatment group displayed a significant decrease in social behavior in both contexts after treatment (see Figure 12–2). Data from the standardized teacher rating instruments supported the superiority of the peer-treatment condition for the withdrawn, maltreated preschoolers over the adult-treatment condition. The children in the peer-treatment condition showed decreases in problem behavior from pre- to posttreatment assessment on indices of psychological adjustment, while subjects in the adult-treatment and control conditions actually evidenced significant increases in problem behavior over time.

The third study (Davis & Fantuzzo, 1989) was designed to determine if these peer and adult treatments would have a similar effect on different populations of socially ineffective, maltreated preschool children. The relative impact of peer and adult treatments were assessed for (1) withdrawn, maltreated; (2) withdrawn, nonmaltreated; and (3) aggressive, maltreated preschool children. Seven preschoolers (two withdrawn, neglected; two withdrawn, nonmaltreated; and three aggressive, physically abused) served as subjects. An alternating treatment design was used to compare the effects of the peer and adult interventions (Barlow & Hersen, 1984). This design involved exposing each subject to each treatment condition in a counterbalanced order to determine the relative impact of the treatment conditions. Observational measures of the social behavior of the subjects were collected across baseline, treatment, and follow-up phases. For the duration of this study each subject attended a play session with a resilient peer and a play session with a familiar adult once a day. The order of the play sessions was alternated on a daily basis for each subject. Three preschool children identified as engaging in high levels of positive social interaction in their respective classrooms served as resilient peers, and two adults involved in the Headstart center served as adult-treatment agents. Play sessions took place in two playrooms equipped with similar furnishings, materials, and toys. During the baseline phase of this investigation peer- and adult-treatment agents responded positively to all play overtures made by the subjects in the context of the play sessions but made no positive social initiations; during the treatment phase peers

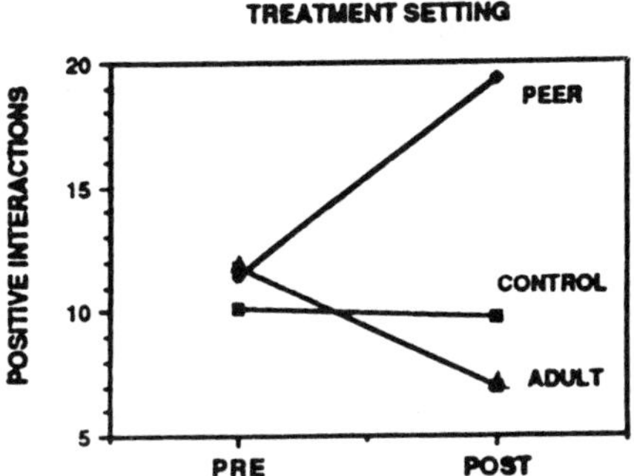

Figure 12–2
Average number of positive interactions for peer (circle), control (square), and adult (triangle) groups at pretest and posttest.

and adults responded positively to all play overtures of the subjects and additionally made specific attempts to involve the subjects in their ongoing play activity; and during the follow-up phase the behavior of the peers and adults was identical to that displayed during the baseline phase.

Results indicate a different pattern of social behavior for these three groups of socially ineffective children. Figure 12–3 presents the findings for one child belonging to each group that clearly elucidates the distinct patterns. The withdrawn, nonmaltreated preschoolers demonstrated equal levels of interaction with the peer and adult across all phases of the investigation. The withdrawn, neglected children evidenced a clear preference for interaction with the peer over the adult. They initiated play more frequently with the peer across all phases. Also, while exposure to the peer resulted in increased reciprocal play behavior during the treatment phase, exposure to the adult only resulted in very brief positive responses. Moreover, during the follow-up phase, treatment gains continued to be made when the peer was present, while social interaction returned to baseline level with the adult. It is important to note, however, that moderate increases in negative play behavior accompanied the increases in prosocial behavior seen during the treatment phase. In contrast to the withdrawn, neglected children, the aggressive, abused preschoolers favored interaction with the adult.

They initiated play more frequently and displayed less negative play with the adult confederate across all phases of the study. Hostile aggressive responses occurred only when subjects were in the company of a peer. Interestingly, the treatment phase that consisted of exclusively positive overtures had a paradoxical effect on the social behavior of the aggressive, abused children. In response to the positive initiations of both the peer and adult confederates, these children evidenced an overall decrease in prosocial behavior and an increase in negative social behavior. Following the treatment phase, this pattern was reversed with the adult (i. e., positive behaviors increased and negative behaviors decreased) but was maintained with the peer.

The different response patterns of the withdrawn and aggressive maltreated children to the peer and adult play partners suggest that the RPT strategy is effective for withdrawn maltreated children but is ineffective in its present form for treating aggressive maltreated children. Modifications to this strategy that would enhance its effectiveness for aggressive children should be considered. Quite possibly for these children the presence of both adult and peer play partners might facilitate more positive play. In general, these findings illustrate that it is important not to overgeneralize the effectiveness of a particular strategy but to evaluate empirically the effects with different groups of children.

NEXT STEPS

The three studies considered above represent initial steps in the complex process of developing and testing intervention strategies for child victims of maltreatment. The differences found between the withdrawn neglected children and the aggressive, physically abused children coupled with reports of numerous family stressors faced by these maltreated children suggest that the next steps include a more complete assessment of the cumulative impact that types of maltreatment and other family stressors have on child victims' social functioning

A detailed analysis of child victims' maltreatment history and family environment should be taken into account in evaluating the outcome of treatment programs for abused and neglected children.

Maltreatment characteristics (e.g., type of maltreatment, sex of the perpetrator, relation to the perpetrator, frequency of the maltreatment, severity of the maltreatment, amount of time from first to last reported incident, and time since last incident) and family factors (e.g., marital dysfunction, conjugal violence, substance abuse, parental psycho-pathology, health problems, financial difficulties, unemployment, and social isolation) may differentially mediate treatment effective-ness, and thus it is imperative that they not be overlooked.

The next steps in researching treatment alternatives should also involve more comprehensive assessment of the social functioning of maltreated children. Researchers must broaden their definitions of social functioning. Instead of narrowly conceptualizing preschoolers' social competency as the number of positive social initiations and responses, investigators should recognize that for preschool children to be socially effective they not only must be able to make appropriate social initiations and respond adaptively to the initiations of others, but they additionally must be able to read social cues accurately, regulate and express emotion in a manner that does not interfere with social relationships, and have a sufficient repertoire of skills to sustain rewarding social interchange.

In addition, research in this area would be greatly enhanced by a careful consideration of how preschool children process the trauma of their maltreatment (Grych & Fincham, 1990). Once we identify different modes of processing these types of traumatic events, we could assess their relative effect on the child victims' social functioning and overall psychological adjustment. Findings from this research would help us differentiate adaptive and maladaptive strategies that would have direct assessment, treatment, and prevention implica-tions.

At the heart of the RPT approach is the recognition of the thera-peutic potential of the play interactions of resilient peer. Although the above-mentioned studies underscore the resource potential of resilient peers, they provide no analyses of the effective strategies used by the resilient peers. A direct investigation of the potent play tactics used by these competent players would greatly enhance the effectiveness of this strategy. For example, we need to identify what play themes, play styles, and modes of verbal and nonverbal play communication differentiate socially successful from unsuccessful

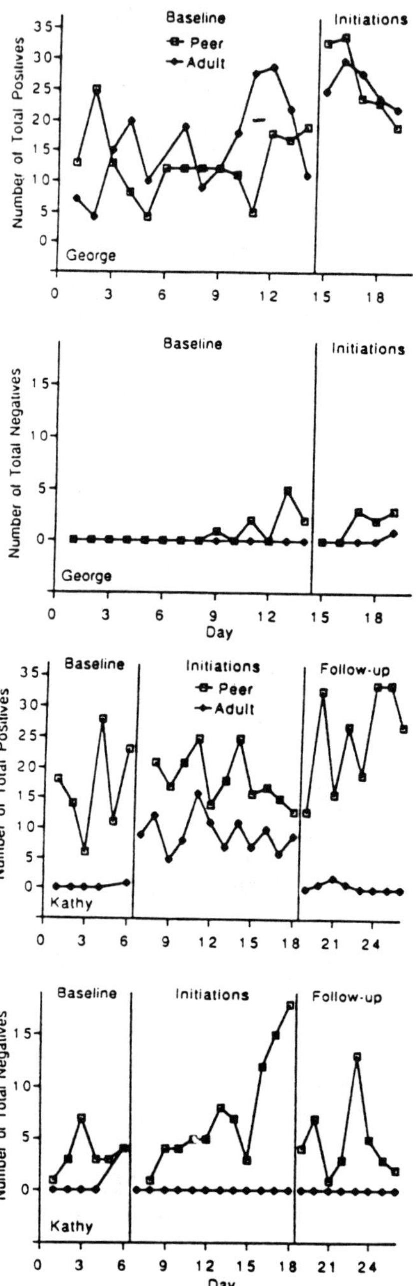

Figure 12–3

Total number of positive and total number of negative interactions across experimental phases. George was a nonmaltreated, socially withdrawn child who served as a control child in this study. Kathy was a maltreated, socially withdrawn child. Angela was a maltreated, socially aggressive child.

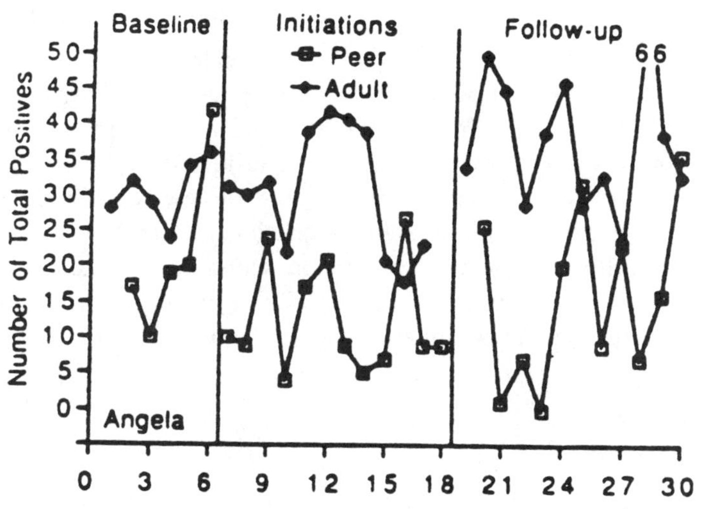
Baseline
Initiations
Follow-up
Peer
Adult
66
Number of Total Positives
Angela
50
45
40
35
30
25
20
15
10
5
0
0 3 6 9 12 15 18 21 24 27 30
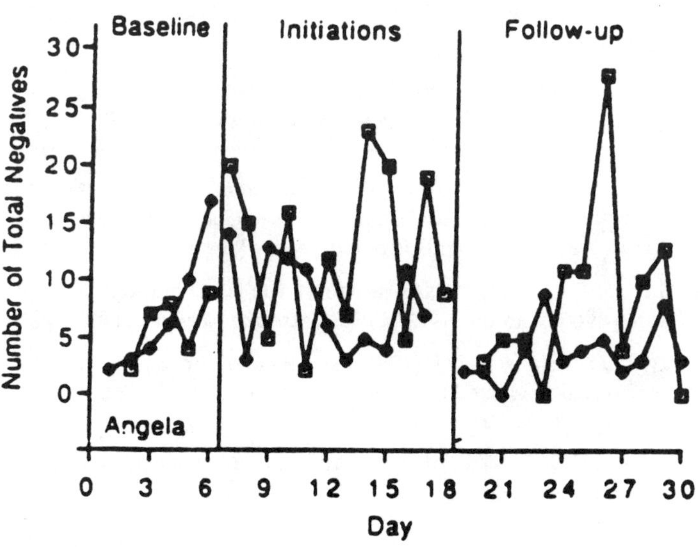
Baseline
Initiations
Follow-up
Number of Total Negatives
Angela
30
25
20
15
10
5
0
0 3 6 9 12 15 18 21 24 27 30
Day

children (Rubin, Fein, & Vandenberg, 1983). If this information is discerned, it is possible that socially ineffective preschoolers could be taught through RPT procedures the adaptive play techniques of their socially successful peers. This, in turn, should enhance the unsuccessful children's overall social competency.

It is obvious that we are in the very early phases of our development of a treatment technology for child victims. The provocative nature of this social problem and the complexities are real obstacles for researchers. The magnitude of the need and the research difficulties will require greater multidisciplinary collaboration and more systematic and programmatic investigation. Our aim in this chapter was to outline and illustrate our approach in hopes that it would stimulate further efforts and encourage colleagues to join in these efforts.

REFERENCES

American Humane Association (1988). *Highlights of Official Child Neglect and Abuse Reporting 1986*. Denver: The Association.

Anthony, J.E., & Cohler, B.J. (1987). *The Invulnerable Child*. New York: Guilford Press.

Barlow, D.H., & Hersen, M. (1984). *Single Case Experimental Designs: Strategies for Studying Behavior Change*. 2nd ed. New York: Pergamon.

Cicchetti, D., & Carlson, V. (1989). *Child Maltreatment: Theory and Research on the Causes and Consequences of Child Abuse and Neglect*. New York: Cambridge University Press.

Cohn, A.H., & Daro, C. (1987). Is treatment too late: what ten years of evaluative research tells us. *Child Abuse and Neglect* 11: 433–442.

Conaway, L.P., & Hansen, D.J. (1989). Social behavior of physically abused and neglected children: a critical review. *Clinical Psychology Review* 9: 627–652.

Corasaro, W.A. (1981). *Friendship and Peer Culture in the Early Years*. Norwood, N.J.: Ablex.

Cowen, E.L.; Pedersen, A.; Babigian, H.; et al. (1973). Long-term follow-up of early detected vulnerable children. *Journal of Consulting and Clinical Psychology* 41: 438–446.

Culp, R.E.; Heide, J.S.; & Richardson, M.T. (1987). Maltreated children's developmental scores: treatment versus nontreatment. *Child Abuse and Neglect* 11: 29–34.

Culp, R.E.; Richardson, M.T.; & Heide, J.S. (1987). Differential developmental progress of maltreated children in day treatment. *Social Work* 32: 497–499.

Davis, S., & Fantuzzo, J.W. (1989). The effects of adult and peer social initiations on social behavior of withdrawn and aggressive maltreated preschool children. *Journal of Family Violence* 4: 227–248.

Fantuzzo, J.W. (1990). Behavioral treatment of the victims of child abuse and neglect. *Behavior Modification* 14: 316–339.

Fantuzzo, J.W.; Jurecic, L.; Stovall, A.; et al. (1988). Effects of adult and peer social initiations on the social behavior of withdrawn, maltreated preschool children. *Journal of Consulting and Clinical Psychology* 56: 34–39.

Fantuzzo, J.W.; Stovall, A.; Schachtel, D.; et al. (1987). The effects of peer social initiations on the social behavior of withdrawn maltreated preschool children. *Journal of Behavior Therapy and Experimental Psychiatry* 18: 357–363.

Fantuzzo, J.W., & Twentyman, C.T. (1986). Child abuse and psychotherapy research: merging social concerns and empirical investigation. *Professional Psychology: Research and Practice* 17: 375–380.

Grych, J.H., & Fincham, F.D. (1990). Marital conflict and children's adjustment: a cognitive-contextual framework. *Psychological Bulletin* 108: 267–290.

Howes, C., & Espinosa, M.P. (1985). The consequences of child abuse for the formation of relationships with peers. *Child Abuse and Neglect* 9: 397–404.

Pelton, L.H. (1981). Child abuse and neglect: the myth of classlessness. In L.H. Pelton (ed.), *The Social Context of Child Abuse and Neglect*. New York: Human Sciences Press.

Roff, M., & Ricks, D.F. (1970). *Life History Research in Psychopathology*. Minneapolis: University of Minnesota Press.

Rubin, K.; Fein, G.; & Vandenberg, B. (1983). Play. In P.H. Mussen (ed.), *Handbook of Child Psychology*. Vol. 4: *Personality, Socialization, and Social Development*. 4th ed. New York: Wiley.

Strain, P.S.; Guralnick, M.J.; & Walker, H.M. (1986). *Children's Social Behavior: Development, Assessment, and Modification*. New York: Academic Press.

U.S. Department of Health and Human Services. (1988). *Study Findings: Study of National Incidence and Prevalence of Child Abuse and Neglect*. Washington, D.C.: The Department.

Walker, C.E.; Bonner, B.L.; & Kaufman, K.L. (1988). *The Physically and Sexually Abused Child: Evaluation and Treatment*. New York: Pergamon.

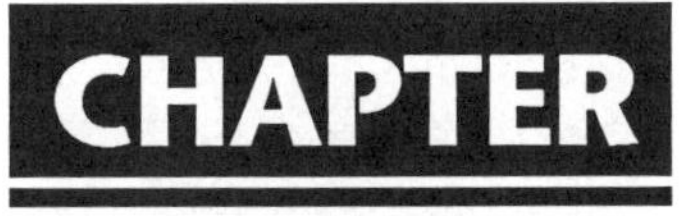

CHAPTER
13

Intergenerational Family Processes in the Treatment of Incest

Margaret Cotroneo
Helene Moriarty

INTRODUCTION

A number of theories have been proposed to explain intrafamilial child sexual abuse and these include some understanding of problematic family systems. What is lacking are well-developed family systems conceptualizations that describe intergenerational family processes that can develop into a maladaptive functioning that focuses on children. Family loyalty conflict is one relational process that increases the risk that children can become the foci of maladaptive interactions among members of a family unit. This chapter draws on clinical findings from contextual family therapy to describe assessment and intervention in family loyalty conflicts.

INTERGENERATIONAL FAMILY PROCESSES IN THE TREATMENT OF INCEST

The negative effects of incest, alarming as they are, are not limited to the present sufferings of victims and their families. These effects persist into adulthood and include relationship difficulties, poor self-concept, impaired cognitive and emotional skills, and the development of psychopathology (Finkelhor, 1986; Gelinas, 1983). A number of theories have been proposed to explain intrafamilial child sexual abuse. These include some understanding of problematic family systems (Finkelhor, Galles, Hotaling, & Straus, 1983; Giaretto, 1982; Kempe & Kempe, 1984; Sgroi, 1982). However, the field of family violence lacks well-developed conceptualizations of family systems that describe intergenerational family processes that can develop into a pattern of maladaptive functioning focusing on children. Family studies to this point have examined the problem of child maltreatment from the perspective of the nuclear family, specifically the parent-child dyad. The histories of maladaptive relating in the backgrounds of those persons who perpetrate intrafamilial abuse indicate that the problem exists in a wider relational context than the nuclear family unit or the two person system.

This chapter seeks to draw on clinical findings from intergenerational family treatment of intrafamilial abuse to describe family loyalty conflicts as one process that increases the risk that children can become foci of maladaptive interactions among members of a family unit. The authors' work with intrafamilial sexual abuse derives from the theory and practice of contextual theory and therapy as it has been developed by Ivan Boszormenyi-Nagy and his associates (Bernal, Flores-Ortiz, Rodriguez, et al., 1990; Boszormenyi-Nagy & Spark, 1973; Boszormenyi-Nagy & Ulrich, 1981; Boszormenyi-Nagy & Krasner, 1986; Cotroneo, 1982; Grunebaum, 1987; Hibbs, 1987; Karpel, 1986). The theory identifies trustworthiness as basic to the quality and continuity of relationships. Trustworthy behavior emerges from responsible caring about oneself and others. It is rooted in the ability of family members to learn how to live and grow as separate persons while at the same time remaining available to each other as resources. Within this framework, the family is viewed as an ongoing configuration of relationships that includes the nuclear family system, the extended family, and the social network of the family.

Contextual theory is organized around four core dynamics that have been identified in treatment families: loyalty, justice, entitlement, and trust. These dynamics are highly visible in families who present with incest. They are said to motivate and shape a person's mode of relating, commitments, and expectations largely through the interactive process of giving and receiving care. A fundamental premise of this theory is that living in a family requires balanced giving and receiving. According to contextual theory, victimization of family members is rooted in an intergenerational matrix of loyalty. It is theorized that loyalty plays a key role in the motivation of adult family members to extend reliable care and protection to dependent children. Loyalty also plays a key role in the children's ability to assert themselves in terms of self-care and self-protection. Conflicts emerge when family members are caught between two or more competing objects of loyalty or competing self-interests. An assessment of at least three generations of family relating is required in order to understand how loyalty manifests itself among members of a family unit. Intervention in loyalty conflicts emphasizes change in individual behaviors and change in patterns of relating.

FAMILY LOYALTY

The authors operate on the assumption that family systems are conservative systems, systems that are highly reactive to gain or loss of members. Disclosure of incest threatens the family unit and activates the family loyalty dynamic; i.e., it activates all those processes by which family members are bound to each other for good or ill. How this dynamic is addressed and managed can set the stage for whether treatment is effective for both the victim and the family and as well as whether the perpetrator can be held accountable for his or her actions. For example, activation of loyalty dynamics can lead to a closing off of the family system to outside intervention, resulting in retraction by the victim, intensification of denial by the perpetrator, withdrawal of support for the victim by the non-perpetrating parent or siblings, and self-invalidating behavior on the part of the victim.

Loyalty refers to shared commitments and values born of expectations for care, devotion, and fairness that family members hold in common. These commitments and values take the form of expectations that bind members to each other over time, and they can be freeing or enslaving for purposes of growth. For example, in the family, the investments of care that parents make in their children from birth onward form the basis for the parental expectations of filial devotion (Boszormenyi-Nagy & Spark, 1973). When parents can make appropriate investments in parenting, their children are free to reciprocate by caring about their parents and by investing in their own lives. This kind of loyalty is self-validating (positive loyalty). When parents, for whatever reason and regardless of fault, cannot invest appropriately in their children, the children tend to react to this loss or deprivation with greater emotional attachment. Because all children are deeply committed to a continuing relationship to their parents, they take on parental failures as their own and react to them with emotions of shame, guilt, and resentment. Thus emotionally bound, they are not free to invest appropriately in relationships outside the family unless and until they can come to terms with the loss or deprivation they have experienced. This kind of loyalty is self-invalidating (negative loyalty).

Negative loyalty can be manifested by behaviors that are self-defeating or self-destructive, such as promiscuity, substance abuse, or suicide attempts. In another mode of negative loyalty, a relationship to a child may be used as a substitutive context to satisfy the possessive, dependent destructive, or sexual needs of the adults (destructive entitlement). People who are destructively entitled ordinarily feel no guilt since they are rebalancing their own relational injuries, and in subjective terms justice is being done (Boszormenyi-Nagy & Krasner, 1986).

Thus, loyalty forms the basis for family members' obligation to care for one another. In addition, whether or not one receives the care one deserves and how one receives care will construct and shape lifelong obligations toward significant other people outside the family. The expectations for care and devotion that were not met in the family of origin are assigned to mates, partners, and children, tending to overburden these relationships, often distorting their reality.

From a contextual perspective, incest is viewed as a loyalty conflict (Gelinas, 1986). It is a triangular configuration in which the relationship to the victim is a substitutive context for rebalancing relational injuries or losses in the perpetrator's family of origin. In addition, there is evidence of a symbiotic relationship between mother and daughter that involves the mother's rebalancing of injuries and losses that incurred in her own family of origin (Koch & Jarvis, 1987). Thus, the victims are held captive in a situation of competing or split loyalties in which the well-being of the self is subordinated to the well-being of significant others. Moreover, the victim actually absorbs parental hurts, disappointments, and failures as if they were his or her own (parentification). This dynamic has also been described in children of alcoholic parents (Stanton, 1984) and in children of divorcing parents (Heatherington, Cox, & Cox, 1982; Wallerstein, 1985).

As a manifestation of loyalty, incest maintains the family as a unit and regulates behavior having to do with closeness and distance in the marital couple and in the parent-child relationship. It carries with it the injunction against harming the family, thus setting up an intrinsic conflict between a family member's self-interests and the maintenance of a significant relationship or set of relationships. Children are especially vulnerable to these conflicts on account of their need for parenting. The denial and loyal protectiveness so evident in incest families is an attempt to avoid the threatened loss of relationship.

While incest presents as a sexual act, its motivational core is relational. The needs and wants of children are subordinated to those of the adults in a way that renders the child's needs and wants invisible (parentification).

Parentification refers to the process by which one member of the family, often a child, comes to act as an overly responsible caretaker for another member, for several others, or for the family as a whole. Parentification is a normal family process that becomes harmful when it involves prolonged and unilateral use of a child to care for and protect adults without such care being reciprocated and without considering the child's needs and rights. The prolonged, unilateral use of children to care for and protect adults depletes children's reserves of trust and self-mastery, placing them at risk for mental health problems.

Parentification of a child signals the adults' needs for self-validation born of unresolved issues of parentification in their families of origin. The child becomes an unintended captive in the parental self-validating cycle and experiences parentification as a loss or abandonment. It is this pattern of parentification, and not the more obvious "role reversal" commonly associated with incest, that has the most harmful long-term consequences for victims. It leaves the child without any reliable measure of what to expect in future relationships. In addition, relational unfairness and injury in one generation present the next generation with a slate of deficits that need to be rebalanced.

In order to manage family loyalty conflicts, the therapist must be skilled in requiring the various family members to consider the merit of the positions taken by other family members even when those positions may oppose each other. This therapeutic stance is called multilateral advocacy (Cotroneo, 1986; Gelinas, 1986; Grunebaum,1987). It enables the therapist to support the victim and the family and simultaneously hold the perpetrator accountable.

Unfortunately, therapists often attempt to deal with loyalty conflicts by inserting themselves in the triangle and taking one side against the other (unilateral advocacy). This is understandable from the point of view that incest is a crime and sexual contact between an adult and a child is always the adult's responsibility. No offender should be permitted to use the therapy room to justify his or her behavior. However, from the child's side of things, another perspective must be considered. Children are intrinsically loyal to their parents, and that loyalty is intensified when they are threatened with the deprivation or loss of a parent, even a parent who harms them. Therefore, the child's loyalties must be made explicit and supported by the therapist. In addition, the perspectives of both parents and all the siblings must be considered, and attention must be given to each parent's own family of origin. This must be done without endangering the rights or welfare of the children, especially the victim.

The authors use a semistructured interview to elicit the multiple perspectives, needs, claims, and obligations in the family. The basic components of the interview are included in Table 13–1 and some specific questions to help the therapist conceptualize intergenerational processes are included in Table 13–2.

The questions in Table 13–2 are designed to add specificity to the general interview structure in Table 13–1, particularly with regard to sections 2 and 3. They are designed to provide the therapist with items related to entitlement and parentification in the conjoint interview with the family. While the questions are in the mode of assessment, family therapists generally consider assessment and intervention to be inseparable processes.

TABLE 13–1

BASIC INTERVIEW COMPONENTS

I. **Current Family Situation**
a. Response of family members to disclosure of incest
b. Effects on family members
    (I) Efforts to help the victim and siblings deal with the situation.
    (2) Contacts with significant legal, religious, psychological, social, and health care resources

2. **Family Genogram Information**
a. Ways in which parents define and validate themselves in relation to significant others, particularly their own families of origin
    (1) Patterns of expectations and commitments across three generations
    (2) Gender-related issues
    (3) Intergenerational history of losses, relational injuries, and injustices

3. **Exploration of Parenting (Past, Present, and Future) of Children and the Developmental Burdens and Demands Placed on Them**
a. Acknowledgment of the children for their contributions to the family that may have been taken for granted
b. Exploration of the worries that the children may have and how they get help when it is needed
c. Acknowledgement of the parents for the losses, relational injuries, and injustices experienced in their families of origin
d. Exploration of the ways in which family members can work to correct injustices and exploitation in past and present relationships and repair injuries that have already been sustained
e. Consideration of the consequences of any imbalances in giving and receiving care and fairness that exist in the family

4. **Family Task (Conjoint Session)**
a. Describe the family situation as you see it. What are the conflicts for you?
b. In thinking about what to do, what are you considering and why?
c. If you could have things your way (according to your preferences), what would you do now?
d. If you were to put your plan into action, what would happen? Do you think your plan would be successful? Why? Why Not?
e. What would be the consequences of your plan for you, your spouse/partner, and each of the children individually?

TABLE 13–2

QUESTIONS TO HELP CONCEPTUALIZE
INTERGENERATIONAL PROCESSES

1. What are the ethnic, racial, and religious roots of the family?
2.. What significant events mark the family legacy, e.g., births, deaths, marriages, separations, divorces, chronic illness, miscarriages, abortions, stillbirths, suicide, migrations, substance abuse, trouble with the law, physical, sexual, or psychologi cal abuse, cutoffs, psychological problems, successes and failures?
3. Do any of the adults express feelings of being cheated or deprived of parenting they rightfully deserve?
4. Do any of the adults express feelings of being used, unappreciated, or taken for granted in relationships?
5. Do any of the adults expect to receive without reciprocal giving (something is owed to them)?
6. Do any of the adults expect to give without reciprocal receiving (overfunctioning, sacrificial giving)?
7. Do any of the adults withdraw from, abdicate, or abandon a responsible position in times of stress or conflict (taking a position of impotence, powerlessness, or revenge)?
8. Are any of the adults unwilling or unable to consider the consequences of their behavior?
9. What "unfinished family business" exists between the generations?
10. What issues between the spouses rightfully belong to the marriage and what i ssues rightfully belong to their families of origin?
11. Can the parents work together on behalf of the children? Do they allow themselves to be split or does one parent always defer to the other?
12. Are family members stuck in stagnant patterns of unfairness? How?
13. How are decisions made in the family?
14. Who is most willing and able to help the children maintain continuity of their significant relationships, including grandparents, aunts, uncles, peers?
15. Who helps the children handle harsh realities?
16. Are the children unfairly used as messengers between the adults?
17. Describe the path of the children's growth and development?
18. Can the children indicate how they have tried to help their parents, and can the parents acknowledge the children's contributions, particularly their emotional caretaking?
19. Who takes responsibility for teaching the children about their legacy?
20. Do the children know how their parents struggle with trust?
21. Are any of the children unfairly blamed for family problems?
22. Are any of the children either scapegoated or idealized?
23. Do the children hide their own needs, hurts, disappointments in order to gain approval or take care of an adult, or sibling?
24. Do the children attempt to respond to, take care of, attend to, worry about, make up for, or take responsibility for the hurt, disappointment, or anger of a parent?
25. Are family roles and functions strongly organized according to gender?

We recommend that a conjoint interview take place as soon as possible after disclosure, usually after the victim has been interviewed alone. Our work with families points to a significant time factor in the management of intense loyalty conflicts. That is, the closer to the event loyalty conflicts can be made explicit, the more the emotional reactivity can be reduced and family members can be involved in the decision-making process (Cotroneo, Hibbs, & Moriarty, 1990). We work on the essentially preventive premise that when a family can assume greater responsibility for their own situation rather than prematurely abandoning it to social agencies, this serves the long-term best interests of the child, the family, and the community. The contextual approach focuses on developing a new pattern of accountability among family members by seeking to mobilize and conserve family resources for the benefit of the children. The aim is not necessarily preservation of the family as a unit but rather the preservation of whatever relationship resources can be made available to children in an ongoing way.

Mental health professionals are often ambivalent about any kind of conjoint work with these families, citing the pressure on the victim. They do not take into account that protecting the victim from the consequences of loyalty intensifies the reaction to loss or deprivation of relationships. Further, such a protective attitude reinforces the family's own self protective tendencies and serves to close off the family system to intervention. Only when the family system can remain open to internal and external intervention is it possible to generate sufficient trust to render treatment effective. Furthermore, when the family system can remain open, potential resources in the family that might be hidden can be activated.

The expression of anger and conflict has an important healing function in incest families for both the parent-child relationship and the marital relationship. However, the demands of loyalty are such that conflicts in the wider relational context remain invisible, rising to visibility only when they focus on children. When loyalty conflicts can be made explicit, a climate is created in which expression of anger and differences can surface.

In a family in which one of the author's served as a consultant to the therapist, the parents had been in marital therapy four years previously when the father's affair was exposed. The couple worked on improving their ability to communicate more openly. However, both parents continued to deny any strong feelings that might lead to open conflict, especially feelings of anger.

Four years later, the family presented with father-daughter incest. They presented as emotionally disengaged, but this masked a very enmeshed pattern of relating in which conflict continued to be avoided. The family, including the victim's only sibling, met conjointly once a month. In the interim the therapist met with the victim alone, the parents as a couple and individually, and the siblings together without the parents. Family-of-origin work was begun to help the family understand the incest as part of a wider relational context. By linking past relational patterns to the present, incest is treated not as an isolated event but rather as an outcome of a mode of relating. Consequently, maladaptive patterns of parentification can be identified and corrected rather than transmitted in future relationships. Family of origin work also makes family members more expert in their own relational processes, thus increasing the preventive potential of the interventions.

The mother believed the daughter's disclosure, but her support was passive. As she was guided toward an intergenerational exploration of relationships, the mother's anger toward her brother who had physically abused her surfaced. She was also able to surface her caretaker position in her family of origin. The daughter was then able to tell her mother the story of the incestuous relationship and her own thoughts and feelings about it. Mother was able to join with daughter in a more explicit sharing and understanding the reality of each other's lives. She was also able to tell her husband that the affair was unfinished business that continued to be very painful and anger producing for her. Daughter's appropriate moves outside the family system, toward her peer network, were encouraged and supported by her mother, who also began to take charge of her own life.

Daughter was able to say to father that the only way he could help her was to remember what he had done and take responsibility for it. He had acknowledged the abuse, it had been reported to child protective services, and his court hearing was scheduled. However, he maintained that he could not remember any of the details. Both mother and daughter held him accountable for remembering the details of the incestuous relationship, and, as part of the treatment, he was required to join a group for perpetrators to help him remember. In father's exploration of his family of origin, a long-term pattern of denial and avoidance of the consequences of one's behavior became clear. Father also began to have recollections of a brief incestuous encounter with his brother.

The victim's young brother was able to talk about his feelings of sadness at what was happening to his family. He expressed his concern for his father and his anger at his sister. He was helped to sort out and express his thoughts and feelings in the presence of his parents. Meeting together, without their parents, the siblings were able to work on this aspect of their relationship and they were guided into finding ways to help and support each other.

Family treatment functioned to surface loyalty conflicts, claims, expectations, and obligations and make them explicit. Much work on rebalancing relationships was needed, and there was some indication that the marriage might not survive the process. The conjoint sessions provided an opportunity for each perspective to be considered by other family members while simultaneously supporting the victim and holding the perpetrator accountable for his behavior.

The legal process and the treatment process proceeded independently and simultaneously. We believe this is helpful in preventing a blurring of the boundaries that occurs when legal and therapeutic processes are enmeshed. This way of proceeding is only effective, however, when legal agents and therapists understand and acknowledge each other's perspectives and surface their conflicts directly rather than through the family. When loyalty conflicts in incest families are intense, they often hold legal agents and therapists captive in a replication of the family dynamics. In our view, a therapist's skill in managing loyalty dynamics in incest families is greatly enhanced when he or she has done some family of origin exploration of their own families.

CONCLUSION

Intergenerational family processes have a powerful influence on shaping maladaptive behaviors that focus on children. Intergenerational loyalty is a core motivator in shaping attitudes and actions in incest families. Skill in working with loyalty conflicts requires a family system conceptualization of incest. Contextual theory and therapy provides a useful method of eliciting loyalty conflicts and making them explicit in a way that supports the victim, holds the perpetrator accountable, and preserves needed relationship resources.

REFERENCES

Bernal, G.; Flores-Ortiz, Y.; Rodriguez, C.; et al. (1990). Development of a contextual family therapy therapist action index. *Journal of Family Psychology* 3: 322–331.

Boszormenyi-Nagy, I., & Krasner, B. (1986). *Between Give and Take. Clinical Guide to Contextual Therapy*. New York: Brunner/Mazel.

Boszormenyi-Nagy, I., & Spark, G. (1973). *Invisible Loyalties*. New York: Brunner/Mazel.

Boszormenyi-Nagy I., & Ulrich, D. (1980). Contextual family therapy. In A. Gurman & D. Kniskern (eds.), *Handbook of Family Therapy*. New York: Brunner/Mazel.

Cotroneo, M. (1986). Families and abuse. In M. Karpel (ed.), *Family Resources*. New York: Guilford Press.

Cotroneo, M. (1982). The role of forgiveness in family therapy. In A.S. Gurman (ed.), *Questions and Answers in Family Therapy*. Vol. II. New York: Brunner/Mazel.

Cotroneo, M.; Hibbs, B.J.; Moriarty, H. (1990). Uses and implications of the contextual family evaluation in child custody litigation. Unpublished.

Finkelhor, D. (1986). *Sourcebook on Child Sexual Abuse*. Newbury Park, Calif.: Sage.

Finkelhor, D.; Gelles, R.J.; Hotaling, G.T.; & Straus, M.A. (1983). *The Dark Side of Families. Current Family Violence Research*. Newbury Park, Calif.: Sage.

Gelinas, D. (1983). The persisting negative effects of incest. *Psychiatry* 46: 312–332.

Gelinas, D. (1986). Unexpected resources in treating incest families. In M.Karpel (ed.), *Family Resources*. New York: Guilford Press.

Giaretto, H. (1982). A comprehensive child sexual abuse treatment program. *Child Abuse and Neglect* 6: 263–278.

Grunebaum, J. (1987). Multidirected partiality and the "parental imperative." *Psychotherapy* 24: 646–656.

Heatherington, E.M.; Cox, M.; & Cox, R. (1982). Effects of divorce on parents and children. In M. Lamb (ed.). *Nontraditional Families.* Hillsdale, N.J.: Erlbaum.

Hibbs, B.J. (1987). The context of growth. Relational ethics between parents and children. In L. Combrinck-Graham (ed.), *Handbook of Family Therapy with Children.* New York: Guilford Press.

Karpel, M. (1986). *Family Resources.* New York: Guilford Press.

Kempe R.S., & Kempe, H.C. (1984). *The Common Secret. Sexual Abuse of Children and Adolescents.* New York: Freeman.

Koch, K., & Jarvis, C. (1987). Symbiotic mother-daughter relationships in incest families. *Social Casework* (February) 68: 94–101.

Sauzier, M. (1989). Disclosure of child sexual abuse. For better or worse. *Psychiatric Clinics of North America* 12: 455–469.

Sgroi, S.M. (1982). *Handbook of Clinical Intervention in Child Sexual Abuse.* Lexington, Mass.: Lexington Books.

Stanton, M.D. (1984). Breaking away: The use of strategic and bowenian techniques in treating an alcoholic family through one member. In E. Kaufman (ed.), *Power to Change: Family Case Studies in the Treatment of Alcoholism.* New York: Gardner Press.

Wallerstein, J.S. (1985). The overburdened child: some long-term consequences of divorce. *Social Work* 30: 116-123.

Extrafamilial Child Sexual Abuse: Family-Focused Intervention

Carol R. Hartman, Allen G. Burgess, Ann Wolbert Burgess, Susan J. Kelley

There is clinical and empirical evidence that following disclosure of extrafamilial child sexual abuse, parents themselves may experience distressing symptoms (Burgess, Groth, Holmstrom, & Sgroi, 1978) characteristic of posttraumatic stress disorder (Kelley, 1990). As noted in Chapter 9, symptoms of distress in children and parents extend over a long period of time postdisclosure.

The family unit is believed by many to be the context for the healing and recovery from adversity. If this unit remains in a state of chronic tension, the primary source of support and strength to combat the long-term consequences of sexual abuse of a child is compromised. For intervention to be effective, there is a need to understand not only the trauma response in the victim, but also the secondary trauma response of family members. The next step is to examine the potential interactive effects of symptoms and other life stresses of family adjustment over time.

In an effort to explore the relationship of distressed states in parents following disclosure of extrafamilial child sexual abuse, a secondary analysis was performed on a data set of 41 cases involving sexual abuse in day care settings. The objective of the secondary analysis was to discern what factors predicted symptoms in each of the subjects: child, mother, and father. This chapter utilizes the descriptive responses of parents regarding this stressful event and outlines three domains of intervention.

METHOD

Sample

The analysis involved a subsample of 41 families that had equivalent data on child, mother, and father. This subsample was drawn from a pool of 67 families in which children were sexually abused in day care settings. Collection of data was by mailed questionnaires. The time elapsed between the end of the abuse and data collection ranged from 8 to 36 months with a mean of 26 months. In all cases child protective services substantiated the allegations of sexual abuse. Criminal charges were filed in 92% of cases, with a conviction rate of 80% of one or more offenders per day care center case.

Procedures

Items for the secondary analysis consisted of variables identified through correlation studies and analysis of variance that were associated with differences observed between parents and children when grouped by (1) sexual abuse versus ritualistic abuse and (2) whether the child testified or did not testify at a criminal trial against the offender(s). All of these variables differentiated children and parents by severity of symptoms (Kelley, 1990).

Independent variables considered were various life events since disclosure of abuse: marital separations (MS); loss of family income (INCOMEDN); death in the family (DEATHFAM); death of a close friend (DEATHFRD); illness in the family (ILLNESS); number of stressful life events (NOEVENTS); history of sexual abuse in either parent (MOABUSED/FAABUSED); and use of therapy = parents in treatment (PARENTTX); time since parents ended treatment (PATXEND); time since child ended treatment (CHTXEND).

Additional variables concerning the child and the nature of the sexual abuse also examined were length of time of abuse, number of times abused, type of abuse (ritualistic, sexual, physical), number of offenders.

Measurements

In addition to these variables, the symptoms of the parents and child were used in the equation, alternating the respective symptom variables as dependent and independent variables. Symptom scores for the child consisted of subscores on the Achenbach and Edelbrock (1983) symptom checklist. These were the Behavior Problem T Score (BEHROBT); Internalizing T Score (INTT); Externalizing T Score (EXTT).

For the parents, subscores on the Impact of Event Scale were used. These were Avoidance Items Subscale Score (IESAVD); Intrusive Items Subscale Score (IESINTR); and the Total Impact of Event Score ([IESTOT). In addition, subscales on the SCL-R-90 were used. These were General Severity Index T Score (GSIT); Positive Symptom Distress Index T Score (PSDIT); Positive Symptom Total T Score (PSTT). Thus for each parent there were six subscale symptom dependent variables, and for each child there were three symptom dependent variables.

Briefly, the Horowitz Impact of Event Scale (15-item self-report) has been used in numerous studies to explore an individuals response to traumatic events. It attends to the phasic qualities of posttraumatic stress disorder (PTSD)—intrusive (reexperiencing) and avoidant responses (denial) to reminders and thoughts regarding a traumatic event. Trauma victims who meet the criteria for PTSD have been found to have higher intrusion and avoidance scores than those who do not (Weisenberg, Solomon, Schwarzwald, & Mikulincer, 1987).

The Derogatis SCL-90-R (1977) is a 90-item measurement of adult psychopathology and has shown high levels of both internal consistency and test-retest reliability. The General Severity Index is a measure of a constellation of symptoms from the various subscales of symptoms and their severity. Positive Symptom Distress Index T Score is a straightforward index of intensity. The Positive Symptom Total T Score is an accounting of the number of symptoms endorsed by a subject.

Analysis

Individual stepwise multiple regressions were performed for the child, mother, and father using the symptom subscales for child, mother, and father as dependent variables, respectively. The nonsymptom score items and the symptoms of family members were used as independent variables.

Limitations of the Study

There are several limitations to this analysis. The data set is small and drawn from a convenience sample. Given the small sample, we decided not to eliminate reporting variables that appear less strong in their prediction. It is apparent that distribution of scores can lead to spurious conclusions. There can be errors made by the elimination of variables based on sample characteristics and the distribution of responses. The statistic chosen for the analysis was done to give some descriptive basis for variable saliency and for the discussion of interaction among variables. Also, mothers tended to complete the child behavior checklist. The number of child symptoms endorsed may reflect the propensity of the mother to note symptoms both in she and the child, thus strengthening associations between mother symptoms and child symptoms. The noting of parent abuse was by a "yes" or "no," which may underreport the abuse history of parents. Data on therapy was by "yes/no" and length of time but did not detail the therapy itself.

RESULTS

Mother

The results of multiple regression analysis using the mother's psychological test scores as dependent variables and the nonsymptom variables, and the child's and father's psychological test scores as independent variables are shown in Tables 14–1—14–6. On the SCL-90-R measurement, the mother's General Severity Index T Score was found to have three useful predictors as shown in Table 14–1: father's (FA) Positive Symptom Total T Score, child's Internalizing T Score, and injury or illness in the family. Table 14–2 contains comparable information for the predictors of the mother's Positive Symptom Distress Index T Score: father's General Severity Index T Score and illness or injury in the family. Table 14–3 shows the predictors for the mother's Positive Symptom Distress T Score: father's Positive

Symptom Total T Score, child's Internalizing T Score, and parent in treatment.

On the Impact of Event measurement, the mother's Intrusive Item Subscale Score is predicted by the father's General Severity Index T Score and the child's Internalizing T Score as shown in Table 14–4. Table 14–5 contains predictor information for the mother's Avoidance Item Subscale: father's Impact of Event Scale Total Score and father's history of abuse. Table 14–6 contains the predictors for the mother's Total Intrusive Impact of Events Subscale: father's Intrusive Impact of Event Score, father's history of abuse, and child's Internalizing T Score.

In summary, father's Positive Symptom Total T Score is most strongly predictive of mother's symptoms as measured on both the SCL-90-R and the Horowitz Impact of Event. Father's Impact of Event subscores predict both SCL-90-R symptoms subscores as well as Impact of Event subscores for the mother. The child's Internalizing subscore predicts mothers symptoms as measured on both the SCL-90-R and the Impact of Event. Of the other variables, illness and injury were predictive of SCL-90-R sub-scores and parents in treatment were predictive of the total number of symptoms endorsed by the mother. Father's history of sexual abuse predicted lower Impact of Event Subscores for mothers.

Father

Tables 14–7—14–12 include the multiple regression for father's symptoms.

On the SCL-90-R subscore measures, mother's symptoms were the leading predictor for three of father's subscores. Table 14–7 contains the predictors for father's General Severity Index: mother's Impact of Event Scale Total Score, death of a friend, and decrease in income. Table 14–8 contains the predictors of father's Positive Symptoms Distress: mother's Impact of Event Scale Total Score, child's externalizing behavior, child's end of treatment, and number of life events. Table 14–9 contains the predictors for father's Positive Symptom Total: mother's General Severity Index Score, death of a friend, mother's history of abuse, decrease in income, death of a family member, and father's history of abuse.

TABLE 14–1
VARIABLE GENERAL SEVERITY INDEX T SCORE—MOTHER (GSITMO)

Step	Mult R	Rsq	F(Eqn)	Sig F	Variable	Beta in
1	.6158	.3793	24.438	.000	In: PSTTFA	.6158
2	.6925	.4795	17.965	.000	In: INTT	.3287
3	.7291	.5316	14.379	.000	In: ILLNESS	.2324

TABLE 14–2
VARIABLE POSITIVE SYMPTOM DISTRESS INDEX T—MOTHER (PSDITMO)

Step	Mult R	Rsq	F(Eqn)	Sig F	Variable	Beta in
1	.5211	.2716	14.915	.000	In: GSITFA	.5211
2	.6352	.4034	13.188	.000	In: ILLNESS	.3637

TABLE 14–3
VARIABLE AVOIDANCE ITEMS SUBSCALE SCORE—MOTHER (IESAVDMO)

Step	Mult R	Rsq	F(Eqn)	Sig F	Variable	Beta in
1	.6613	.4373	31.082	.000	In: IESTOTFA	.6613
2	.7503	.5630	25.119	.000	In: FAABUSED	-.3546
3	.7790	.6068	19.547	.000	In: EXTT	.2098

TABLE 14–4
VARIABLE INTRUSIVE ITEMS SUBSCALE SCORE—MOTHER (IESINTRMO)

Step	Mult R	Rsq	F(Eqn)	Sig F	Variable	Beta in
1	.5804	.3369	20.320	.000	In: GSITFA	.5804
2	.6618	.4380	15.199	.000	In: INTT	.3270
3	.7201	.5126	13.639	.000	In: IESINTRF	.4629
4	.7160	.5126	20.510	.000	Out: GSITFA	

TABLE 14–5
VARIABLE POSITIVE SYMPTOM TOTAL T SCORE—MOTHER (PSTTMO)

Step	Mult R	Rsq	F(Eqn)	Sig F	Variable	Beta in
1	.6053	.3664	23.131	.000	In: PSTTFA	.6053
2	.6959	.4843	18.311	.000	In: INTT	.3565
3	.7313	.5348	14.562	.000	In: MOABUSED	.2407

TABLE 14–6
VARIABLE TOTAL INTRUSIVE IMPACT OF EVENT SUBSCALE—MOTHER (IESTOTMO)

Step	Mult R	Rsq	F(Eqn)	Sig F	Variable	Beta in
1	.6710	.4502	32.754	.000	In: IESTOTFA	.6710
2	.7558	.5712	25.973	.000	In: INTT	.3484
3	.8115	.6585	24.426	.000	In: FAABUSED	-.2967
4	.8320	.6934	20.918	.000	In: IESINTRF	.5706
5	.8320	.6922	28.483	.000	Out: IESTOTFA	

Note: The abbreviations that follow are used in Tables 14–1 to 14–15: OUT = variable removed from significance after the variable listed; IN = added to regression; Rsq = R squared; SigF = Significance of F; Mult R = value of R as a statistical term/symbol.

For the Impact of Event measurement, Table 14–10 contains the predictors for father's Avoidance Items: decreased income, mother's Impact of Event Scale Total Score, number of life events, and death of a friend. Table 14–11 contains the predictors for father's Intrusive Items Subscale: decreased income, mother's Impact of Event Scale Total Score, father's history of abuse, death of a friend, end of parent treatment, and child's Exterminating Behavior Score. Table 14–12 contains the predictors for father's Impact of Event Scale Total Score: decreased income, mother's Impact of Event Total Score, father's history of abuse, death of a friend, number of events, and end of parent treatment.

In summary, mother's symptoms on both SCL-90-R and the Impact of Event predict father's symptoms on the SCL-90-R and the Impact of Event. The next strong positive predictor of father's symptoms on both measures is loss of income. This is followed by father's history of sexual abuse and number of life events.

There were several variables that predicted in a negative direction, i.e., less symptom response: these were death of a family friend and family member; exterminating symptoms in the child, mother's history of sexual abuse, and parents and the child ending treatment.

Child

Tables 14–13—14–15 include the multiple regression for the child's symptoms. For the Child Behavior Checklist Subscales, Table 14–13 includes the predictor for the child's Behavior Problem T Score: mother's Positive Symptom Total Score. Table 14–14 indicates the predictors for the child's Internalizing T Score: mother's Positive Symptom Total and the child's end of treatment. Table 14–15 indicates the predictors for the child's Externalizing T Score: child in treatment and mother's Positive Symptom Total.

Beside the importance of the interaction of symptoms between mother and child, treatment predicts externalizing symptoms.

DISCUSSION

This secondary analysis suggests an interaction between mother's symptoms and the child's symptoms. However, the strongest interaction is between the mother and father with the child having a

TABLE 14–7
VARIABLE GENERAL SEVERITY INDEX T SCORE—FATHER (GSITFA)

Step	Mult R	Rsq	F(Eqn)	Sig F	Variable	Beta in
1	.6293	.3961	26.231	.000	In: IESTOTMO	.6293
2	.7198	.5181	20.966	.000	In: DEATHFRD	-.3555
3	.7621	.5808	17.552	.000	In: INCOMEDN	.2888
4	.7913	.6261	15.492	.000	In: GSITMO	.3100
5	.7832	.6134	20.101	.000	Out: IESTOTMO	

TABLE 14–8
VARIABLE POSITIVE SYMPTOM DISTRESS T SCORE—FATHER (PSDITFA)

Step	Mult R	Rsq	F(Eqn)	Sig F	Variable	Beta in
1	.4626	.2140	10.891	.002	In: INCOMEDN	.4626

TABLE 14–9
VARIABLE POSITIVE SYMPTOM TOTAL T SCORE—FATHER (PSTTFA)

Step	Mult R	Rsq	F(Eqn)	Sig F	Variable	Beta in
1	.6158	.3793	24.438	.000	In: GSITMO	.6158
2	.7063	.4989	19.413	.000	In: DEATHFRD	-.3538
3	.7858	.6175	20.447	.000	In: MOABUSED	-.3546
4	.8179	.6690	18.697	.000	In: INCOMEDN	.2393
5	.8400	.7056	17.257	.000	In: DEATHFAM	-.2045
6	.8648	.7479	17.304	.000	In: FAABUSED	.2265

TABLE 14–10
VARIABLE AVOIDANCE ITEMS SUBSCALE SCORE—FATHER (IESAVDFA)

Step	Mult R	Rsq	F(Eqn)	Sig F	Variable	Beta in
1	.6214	.3861	25.160	.000	In: INCOMEDN	.6214
2	.6923	.4793	17.592	.000	In: IESTOTMO	.3505
3	.7324	.5364	14.658	.000	In: NOEVENTS	.2544
4	.8084	.6535	17.443	.000	In: DEATHFRD	-.4126

TABLE 14–11
VARIABLE INTRUSIVE ITEMS SUBSCALE—FATHER (IESINTRFA)

Step	Mult R	Rsq	F(Eqn)	Sig F	Variable	Beta in
1	.6800	.4625	34.413	.000	In: INCOMEDN	.6800
2	.7821	.6116	30.712	.000	In: IESTOTMO	.4435
3	.8357	.6985	29.339	.000	In: FAABUSED	.3136
4	.8628	.7445	26.950	.000	In: DEATHFRD	-.2193

Note: The abbreviations that follow are used in Tables 14–1 to 14–15: OUT = variable removed from significance after the variable listed; IN = added to regression; Rsq = R squared; SigF = Significance of F; Mult R = value of R as a statistical term/symbol.

slight negative interaction with father's symptoms. Of particular significance is the highly predictive nature of the Impact of Event Subscales. The difficulty of dealing with the abuse event underscores the probability of parents suffering from secondary posttraumatic stress disorder, also termed vicarious traumatization (McCann & Pearlman, 1990). This trauma may result in a continuous state of unresolved stress and maladaptation within family structures over time. In turn, this can lead to an inaccurate understanding of the etiology of dysfunctional family processes.

Fathers were more symptomatic than mothers, especially those whose children had been victims of ritualistic abuse (Kelley, 1990). It appears that the mother is the central recipient of both the distress of the child and that of the father. This does not mean that the father is not affected by the child's symptoms, but, rather, the interaction effect between mother and father is in the areas of processing the traumatic event as evidence by the strong predictive associations of the Impact of Event Subscales. However, it is complicated in that the interaction between symptomatic mother and father is driven by not only the traumatic event but also other life stresses.

While the parents are managing the sequelae of their child's sexual abuse, there is the demand to manage other life stresses, some of which have been generated by the event itself. In particular, we see that the father is most sensitive to the loss of income. As mothers decided to stay at home after their child was abused, the family's changed economics added pressure on the father. For mother, additional illness in the family represents a pressure, blocking resolution of parental symptoms associated with the abuse itself.

The results also identified the negative effect of family and friendship death and a history of childhood sexual abuse on father's symptoms. It may be speculated that prior trauma and losses affect the meaning structure of the father differentially, shielding him from the impact of trauma (Flannery, 1990). We hypothesize that fathers, when comparing two competing emotional demands, displace emotion and concern for something perceived to be more manageable. Self-efficacy, a sense of control and management, and a commitment to another are often behaviors that appear to buffer people from the impact of trauma.

TABLE 14–12
VARIABLE TOTAL INTRUSIVE ITEMS SUBSCALE SCORE—FATHER
(IESTOTFA)

Step	Mult R	Rsq	F(Eqn)	Sig F	Variable	Beta in
1	.7011	.4915	38.662	.000	In: INCOMEDN	.7011
2	.7050	.6320	33.494	.000	In: IESTOTMO	.4304
3	.8320	.6922	28.485	.000	In: FAABUSED	.2610
4	.8575	.7353	25.692	.000	In: DEATHFRD	-.2122
5	.8814	.7769	25.071	.000	In: NOEVENTS	.2599

TABLE 14–13
VARIABLE BEHAVIOR PROBLEM T SCORE—CHILD (BEHPROBT)

Step	Mult R	Rsq	F(Eqn)	Sig F	Variable	Beta in
1	.4196	.1761	8.547	.006	In: PSTTMO	.4196

TABLE 14–14
VARIABLE INTERNALIZING T SCORE—CHILD (INTT)

Step	Mult R	Rsq	F(Eqn)	Sig F	Variable	Beta in
1	.4934	.2434	12.871	.001	In: PSTTMO	.4934

TABLE 14–15
Variable Externalizing T Score—Child (EXTT)

Step	Mult R	Rsq	F(Eqn)	Sig F	Variable	Beta in
1	.3594	.1291	5.931	.019	In: PSTTMO	.3594

Note: The abbreviations that follow are used in Tables 14–1 to 14–15: OUT = variable removed from significance after the variable listed; IN = added to regression; Rsq = R squared; SigF = Significance of F; Mult R = value of R as a statistical term/symbol.

Did treatment affect symptoms? Yes, treatment tended to predict symptom profiles in an expected way. First, there were fewer symptoms at completion or termination of treatment for both parents and the child, and, second, children manifested more acting- out symptoms while in treatment.

Although parental reactions to childhood illness and injuries have been studied (Baskin, Forehand, & Saylor, 1985; Boldberg, Morris, Simmons, et al., 1990; Cella, Perry, Poag, et al., 1988) few researchers have examined parent reactions to child sexual assault. Those who have done so noted initial stage reactions of disbelief, alarm, embarrassment, anger, fear, grief, and guilt (Burgess, Groth, Holstrom, & Sgroi, 1978; De Jong, 1986; De Vine, 1980; Finkelhor, 1984; MacFarlane & Waterman, 1986; Regher, 1990). The foregoing studies suggest that we have to consider recovery within the context of the effects of prolonged traumatic responses of the child victim and the parents. For parents, the trauma is generated through indirect exposure to information of what happened to the victim—in this case, children sexually abused in a day care setting—and their own (parental) imagining and processing of their internal reactions.

Several studies have examined the child victim's response as a function of parental reaction. Gomes-Schwartz, Horowitz, and Sauzier (1985) found that when mothers reacted to disclosure of sexual abuse with anger and punishment, children manifested more behavioral disturbances. Supportive relationships within the family have been noted to be associated with positive recovery from sexual abuse (Conte & Schuerman, 1987; Finkelhor, Williams, & Burns, 1988). But as yet we have no systematic investigation of family approaches. Based on the mounting evidence that the family response may well affect the child victim and now with greater insight into parental symptomatology associated with the disclosure of abuse and its extension well beyond criminal prosecution, we have a basis for identifying domains of treatment for the individuals as well as the family unit.

LEVELS OF FAMILY-FOCUSED INTERVENTION

Family responses that are considered to be characteristic of an adaptive parental response consist of believing the child, protecting the child, focusing on the child's well-being, accepting the child's feelings, and maintaining an image of the child as a survivor. These responses are thought to help the child acknowledge feelings and integrate the experience. Esquilin (1987) has identified the following parental responses as maladaptive and impeding the process of recovery: denial, blaming the child, persistent parental guilt, rage at assailant, and an image of the child as damaged. Conte and Schuerman (1987) found that child victims who were judged by their therapists to have supportive relationships with nonoffending adults of siblings were less affected by the abuse than children lacking social supports.

Friedrich and Reams (1987) suggest that the symptoms seen in sexually abused children may reflect not only the trauma they have experienced directly, but also their family environment, the amount of support the child feels, and the level of disruption that follows the disclosure of abuse. According to Finkelhor, Williams, and Burns (1988) recovery from sexual abuse in day care was closely related to the support children received from their parents. Thus, based on the available data, it appears that the reactions of parents to their child's victimization critically influences the child's reaction.

The data analysis of this preliminary study notes the interaction of parent and child symptoms and suggests the need for clinicians to monitor symptoms carefully. A goal of treatment is to decrease symptomatology and to increase information processing of trauma. If not, there will be symptom interaction between the parents that will keep all three family members highly symptomatic. One way to reduce the abused child's symptoms is to reduce parent symptoms. The following outline of a family-focused intervention program includes the descriptive comments by study parents to questions posed regarding their experiences with the recovery of their child. The three levels to be discussed include family crisis intervention, individual trauma therapy, and group treatment.

LEVEL 1: FAMILY CRISIS INTERVENTION

Active crisis intervention is recommended for the parents as well as the child victim. As one parent said, " When a sexually abused child is being treated, the parents and the other members of the immediate family need to be in treatment too."

Traditional crisis intervention is a short-term therapy of up to 12 sessions. The client prioritizes the content to be discussed, and the focus is present oriented and generally on day-to-day issues. The goal is to stabilize the biopsychosocial equilibrium of the child and family following disclosure of sexual abuse. The crisis intervention assists the family with their reactions to the interface of the various disciplines called upon to help, such as nursing and medical staff, law enforcement agents, and victim-witness staff in the criminal justice system. Therapeutic strategies include anchoring for safety and building personal client resources (Hartman & Burgess, 1988).

In the crisis phase the family experiences a wide range of mood dysregulation, cognitive confusion, and autonomic nervous system arousal specific to limbic system involvement (see Chapter 3). Symptoms include hyperstartle reflex, generalized anxiety, sleep and appetite disturbance, sexual and aggressive dysfunction, and emotional numbing.

The clinician first deals with the parents' initial reactions and the knowledge that their child was abused. Self-blame and fears need to be discussed and detailed. The high emotional intensity of this early period often solidify the thought structures that contribute to further anxiety and depression. Examples of parent comments as well as their symptom patterns reveal that the parents can experience secondary posttraumatic reactions. The abuse information stimulates images and emotions within each parent. As one mother wrote:

> *I can visualize what happened to my boy in my head. I also have a flashback to my boy laying on the classroom floor, totally destroyed, broken.*

Study parents' initial reaction to the knowledge that their child had been sexually abused included shock, disbelief, rage, a sense of betrayal, and self-blame. Two quotes illustrate the range of distress including relief and identification.

> *I was unable to react for 24 hours. I felt emotionally numb. I laughingly told my husband what my son had said. When the horror began to set in, I felt deeply sad for my son, and myself as well. I felt that I had failed him, and that his babyhood had been destroyed. I felt guilty. Later, I had many fantasies of killing the perpetrators.*

> *My initial reaction was relief. I thought that I had done something wrong in raising this child to make him the "monster" that he was. I was ready to get counseling for me and for him.*

> . . . .

> *I was at my wits end with him. After my relief, I was filled with grief and an overwhelming sense of needing to help him. I wanted to know what I could do to help him overcome this. I also felt a sense*

> *of identity having been abused myself. I wanted to*
> *withdraw from everyone and totally protect him from*
> *everyone. I also felt rage for the abuser. I wanted to do*
> *to him everything he did to my son and more. I feel*
> *concern for the parents who seemed to be torn apart*
> *emotionally. I needed to talk about it a lot to someone*
> *who loved me and understood my need to express my*
> *fears and feelings. I also felt fear for my son, fear that*
> *he maybe would not ever be normal again or become*
> *an abuser himself. I had anger toward God and a lot*
> *of questions of why.*

These examples reveal the range of thoughts of past, present, and future. A cursory interpretation reveals the internal dissonance set into motion. We note parental shifts in attention from self to the child, to the environment, to the perpetrator. These thoughts are discontinuous fragments of strong imagery, emotion, and meaning. There are hints of despair and doom as well as strength and mastery. There is note of physical pain and numbing, intensity, and fear.

The crisis intervention is directed to this information processing of parental disturbance. The therapeutic task is to reduce the symptoms of distress. In addition, there most often are other family members, such as siblings, grandparents, who are confused and upset. The clinician can ask how all family members are managing the information and plan for their needs accordingly.

We suggest that the parents be prepared to deal with their child and with themselves. They need to be educated that they too will experience posttrauma symptoms similar to their child. The task is to build a foundation for processing and integrating a negative event that cannot be undone.

As can be seen from the quotes, a time dimension is imprinted at the onset of awareness. The greatest sustainer to negative ruminations is parental desire to "set the clock back" and to eliminate the event from ever happening. This desire reveals regressed presuppositions regarding expectations, cause and effect, and probability. Such ideas that "It shouldn't have happened to my child!" "How can these things happen when I have done everything to protect my child!" reveal belief structures of fear and anxiety that deny the reality of crime.

These beliefs are compelling and activated at the sensory level as the child begins to detail the abuse event. The parents will register visual, auditory, olfactory, kinesthetic experiences as they build personal structures of "understanding" what happened to their child. People are not usually aware of these psychological processes being the source of their emotional distress. While they can say they see their child "broken, crushed, on the floor," they regard their comments as a figure of speech. Consequently, the self-generated traumatic stimuli and the underlying presuppositions remain out of awareness and not amenable to self-correction. In fact, the emotional arousal can be so great that it alters basic structures of informational processing for extended periods of time. For example, the mother who did not want to leave her child out of her sight.

When parents understand how their own reactions to the abuse is elaborated and sustained in their thinking, they can begin to decide their needs in the areas of treatment. One decision regards individual trauma therapy. Evaluation of the individual and the family unit now become a natural outcome of the initial crisis work. It is at this point that parents make their first decisions regarding whether they will move with their child from the clinical documentation of sexual abuse to a therapeutic process that is aimed at (1) moving the family unit through the criminal justice system, (2) dealing with acute and recurrent reactions with individuals, and (3) evaluating alterations in family adaptation.

LEVEL 2: INDIVIDUAL TRAUMA THERAPY

Once the family has been mobilized and symptoms evaluated, an individual therapy-focused plan may be made. In this modality there is careful monitoring and managing of symptoms. A formula from the data analysis is provided for determining who might best benefit from in-depth individual work, e.g., the child, the parents, and/ or both.

Child Trauma Therapy

For the traumatized child the aim of individual efforts is to process the trauma as one step in restoring the child to a prior state of psychological equilibrium. The therapeutic framework for the model is the information processing of trauma (see Chapter 3). In brief, the model assumes the basic constructs of information processing of a living system. These propositions state that experiences are processed on a sensory, perceptual, cognitive, and interpersonal level. The sensory level is the basic registrant of experience in the individual. The perceptual level is the beginning classification of the sensory processing. The cognitive level is the larger organization of experience into meaning systems, and the interpersonal level includes the persons involved in the traumatic event and those with whom there is interaction following. The effect of memory applies at each level of information processing. Based on Horowitz's work (1976), the presumption is made that traumatic information is kept in active awareness until it can be placed in distant memory and that trauma resolution occurs when there is sufficient processing for the information to be stored, i.e., when the event is remembered, the attendant feelings are neutralized, and the anxiety generated by the event is controlled. When a traumatic event is not resolved and either remains in active memory or becomes defended by a cognitive mechanism—such as denial, dissociation or splitting—the diagnosis is generally posttraumatic stress disorder (PTSD). The central feature of PTSD, which is the stress pattern resulting from traumatization, is that the individual reexperiences the original trauma both unconsciously and consciously.

Addressing trauma-specific information is a key step in information processing of trauma. Techniques can be employed that address the domains of personal and interpersonal experience, i.e., sensory, perceptual, cognitive, and interpersonal. Methods such as drawing, writing out memories, self-monitoring skills, symptom management skills (such as relaxation, exercise, and creative games) can be used not only to elaborate information but also to build resources and manage symptoms without total denial of the event.

Trauma therapy is issue-oriented, in this case, the child's sexual abuse. With permission of the client, the trauma is surfaced, e.g., discussed at the sensory, perceptual, cognitive, and interpersonal domains. Duration of treatment averages weekly or bimonthly. The goal of therapy is to process the trauma, neutralize the attendant emotions and symptoms, integrate the trauma, and transfer the trauma into past memory as a life experience.

Parent Trauma Therapy

For the parents trauma therapy involves debriefing of parents regarding their own personal reactions. Specific information from the child can increase parents' symptoms and interfere with their ability to soothe and comfort their child. At the same time parents have to deal with their reactions of disbelief, horror, blame, and rage.

This intervention will help the therapist to monitor symptoms and address the issues and conflicts that emerge between the parents. For the most part, the response of the mother to the sexual abuse is different than that of the father, particularly in the initial stages. Clinical documentation of sexual abuse becomes a traumatic experience for parents. They are often at the front line of the child's revelations of what has happened to them. They are the key in learning how the return of memories is heralded by symptomatic responses in the child and then by the traumatic memories brought forward.

Strategies to deal with the ongoing trauma responses and to attend to the emergence of meaning systems that can impede resolution of personal distress can be assessed through the use of the standardized measures described in this chapter: the Derogatis SCL-90-R, the Horowitz IES Scale, and the Achenbach and Edlebrock CBCL.

If father, mother, and child score in the clinical range, as in this study, individual trauma therapy is recommended for father, mother, and child to begin to decrease their symptomatology. When the symptoms decrease, a level-3 intervention such as family or group therapy is indicated. A formula to consider would be the following. If father's scores are high, expect mother's symptoms to increase. Mother's symptoms are driven by father and child. A decrease in mother's scores should decrease father and child.

LEVEL 3: GROUP PROGRAMS AND TREATMENT

The goal of group intervention is to strengthen and augment trauma therapy by linking the child and family to a group modality. The timing of group work is decided by parent and therapist. There are a variety of group programs to select from including psychoeducational programs, marital counseling, parents group, sibling groups, family therapy, and sports and group activities for children.

Psychoeducational Groups

Psychoeducational groups focus on informing the parents of the trauma response in their child and within themselves. The objectives of this contact is to emphasize that safety is the first order of business. Then there is exploration of resources to stabilize the family unit.

Basic information as to the neurobiology of trauma and information processing can be important knowledge for parents. Parent education can occur on an informal or formal basis. Informally, the initial contact and expressions of the child and parent are accepted, and brief explanations as well as encouragement are given to accept personal reactions. Formal psychoeducational information can be provided through written information, group meetings with experts or informed providers of clinical, investigative services, and legal services.

Marital Counseling

One type of group treatment is marriage counseling. In the study some marriages were strengthened, others were destroyed. Lack of sexual desire on the part of the mothers was noted. Father were often silent regarding what was happening and differed from mothers regarding open discussion with their child as to what had happened. Below follow examples of responses to open-ended questions provided by parents.

> *1. Has the abuse of your child affected your marriage (or other close relationship)?*

> *"Yes. At first there was a lot of tension because we were not dealing with it the same way. I needed to talk a lot; he needed to handle little bits at a time. When we saw that and accepted that in each other, I felt free and good about receiving my emotional support elsewhere. Now we are able to handle it as a team."*

*"Definitely. We both coped differently and didn't
understand why the other did what they did. I became
sexually dysfunctional for at least six months.
Emotional intimacy became painful so we withdrew
from each other. We have had marital therapy, but
the relationship still suffers."*

*"My marriage had its ups and downs but this was
the straw that broke the camel's back. My husband
found it hard to live with the fact that our daughter
was abused. He drank and drugged and stayed out
late so that it affected our marriage, which ended in
divorce."*

Sibling Groups

Parental guidance is needed to focus on the management of the
abused child's behavior as well as the sibling group. Noninvolved
siblings need a place to talk also. The impact on siblings in this
study revealed that they felt jealous, lacked attention from the parents
preoccupied with the abused child, had to mediate acting-out behavior
and withdrawn behavior, felt perplexed dealing with anger and
sexually aggressive behavior.

*2. Has the abuse affected any of your other
children?*

*"Daughter attended school also—has her own
things to deal with. Has to deal with brother's anger,
which is often directed at her."*

*"Yes. It had a drastic effect on my second son, who
was born several days before my first son disclosed the
abuse. For the first year of his life, I was totally
preoccupied with the older boy. As a result, my second
son was withdrawn as an infant, shy, too quiet.
Later, he learned to scream in order to get attention.
He needs special attention now, I feel, in order to
make up for what he didn't get as an infant."*

*"Yes. Her sister was 2, my daughter was almost 5.
The younger child was evidently getting disclosure
long before I was. She is expressing fears now that she
was unable to express then. She had a strong need to
be the 'good' child and was torn between resenting her*

*sister and protecting her. Since my older child has
become more competent, we have experienced a
'backlash' from the younger. She has been fearful this
summer that she would be hurt. She is now 5. She
recently had a nightmare from which I could barely
awaken her. She said they were shooting her sister.
Then she talked about grandpa holding her up so she
could see her sister in the courtroom. She wondered
why we let her sister in the court with the bad people
and talked about being afraid they would kill her
sister. She was 3 when that happened—two years ago.
The dream about them shooting her sister was during
the same month the trial started. A sibling's anniver-
sary reaction."*

Family Therapy

Group interaction is important for families who wish to participate in them. The group would include the entire nuclear family. At
times, other key family members, including grandparents, would be
invited to discuss issues relevant to the child abuse. Issues to be
worked on include identifying supportive people and reactions to
the offender.

*3. Who has been your greatest source of emotional
support since the discovery of your child's abuse?*

*"A dear friend of my son, when his parents heard
they immediately came over and talked with us and
prayed for protection and healing. They did this
without knowing us——only that our sons loved each
other——and they did this while they struggled over
their own pain as their son was involved as a victim. "*

*"There were several parents——especially other
mothers who were there going through the same
experience. There was a close relative who gave quite
a lot of support in the beginning. In the very initial
stages our family physician gave good support."*

Mothers noted that their child mentioned the offender either to
tell aspects of what the offender did to the child or to inquire if the
offender would remain locked up and that the child and the family

was safe. Some children talked about the offender frequently, others not at all.

4. Does your child talk about the offender(s)?

"Yes. She wants to know if they are locked up and if they can hurt her or anyone else again."

"Once in awhile when something triggers her memory."

"Occasionally expresses anger; sometimes points out the good things about him."

"Yes. He once in awhile will say something about the abuser or about the abuse. He's pretty open and talks about it freely. But he mentions it less and less. This is good; it means he's finding a way to be done with it and file it in the back of his consciousness. It used to be in the front of his mind all of the time. So I am encouraged that he is dealing with it."

Parent Groups

Parent groups can include mothers only, fathers only, or both parents only. A major issue in parent groups is dealing with the abused child. Parents need support dealing with symptomatic children. These parents struggle with their child's present behavior and their anxiety of the long-term consequences to their child. It is helpful to hear how other parents are coping with traumatized behavior; thus, parent group work is a useful intervention. Parents noted their child being shy and withdrawn or aggressive and acting out. Some mothers noted a drop in the child's interest in the outside world—lack of being inquisitive. Clinging behavior was frequently mentioned.

5. Have you observed any major changes in your child since he/she was abused?

"My child changed dramatically after the abuse. Part of the therapeutic process was to help her redefine who she was before, which we did with pictures, with stories, with old friends. Her need for her history was so strong, I wrote her a book so she could read it whenever she wanted. She also comes from us, and

*her need to identify with us—particularly me—was
very strong."*

*"Yes. My daughter is hyperactive. She has very poor
impulse control. She is aggressive toward others. She
has a great deal of trouble sleeping (suffers from night
terrors and sleepwalking). She is very frightened in
regard to her safety and her family's."*

*"Requires constant reassurance that he is loved;
much more frustrated; masturbates quite frequently;
uses certain language and shock effects; afraid to be
left alone even for short periods of time."*

*"My daughter is more protective of me because she
knows I was hurt emotionally. She is shy around
others, and I feel it has taken her a long time to learn
to trust others again. Sexually, I just don't know what
will happen with her or the boys."*

*6. What has been the most difficult aspect of the
abuse for your child?*

*"I would say not so much the sexual things. More
the horrible fears they instilled in her. Their threats of
killing us or burning down our home. It will take
many years to erase those awful memories from her
mind.*

*"Being forced to perform and being scared to tell
us.He is also afraid to think of the abuser's hands on
his body. He quivers, cries, and has a hard time
talking about it in detail."*

*"It has taken her two to three years to come to the
most gruesome aspects of the abuse for her in
therapy—the infanticide and cannibalism."*

Some parents made specific reference to aspects of their child's abuse,
such as the ritualistic aspects. Others noted extreme guilt in themselves for not recognizing and responding to the behavior of their
child prior to the disclosure. Parents were uncertain about the future

for their child and fearful of the sexual development and gender orientation of their child.

7. What has been the worst aspect of your child's abuse for you?

> *"Worst for the child: the emotional torture. . . . It is still difficult for me to comprehend how anyone could be so deliberately and systematically cruel and destructive. Worst for me, the uncertainty. The struggle to understand what the real issues were as disclosure and behavior was presented . . . not knowing if things were getting better or worse . . . not knowing where we were going or where it would end."*

> *"The guilt I feel about having sent her there and having ignored or misinterpreted symptoms has been hard to work through. At times I worry that the abuse has permanently altered how my child and I relate to each other. She blamed me, and I blamed myself for a period of years. I also feel a tremendous need for validation."*

Parents harbor great anxiety around the future outcome for their child. Some admitted to fears of very long-term consequences; others hoped that none would occur and saw their sense of hope intimately attached to the belief that in time the child would get over what happened to him or her.

> *8. Do your think that the abuse will have any long-term effects on your child?*

> *"Yes. But I feel we may not see some of them until she reaches puberty and begins to date. I feel she may always carry some of the betrayal of trust issues with her."*

> *"I don't know what the future holds for all three. I do know they avoid anything that deals with sex and sex education. My daughter claims (at 7) that she'll never marry. I hope that with time and therapy she"ll regain the trust of men, and she'll learn that sex can be beautiful and rewarding as an adult. Not the horror she encountered."*

"Yes. This is something he will never forget. He will always have to deal with his sexuality. He will need to be more open with us as he goes through his teen years, needing help to understand his reactions and responses to things that seem abnormal. He will be easier to stimulate sexually. He'll have to be careful that he doesn't get caught in anger or self-destructive behavior. Yes, I think he'll have lifelong effects. Not all negative, but different than most children."

"I don't know how it could not effect her. It is part of her. I hope that because we are willing to talk with her and she knows we love her that it will be no more than a real bad memory. So far almost everything that she was doing that made us aware of it bothering her has changed for the better."

Group Termination

In the termination of group treatment, the saying goodbye is important and the process of reflecting on what changes have occurred and where do they lead in the future.

Responses to question 9 below ranged from a lack of trust in others, a change in feelings and thoughts toward others, distrust, and symptomatic changes, such as increased depression. There were also positive changes noted, such as more empathy toward others, a renewed faith in God.

9. Have you experienced any major changes in yourself since the abuse was discovered?

"Yes. My view of the world has changed drastically. I no longer see people as good and kind, or trust that others are like myself in basic ways. I am very suspicious and watchful of anyone I meet, and even of people whom I think I know well. I am less shy or self-involved than I used to be—I don't have time for that anymore. I am committed to taking action on behalf of my child."

"I have learned a lot of patience and am more aware and discerning of my children's emotional

> *needs. I have learned to listen to my children with not*
> *only my ears but with my senses. I do not feel that I*
> *have changed in any major way, but I have grown as*
> *a person because of it. I have had to learn to trust*
> *God more and realize that my 'perfect' little family*
> *isn't less perfect because the evil in this world has*
> *touched us."*

The world view now created provides a basis for future resiliency in parents, child, and family unit. Life, death, the meaning of adversity and its probability of occurrence are open areas for discussion. Renewed spirituality, movement outward, and a construction of a positive future are most important in turning adversity into less devastating experiences. The potential to have these life-enhancing processes disrupted through trauma is apparent from the personal struggles revealed by the study parents. When we can envision outcomes, we can than focus on how to get there.

CONCLUSION

Sexual abuse of children demands action from all those charged with the protection of children. The questions are how to help the child and how to prevent further perpetration of sexual abuse. The parent is confronted with the fact that these questions cannot be answered in a definitive manner. Thus parental decision making includes uncertainty, which in itself has an unnerving effect. Research has not answered the question of who benefits from in-depth discussion of traumatic events and who is further traumatized by such discussion. Clinically, we offer arguments as to the therapeutic intention, and we are evolving guidelines for intervention steps of anchoring for safety, resource building, and specific trauma processing. However, parents are not expert in this effort and are guided by their own observations, sensitivity, and tolerance for stress and disorganization as well as belief or trust in mental health counseling.

In summary, the secondary analysis of data on the study of 41 families in which parents scored in the clinical range for being symptomatic has revealed a dynamic stressful interaction of symptoms between child and parents. Following from this information and documented statements of parents, a trilevel intervention program was explored. Hopefully, this can advance an examination of the positive and negative effects of therapeutic efforts with children and families suffering the consequences of sexual abuse.

REFERENCES

Achenbach, T.M., & Edelbroch, C.S. (1983). *The Child Behavior Checklist Manual.* Burlington: The University of Vermont.

Baskin, C.H.; Forehand, R.; & Saylor, C. (1985). Predictors of psychosocial adjustment in mothers of children with cancer. *Journal of Psychosocial Oncology* 3 (3): 43–54.

Burgess, A.W.; Groth, A.N.; Holmstrom, L.L.; & Sgroi, S. (1978). *Sexual Assault of Children and Adolescents.* Lexington, Mass.: Lexington Books.

Cella, D.F.; Perry, S.W.; Poag, M.E.; et al. (1988). Depression and stress responses in parents of burned children. *Journal of Pediatric Psychology* 13 (1): 87–99.

Conte, J., & Schuerman, J. (1987). Factors associated with an increased impact of child sexual abuse. *Child Abuse and Neglect* 11: 201–211.

De Jong, A.R. (1986). Childhood sexual abuse precipitating maternal hospitalization. *Child Abuse and Neglect* 10: 551–553.

De Vine, R.A. (1980). The sexually abused child in the emergency room. *Sexual Abuse of Children: Selected Readings.* Washington, D.C.: U.S. Department of Health and Human Services.

Esquilin, S.C. (1987). Family response to the identification of extra-familial child sexual abuse. *Psychotherapy in Private Practice* 5 (1): 105–113.

Finkelhor, D. (1984). *Child Sexual Abuse: New Theory and Practice.* New York: Free Press.

Finkelhor, D.; Williams, L.; & Burns, N. (1988). *Nursery Crimes: Sexual Abuse in Day Care.* Newbury Park, Calif.: Sage.

Flannery, R.B. (1990). *Becoming Stress-Resistant.* New York: Continuum.

Friedrich, W.N., & Reams, R.A. (1987). Course of psychological symptoms in sexually abused children. *Psychotherapy* 24 (2): 160–170.

Goldberg, S.; Morris, P.; Simmons, R.J.; et al. (1990). Chronic illness in infancy and parenting stress: a comparison of three groups of parents. *Journal of Pediatric Psychology* 15 (5): 503–508.

Gomes-Schwartz, B.; Horowitz, J.; & Sauzier, M. (1985). Severity of emotional distress among sexually abused preschool, school-age, and adolescent children. *Hospital and Community Psychiatry* 36 (5): 503–508.

Hartman, C.R., & Burgess, A.W. (1988) Information processing of trauma: application of a model. *Journal of Interpersonal Violence* 3 (4): 443–457.

Horowitz, M. (1976). *Stress Response Syndrome*. New York: Aronson.

Kelley, S.J. (1990). Parental stress response to sexual abuse and ritualistic abuse in day care centers. *Nursing Research* 25 (1): 502–513.

MacFarlane, K., & Waterman, J. (1986). *Sexual Abuse of Young Children*. New York: Guilford Press.

McCann, I.L., & Pearlman, L.S. (1990). Vicarious traumatization: a framework for understanding the psychological effects of working with victims. *Journal of Traumatic Stress* 3 (1): 131–150.

Regher, C. (1990). Parental responses to extrafamilial child sexual assault. *Child Abuse and Neglect* 14 (1): 113–120.

Sesan, R.; Freeark, K.; & Murphy, S. (1986). The support network: crisis intervention for extrafamilial child sexual abuse. *Professional Psychology, Research, and Practice* 17 (2): 138–146.

Winton, M.A. (1990). An evaluation of a support group for parents who have a sexually abused child. *Child Abuse and Neglect* 14 (3): 397–405.

Weisenberg, M.; Solomon, Z.; Schwarzwald, J.; & Mikulincer, M. (1987). Assessing the severity of post-traumatic stress disorder; relation between dichotomous and continuous measures. *Journal of Consulting and Clinical Psychology* 55: 432–434.

CHAPTER 15

Sexual Abuse Prevention Programs for Children

Jon R. Conte
Linda Fogarty

A version of this chapter was printed in *Education and Urban Society* (22 (3): 270–284, 1990.

Public and professional awareness of the extent and effects of childhood sexual victimization has increased over the last decade or so. Over this time period there has been a steadily increasing interest in how sexual abuse can be prevented. Our aim in this chapter is to review current efforts to prevent sexual abuse of children. In doing so we will discuss the nature of sexual abuse and what an understanding of that nature implies for programs to prevent sexual abuse of children, summarize the effects of sexual abuse prevention programs, and outline some of the major policy implications of this material.

THE NATURE OF SEXUAL ABUSE

Definition

Sexual use of younger persons by older persons may involve a wide range of specific behaviors. A popular definition of sexual abuse is forced, tricked, or coerced sexual behavior between a young person and an older person. Although generally there is agreement in the field that an age of at least five years between victim and offender is one of the criterion for sexual abuse, the element of force is a key dynamic. The sexual behaviors may involve direct body to body contact as in fondling, penetration of the child's body by nonsexual objects of the offender's sexual organs, and noncontact behaviors such as voyeurism or pornography.

In a comprehensive and thoughtful review of studies on the incidence and prevalence of child sexual abuse, Peters, Wyatt, and Finkelhor (1986) report that estimates of the prevalence range from 6% to 62% for females and from 3% to 31% for males. As they point out, this variation may be accounted for by a number of methodological factors, such as differences in definitions of abuse, sample characteristics, interview format (e.g., in-person versus phone interview), and number of questions used to elicit information about abuse experience. Whatever the number, it is clear that sexual abuse is a problem that effects large numbers of children. The only question is how large that number is in a particular community.

Risk Factors

Two key questions with policy implications are whether all children are at risk for sexual abuse or whether some children, because of some specific characteristic (e.g., age or poverty status), are at greater risk. If risk factors could be identified, greater precision could be undertaken in direct prevention where it is most needed. In their review of studies on prevention, Finkelhor and Baron (1986) conclude that it is currently not clear what factors increase children's risk for sexual abuse. It appears that girls are at greater risk, although boys are also victimized. Girls are more likely to be victimized if they have somehow been separated from their mothers (e.g., ever lived away from mother or mother is ill or disabled) or if they report poor relationships with their mothers. As the authors note, these factors may be consequences of sexual abuse as much as risk factors.

Several studies have recently focused on what sexual offenders tell about prevention. For example, Conte, Wolf, and Smith (1989) interviewed a sample of sexual offenders treated in the community about the victimization process. These offenders claim an ability to identify and use vulnerabilities in a potential victim to gain sexual access to and maintain control over the child. Vulnerabilities were defined in terms of status conditions (e.g., living in a single parent family), emotional characteristics (e.g., needy, unhappy, shy), and situational factors (e.g., child was alone and unprotected, child was young). It is not clear if sexual offenders differ from other adults in that they have a special capacity to identify vulnerable children or if they are simply willing to use this knowledge against children (see also Budin & Johnson, 1989).

What Abuse Involves

While we are not sure if all children are at equal risk for sexual victimization, we are increasingly sure of what sexual abuse involves. Sexual abuse consists of specific actions employed by the offender to engage a victim and maintain that victim in an abusive situation; it also includes the specific sexual behaviors and practices of the offender. The elements of sexual abuse that make up these actions include manipulation of the child (e.g., psychologically separating the child from his or her mother), coercion (e.g., using adult authority or size differential), force (e.g., holding the victim or showing a weapon), threats (e.g., "If you tell, I will kill your mother" or "I will go to jail"), and virtually every kind of sexual behavior.

For many reasons, and some only partly understood, sexual abuse inherently involves elements that directly function to keep the child from disclosing the abuse, such as offender threats or bribes, and involves some elements that indirectly serve the same function. Indirect functions may not be present in every case and are only beginning to be understood. For example, a child may have a sense of duplicity with ongoing abuse because he or she did not tell about the first abuse incident, or the child may have feelings of guilt generated from an irrational belief that going along with the behavior implies responsibility. Some of the effects of sexual abuse (e.g., fear, emotional or physical separation from adults who could protect the child, diminished self-esteem, unassertiveness, dissociation) also work against a child's disclosing abuse. Other children will not report because they wish to protect a parent from the pain associated with sexual abuse. Other children may be indoctrinated by offenders into not telling, for example, by being forced to abuse other children, thereby convincing them that they too are offenders. Some children, especially young ones, appear not to know that sexual abuse is something to tell anyone about (Berliner & Conte, 1989).

Who Offenders Are

Prevention efforts would be greatly aided if it were possible to identify older persons more likely to use children sexually. A large literature has developed on sexual offenders. This literature includes information about the nonfamily offender (i.e., pedophile) (for review, see Quinsey, 1984; Quinsey,1986). Pedophilia involves recurrent, intense, sexual urges, and sexually arousing fantasies, of at least six months' duration, involving sexual activity with a prepubescent child (American Psychiatric Association, 1987). Literature also has focused on the family or incest offender (for review, see Conte, 1986). Definitions of incest vary, but incest is generally recognized as sexual contact between persons who are biologically related (e.g., father-daughter, mother-son, grandparent-grandchild, or brother-sister) or between stepparents and stepchildren. Clinical reports indicate that most children are abused by someone known to them and in about half of cases by members of their own families. Much of the professional literature to date has focused on father or stepfather and daughter abuse.

Recent data tend to raise questions about the validity of characteristics used to describe differences between types of sexual offenders. For example, Abel, Becker, Cunningham-Rathner, et al. (1988) indicate that 49% of the incestuous fathers and stepfathers referred for outpatient treatment at their clinics, also abused children outside of the family, and 18% of these men were raping adult women at the same time they were sexually abusing their own child. While these data are preliminary and replication is critical in understanding how generalizable they are, they do raise concern about the popular notion that incest and nonincestuous offenders represent different classes of offenders.

Some research has detected differences in sexual arousal patterns of different types of offenders. For example, Quinsey and Chaplin (1988) have reported that child molesters who have injured their victims are more sexually responsive in laboratory assessments to audiotape descriptions of violent sex depicting gratuitous infliction of physical violence than were child molesters who had not inflicted injury. Laboratory assessments of sexual arousal patterns are of limited usefulness in screening large numbers of men, both because it is unlikely that most communities will support widespread laboratory assessments and because such assessments are far from 100% reliable (see Earls & Marshall, 1983).

Current research has failed to identify characteristics, especially demographic, social, or psychological characteristics, that discriminate between older persons who have or are likely to have sex with younger persons and those who have not and are not likely to (Conte, 1985; Conte, 1986; Conte 1989; Quinsey, 1984; Quinsey, 1986).

PREVENTION PROGRAMS

Implications for Prevention

The ideas outlined above suggest that sexual abuse is a childhood experience that affects a large number of children, although the exact number is not completely clear. Current knowledge indicates that female children are at greater risk, although male children are also abused. It is not clear what other risk factors for sexual abuse are, although certain characteristics of children's condition (e.g., social environment, psychological makeup, status condition) are hypothesized to be associated with an increased risk for sexual abuse. Current knowledge has failed to identify psychosocial characteristics of adults likely to have sexually abused a child or at risk to do so. Sexual abuse is a complex situation inherently involving actions (e.g., threats), psychological processes (e.g., a child's fear or guilt), and social influences (e.g., an offender's separation of a child from adults who can protect the child) that reduce the likelihood that a child will disclose abuse.

These ideas underlie a set of core assumptions behind sexual abuse prevention programs directed at children. These assumptions include that many children do not know what sexual abuse is, that sexual touch need not be tolerated, that adults want to know about sexual touching by older persons, and that it is possible to tell about sexual abuse to have it cease. Children can be taught knowledge (e.g., the difference between a safe and unsafe touch or who to tell about abuse) and skills (e.g., how to assertively say "no" to unwanted touch) that will be useful in preventing or escaping their own abuse.

These assumptions underpin a large number of programs and materials designed to help children prevent or escape sexual abuse (for reviews see Kolko, 1988; Tharinger, Krivacska, Laye-Donough, et al., 1988; Wurtele, 1987). There are differences among these programs and materials in terms of the range of material presented, the time it takes to deliver the message to the child, the concepts or words used to describe the concepts, the location in which the material is presented (e.g., home or school), the format of presentation (e.g., video, instruction by adult trainers, printed matter), the degree to which the child interacts with the materials (e.g., reads a book, listens to and asks questions of an instructor, observes a model demonstrating a prevention behavior and then role plays the skills), and occupation of the trainer. With the exception of the value of modeling and rehearsal of skills, little is known about how important these alternatives are in the prevention effort.

Notwithstanding this variation, most prevention material consists of the key concepts outlined by Conte, Rosen, and Saperstein (1986). These include the concept that children *own their own bodies* and therefore can control access to their bodies; the *touch continuum*, which recognizes that there are different kinds of touches (e.g., safe and unsafe); *secrets about touching* can and should be told; children have a range of individuals in their *support systems* whom they can tell about touching problems; some programs encourage children to *trust their own feelings* so that when a situation feels uncomfortable or strange they should tell someone; and *how to say "no!"*

RESEARCH ON PREVENTION TRAINING

Program Effectiveness

An expanding research literature is available answering questions about prevention program effectiveness. Among the initial questions are "do children learn the prevention concepts, are they able to generalize this knowledge to new situations, and can they apply the prevention strategies in potentially dangerous situations in the 'real world.'" Program developers and researchers also want to know what approaches to prevention education are most effective (for reviews, see Conte, 1984; Finkelhor & Strapko, 1987; Kolko, 1988; Tharinger, Krivacska, Laye-McDonough, et al., 1988; Wurtele, 1987).

The goals of sexual abuse prevention education curricula and many of the underlying concepts are shared by most, if not all, programs. Although the goals are straightforward—empowering children to help prevent their own sexual victimization and providing an opportunity for disclosures—the degree to which these goals are met is not easily evaluated. Program evaluators have settled for assessing knowledge gains, skill acquisition, and, in some cases, application of the prevention skills and knowledge. It is recognized that outcomes measured in this way may not describe a child's ability to escape assault or report abuse.

Knowledge Gains

Evaluation measures designed to assess knowledge gains typically ask children questions such as what is sexual abuse, who sexually abuses children, whose fault is abuse, and what should a child do if touched inappropriately. Many assessments include questions about strangers, secrets, social supports, and body ownership. Knowledge gains have been found in evaluations of several different programs using a variety of training formats (Binder & McNiel, 1987; Conte, Rosen, Saperstein & Shermack, 1985; Downer, 1984; Garbarino, 1987; Harvey, Forehand, Brown, & Holmes, 1988; Plummer, 1984; Ray & Dietzel, 1984; Wolfe, MacPherson, Blount, & Wolfe, 1986; Wurtele, Kast, Miller-Perrin, & Kondrick, 1989; Wurtele, Marrs, & Miller-Perrin, 1987). Typical of these results, Kenning, Gallmeier, Jackson, and Plemons (1987), evaluating the effectiveness of child assault prevention (CAP), found a significant difference in posttest scores for 72 first and second graders on a 25-item knowledge questionnaire.

In another study of 71 kindergartners, children receiving a three 1/2-hour-session prevention program, scored significantly higher on a knowledge test than children in a control group (Harvey, Forehand, Brown, & Holmes, 1988). Wolfe and colleagues (1986) also found knowledge gains in a sample of 290 fourth and fifth graders who viewed skits on sexual abuse prevention and participated in guided class discussions on the topic. Children participating in the prevention program scored significantly higher on a 7-item true/false evaluation questionnaire than controls.

Most evaluations assess learning directly following the education program, but only a few have instituted a follow-up test to look at "long-term" retention and knowledge drop off. Harvey and colleagues (1988) found that at a seven-week follow-up children in the treatment condition had retained the knowledge gains found at posttest and scored significantly higher than controls at the follow-up assessment. Ray and Dietzel (1984) tested children immediately following a sexual abuse prevention presentation, which consisted of a slide show, a film, a brief discussion and workbook to take home, at one-month and six-month follow-ups. No decrease in knowledge was found at the six-month follow-up. Wurtele and colleagues (1987) found that kindergartners in both training groups—"participant" and "symbolic" modeling—had retained their knowledge gains six weeks following the program implementation. One method of maximizing the effectiveness of programs and aiding in retention of information may be with the use of additional booster sessions to review program messages. Third graders receiving a one-hour training session followed two weeks later by a booster session with the film *Better Safe Than Sorry II* (1980) score significantly higher on a 12-item knowledge test at a one-month follow-up than those receiving the one-hour training alone. This difference was maintained at a six-month follow-up (Ray & Dietzel, 1984).

Although evaluations have generally found overall knowledge gains following prevention program implementation, there is evidence that some concepts are more difficult to learn than others. For example, at least one study empirically supported the notion that children have an easier time learning concrete than abstract concepts (Conte, Saperstein, & Shermack, 1985). Similarly, Gilbert and his colleagues report that preschoolers had difficulty explaining the abstract idea of why specific touches would create specific feelings and that they could not give examples of why feelings about a touch might change (Gilbert, Daro, Duerr, et al., 1988). These same children had difficulty learning which secrets to keep (e.g., secrets about a surprise party) and which to report (e.g., secrets about touching).

Another difficult concept included in most prevention curricula is that someone familiar to the child can be the perpetrator of sexual assault. Some evaluations have found that even after training, children have a difficult time understanding that a family member or someone they know could try to abuse them (Wurtele, Marrs, & Miller-Perrin, 1987) and have difficulty knowing what to do if approached by someone known (Plummer, 1984). Although Ray and Dietzel (1984) found that the percent of incorrect responses to the question "do kids ever have touching problems with people they know and like" decreased from 62% at pretest to 11% after training, this was still the most difficult item at posttest. Other studies have also found substantial posttraining increases on this concept (Kenning, Gallmeier, Jackson, & Plemons, 1987; Swan, Press, & Briggs, 1985), but it continues to be a difficult one for children and adults in our society. Another concept found difficult to learn in two studies is that the victim is not to blame (Plummer, 1984; Wolfe, MacPherson, Blount, & Wolfe, 1986). This is understandable following a program in which we are at once describing sexual touch as "bad" or "inappropriate" and inviting children to take responsibility for their bodily integrity, while presenting sexual touch as the "adult's fault." The implied message may be "it is your fault" if sexual touching occurs because you should know it's bad and now you should know how to escape it.

Touch Discrimination

A key component to program assessments is the touch discrimination task. This type of measure attempts to assess the child's ability to discriminate between "good," appropriate, or nurturing touch and "bad," inappropriate, or sexually exploitative touch. Several evaluations have found that older children are typically quite good at judging good and bad touches, even before attending a prevention education (Blumberg, Chadwick, Fogarty, et al., 1988; Miltenberger & Thiesse-Duffy, 1987; Swan, Press, & Briggs, 1985; Thiesse-Duffy, Miltenberger, Kozak, & Suda, 1987). For example, on a nine-picture touch discrimination task used in one study, children in third grade made correct discriminations 97% of the time before the prevention training (Thiesse-Duffy et al., 1987). In another study 8- to 11-year-old children made correct discriminations 92% of the time at pretest (Swan, Press, & Briggs, 1985). Because children score so high on these tasks before training, it is impossible to know what they learned from the program.

Although discriminating inappropriate from appropriate touch may not be difficult for older children, there is reason to believe very young children may have more difficulty, especially when asked to make this judgment based on intuition. Children under age 7 are in what Piaget referred to as the preoperational stage of moral development (Piaget, 1963). During this period children determine what is "right" or "wrong" based on the outcomes of the action or according to the characterological attributes, or "goodness," of the actor and not according to the motives of that person. Some prevention curricula teach children to listen to their feelings about touch to make decisions about the appropriateness or inappropriateness of a touch. If a "bad" touch comes from a "good" person, the child may be inclined to interpret the touch as "good" or appropriate in synchrony with the child's beliefs about this person. At the same time, if a sexual touch by an adult feels good to a child, the child is likely to label the touch a "good touch" if a child is taught to discriminate based on their feelings (de Young, 1988). Therefore the attributional styles of preschool-age children may prevent them from learning that a bad touch can come from a "good" person and can feel pleasant. Especially among young children, it is essential that program messages are developmentally appropriate both so they are maximally effective, and so they do not harm children.

From victims' reports it is clear that often the sexual touch is not considered bad or inappropriate (Berliner & Conte, 1988). This could be because the gradual progression of touch from nonsexual to sexual desensitizes the victim. In addition, if the only clear message a child receives about sexual behavior comes from the perpetrator (e.g. "He told me he needed some love and this is the way people show their love," Berliner & Conte, 1988), the more subtle and mixed messages from a society reluctant to address the topic will be misinterpreted. Creating touch discrimination tasks complex enough to include the difficult and ambiguous situations victims can face is a major challenge.

In spite of the often high pretest scores, and the sometimes abstract presentation of the concept, many evaluations have found a significant increase in children's abilities to discriminate between appropriate and inappropriate touch after training (Blumberg, Chadwick,

Fogarty, et al., 1988; Harvey, Forehand, Brown, & Holmes, 1988; Kolko, Moser, Litz, & Hughes, 1987; Wurtele, Kast, Miller-Perrin, & Kondrick, 1989). A recent study compared the effectiveness of two approaches to teaching preschoolers how to distinguish between appropriate and inappropriate touch (Wurtele et al., 1989). Both approaches taught prevention concepts using interactive roleplaying and rehearsal, but explanations of a "good" touch and "bad" touch varied. The first approach, the "feelings" approach based on the touch continuum (Anderson, 1986), required that children rely on their intuition and feelings to judge the appropriateness of touch. The second approach—the Behavioral Skills Training program— focused on the behavior of others, and established clear rules for touching and clear exceptions to the rule (e.g., touch for hygiene purposes). Children in the "feelings" group were more likely to label an appropriate touch that made them feel bad as inappropriate touch and more likely to mislabel an inappropriate touch that made them feel good than those in the Behavioral Skills Training group.

Another study compared a role-play-based one-hour prevention program, a multimedia presentation, and a control group in a sample of 264 kindergarten through third graders. Definitions of inappropriate touch differed in the two prevention approaches. The role-play presentation defined an "uh-oh" touch as "an older person touching you in your private places when you don't need help in a way you don't like." The multimedia program defined confusing touch as "the kind of touch where you don't know what to do. It doesn't feel good, but it doesn't hurt. You sort of get the feeling in your stomach, and if that feeling could talk it would say 'uh-oh'." Children receiving the role-play-based program scored higher on a touch discrimination task than controls at posttest, while the group receiving the multimedia-based presentation did not score higher than controls (Blumberg et al., 1988). Like in the Wurtele and colleagues study above (1989), the definition in the multimedia presentation was more abstract and called upon children to make more inferences than the definition in the role-play-based program, which stated more concretely rules for judging inappropriate touch. (See also Harvey, Forehand, Brown, & Holmes, 1988; Kolko, Moser, Litz, & Hughes, 1987.)

Behavioral Strategies: Say "No," Get Away, Tell Someone

Prevention education programs typically teach children to follow three strategies in a "dangerous" or sexually abusive situation. Children are taught to say "no," get away from the assailant or dangerous situation, and report the incident to a trusted adult. Many evaluations have assessed the learning of these skills using multiple choice, true/false or yes/no questions such as "If an older child touched your private parts, would you tell?" (Binder & McNiel, 1987; Conte, Rosen, Saperstein, & Shermack, 1985; Plummer, 1984; Wolfe, MacPherson, Blount, & Wolfe, 1986).

Another method of assessing the three behavioral rules has been presenting scenarios including appropriate and inappropriate touch and asking the child what should be done in such a situation (Borkin & Frank, 1986; Harvey et al., 1988; Hill & Jason, 1988; Kenning et al, 1987; Kolko, Moser, Litz, & Hughes, 1987; Thiesse-Duffy et al., 1987; Wurtele et al., 1987; Wurtele et al., 1989). For example, in one study children were asked, "What if you are having fun wrestling with your cousin, and all of a sudden your cousin starts grabbing and feeling your private parts. Is there anything wrong with this situation?" (from the WIST, Wurtele, Marrs, & Miller-Perrin, 1986). Assessments of this kind have the advantage of requiring a child to apply prevention knowledge rather than just reciting it. Again, although it is not certain that success on such measures is correlated with prevention behaviors in real-life situations, results of these behavioral assessments have been promising. Sandy Wurtele and her colleagues (1987) using the What If Situations Test (WIST), presenting a hypothetical touch situation, found that in response to the question "What would you do?" the percent of children with perfect scores, requiring that they apply the strategies—say "no," get away and tell someone—increased from 19% at pretest to 79% at posttest for both experimental groups. When a similar procedure was used—reading a vignette to a child—children were better able to take appropriate action at posttest when the stories involved strangers and exploitative touch and nonexploitative requests from known adults (Kenning, Gallmeier, Jackson, & Plemons, 1987). In another study children in the experimental group were more likely to report using all three strategies (i.e., say "no," get away and tell someone) in response to the question, "What would you do if an adult tried to play secret or private games where he/she touched your body in a way that made you feel uncomfortable?" (Kolko, Moser, Litz, & Hughes, 1987), while those in the control group were more likely to report engaging in an emotional, physical, or miscellaneous response.

Although measures describing children in various touching situations require that children begin to apply their knowledge to new situations, such vignettes may fall short of capturing the power differential between a child victim and adult offenders or the subtle coerciveness of a conscious grooming process by the offender. Using a videotape of a dramatized set of vignettes describing potentially abusive or dangerous situations may be one way of creating more realistic scenarios, which describe the dynamics between the child and offender and thereby display more of the complexity of abusive situations. A videotaped set of five stories describing positive, negative, and sexually abusive touch situations was presented to assess skill learning in one study, and children were asked, "What should a person do who is touched in this way?" Children reported that they would tell someone about the abuse significantly more often after the prevention education although no increases in touch discrimination were found (Swan, Press, & Briggs, 1985).

In an attempt to design a behavioral skills measure that approximates reality more closely, some researchers have created "stranger abduction situations," where a child is approached by a confederate of the experiment, unknown to the child, and the child's help is solicited (Fryer, Kraizer, & Miyoshi, 1987; Miltenberger & Thiesse-Duffy, 1988). In a sample of 44 kindergarten through second graders, children in the education program were more likely to refuse to help from the unknown confederate than those in a control group (Kraizer, Fryer, & Miller, 1988). Although these findings are encouraging, considerations arise in the use of such procedures because of the possibility of desensitizing children to abduction situations and incomplete subject debriefing (Conte, 1987). At the same time these measures do not assess responses to approaches by nonstrangers, who are the majority of offenders.

Learning Assertiveness

A central theme in many sexual abuse prevention curricula, as well as drug and gang prevention curricula, is teaching children to respond assertively to other children and to adults. In one assertiveness measure developed by Ann Downer (1984), children's responses to a puppet acting out a situation, (e.g., a woman drives up and asks for help holding her sick dog while she drives to the vet) are scored according to the child's assertive tone of voice, body language, and the actual verbal message employed by the child while resisting the pleas, promises, cajoles, bribes, and threats of the puppet. Children receiving the Talking About Touching curriculum (Committee for Children, 1983) scored significantly higher on this assertiveness measure at posttest than children in a control group (Downer, 1984). Hill and Jason (1988), using the measure developed by Downer, also found an increase in assertiveness for one of the two experimental groups evaluated in a day care sample. A third study, using a similar format to assess gains in assertiveness, also found significantly more assertive responses at posttest compared to pretest in a first- and second-grade sample (Kenning, Gallmeier, Jackson, & Plemons, 1987).

Program Comparisons

It is clear that, in general, children learn from well-designed and carefully implemented prevention programs. But what variables maximize program success? With the wide variety of creative programming available, comparisons of programs are needed to delineate maximally effective components. Some promising, well-designed studies have already begun to shed light on differential program effectiveness (Chadwick, 1988; Ray & Dietzel, 1984; Wurtele, Kast, Miller-Perrin, & Kondrick, 1989; Wurtele, Marrs, & Miller-Perrin, 1987). Children in a "participant modeling" prevention program, which incorporated role-play, modeling and rehearsal, scored significantly higher on the WIST than did children in a "symbolic modeling" program, which taught the same skills but the child watched the experimenter model on a video (Wurtele, Marrs, & Miller-Perrin, 1987).

In another comparison of prevention education approaches with a sample of 264 children in kindergarten through third grades, children receiving a role-play-based curriculum with rehearsal and modeling, scored significantly higher on a touch discrimination task at posttest than pretest, while those receiving a multimedia prevention presentation and those in a control group did not score higher at posttest (Blumberg, Chadwick, Fogarty, et al., 1989). Similarly, Miltenberger and Thiesse-Duffy (1988) found that although use of the home-based Red Flag/Green Flag (Rape & Abuse Crisis Center, 1986) curriculum did not significantly increase knowledge or skill scores in a group of 4- to 7-year-old children, the addition of a behavioral skills training (with individual instruction, rehearsal, and modeling) did.

The effectiveness of the film *Touch* (Illusion Theater, 1984) was compared to that of the Behavioral Skills Training (BST) program, also employing modeling and active classroom participation. This comparison also indicated that children in the BST group scored higher at posttest on personal safety skills and prevention knowledge than those viewing the film (Saslawsky & Wurtele, 1986). The results of these comparisons suggest that children learn better when taught in an interactive way including role playing and rehearsal.

Side Benefits: Communication at Home

Many believe one of the positive side benefits of participation in prevention programs is the opening of communication about personal safety issues at home providing parents and children the language to discuss the sensitive topic. Recruiting parents as allies in the prevention effort is an important component to many programs. The Talking About Touching curriculum (Committee for Children, 1983) includes letters to send home to parents during each personal safety unit to inform parents of the specific topics covered in class. It is common for schools to require a parent meeting before program implementations to answer parents' questions and to inform them of program goals and procedures. Unfortunately, these parent meetings tend to be poorly attended (Chadwick, 1988; Gilbert, Daro, Duerr, et al., 1988; Spungen, Jensen, Finkelstein, & Satinsky, 1989), and involving parents is a challenge to program implementors. Even without overwhelming parent involvement, it appears that children bring the information home with them and discuss program concepts with family members. Although few evaluations have included a formal assessment of the topic, some programs seem to have had the effect of increasing discussion at home (Binder & McNiel, 1987; Kolko, Moser, Litz, & Hughes, 1987; Swan, Press, & Briggs, 1985). For example, 47% of parents in one study reported they talked to their children about sexual abuse prevention before the child training (Wurtele & Miller-Perrin, 1987). This number had increased to 80% at posttest.

Prevention programs are expected to create a language and environment for disclosures of abuse that has already occurred or is currently ongoing. Again, very few evaluations have systematically assessed this goal. Gilbert and associates (1988) discovered no disclosures in a study of 118 preschoolers as a result of prevention training. Among 349 third and fourth graders no differences were found in disclosure rates between the two experimental groups and the control group, although approximately 7.5 % of fall subjects did report abuse (Kolko, Moser, Litz, & Hughes, 1987). Systematic record keeping of disclosures during prevention programs is needed to assess the success of this goal of prevention.

Unanticipated Consequences

As attention to programs aimed at empowering children to prevent their own sexual victimization increases, so does the fear that these same programs may be hastily instituted, harmful to children, and may create a false sense of security to members of our society. Researchers have attempted to address concerns that program participation may be harmful to children by evaluating immediate behavioral changes or increases in fear and anxiety. Using these outcomes to measure effects, evaluations have generally found positive results (Binder & McNiel, 1987; Kenning et al., 1987; Miltenberger & Thiesse-Duffy, 1988; Wolfe et al., 1986; Swan et al., 1987; Wurtele, et al., 1987; Wurtele, 1988). Binder and McNiel (1987) found no significant increases in behavior problems recorded by parents' ratings after prevention programs in a 5- through 12-year-old sample, but they did find a decrease in 3 of 18 problem behaviors. Similarly, no significant increases in children's State-Trait Anxiety Inventory scores and the adapted version of the Quay and Peterson's Problem Behavior's Checklist (using four subscales only: conduct disorders, anxiety withdrawal, attention problem, and motor excess) completed by parents were found following implementation of the Talking About Touching curriculum (Kenning, Gallmeier, Jackson, & Plemons, 1987). In another study designed to assess the negative consequences of prevention programs, no increases in the child's fear, as reported by the child and parent, were found (Wurtele & Miller-Perrin, 1987). Three significant changes in pre- to posttest behavior problems were found by parents' ratings, but these three were decreases.

Miltenberger and Thiesse-Duffy (1988) found no new behavioral problems, nightmares, or other lasting emotional reactions according to parent reports, but nearly a third were "a little more scared" and over two-thirds were more cautious. Similarly, after reading the *Spiderman* comic on sexual abuse prevention, Garbarino (1987) found a sizeable minority of children of both sexes and each of three grades reported that the comic worried or scared them (from 17% to 50%). The reason given most often was because they realized "it" might happen to them.

A number of evaluations have assessed children's more general reaction to the program following program implementation. Most children reported feeling "much safer" (64%) or "somewhat safer" and better able to take care of themselves (94%) after a school-based training, while only 3% felt "somewhat more scared" (Binder & McNiel, 1987). When children are asked how they like the prevention programs, most report enjoying them (Swan, Press, & Briggs, 1987; Wolfe, MacPherson, Blount, & Wolfe, 1986). For example, in one study 65% of the second through fifth graders who viewed the "Bubbylonian Encounter" video either "liked the play", or "liked the play a lot" (Swan, Press, & Briggs, 1987).

The possibility that programs could create an exaggerated suspiciousness about all touch has also been explored by researchers. By learning the lessons of the program "too well," children may be inclined to see abuse when there is none or avoid even nurturing touch. Evidence from evaluation studies is mixed. One study found that first through third graders were significantly better at discriminating good touches—i.e., labeling a nurturing, nonsexual touch correctly—after one hour of role-play-based prevention training (Blumberg, Chadwick, Fogarty, et al., 1988). In another study fifth graders did not report feeling more negatively about touch between people at posttest, but "overall, they were less willing to trust in, believe, obey, and rely on any and all adults" (Plummer, 1984). One study reported preschoolers had "an increase in the degree to which they associated ambiguous touches (tickling and bathing) with feeling "sad," and "a decrease in their association of these touches with happy feelings," following training (Gilbert, Daro, Duerr, et al., 1988).

Again, carefully constructed studies comparing two or more programs are needed to explain what makes a program have an oversensitizing effect and what is required in programs to provide realistic information that eases the child's burden rather than intensifying it.

Summary of Effects

Overall it appears that the sexual abuse prevention education programs evaluated to date have generally achieved the goals of teaching prevention knowledge and skill acquisition. It remains to be seen if these gains will be retained over time and will be useful to a child in potential assault situations. It also appears that curricula employing concrete concepts, and an interactive learning experience, including rehearsal and modeling, will be most effective. Many programs seem to have the additional benefit of inspiring discussion about personal safety at home. Although the goal of exposing abuse needs to be more systematically assessed, current data does not support this desired program effect. Fears that prevention programs will have negative consequences on the child, such as increasing anxiety or creating behavioral problems, do not seem to be supported by the data, generally speaking. Still, continuing to assess the possible negative consequences is of primary importance to protect children exposed to these programs.

POLICY IMPLICATIONS

Setting Priorities

It is clear that the demands on teacher and school time are significant and increasing. The demand that schools teach material dealing with social problems, such as teenage pregnancy, AIDS, drugs, and suicide, have to be carefully analyzed in terms of how likely it is that schools are going to be effective in dealing with the problem.

We recognize that schools can do more than teach and that a range of psychosocial interventions may take place in the school context. Nevertheless, it seems clear to us that the current level of support for education will make it necessary to select from a range of worthy goals that, in fact, can be achieved in the school setting. After education in academic subjects it will be necessary to decide what subjects or social problems can effectively be dealt with in school.

In the special case of sexual abuse prevention education we ask that teachers wear many hats. As discussed by Trudell and Whatley (1988), teachers are expected to present sensitive and difficult information to children about the realities of sexual abuse, are expected to be advocate and emotional support to a disclosing child following prevention lessons, are required to report cases of suspected abuse, and still are expected to maintain a traditional alliance with parents who may feel threatened by or suspicious of sexual abuse education being taught at school.

It is not clear to us that all social problems are matters best resolved by teaching children new concepts or skills. Ignorance (e.g., of the danger of taking drugs) appears not to be a key dynamic in many problems.

While we recognize that many aspects of sexual abuse are not a function of children's ignorance (see the next section), it is becoming increasingly clear that certain concepts, such as discriminating between types of touch or knowing who to tell if exposed to an unsafe touch, may be useful to children in preventing or escaping sexual abuse. Additionally, current research indicates that children can learn this content. It remains to be seen how effective the content will be over time in actually preventing abuse.

Mental Health of Pupils Is Key

There appears to be some indication that certain characteristics of the child (e.g., emotional neediness) or the child's environment (e.g., unavailability or inability of adult to protect the child) are associated with an increased risk for victimization. While additional research will be necessary to confirm the role of these characteristics in sexual abuse of children, careful consideration should be given to the importance of mental health services, such as student counseling or school social work, that increase children's self-esteem, increase the capacity of adults to protect children, or otherwise effectively intervene on these vulnerabilities. Such mental health interventions in the schools are also likely to make children better students.

At the same time, it appears that a variety of programs and curricula addressing the prevention of AIDS, suicide, pregnancy, drug abuse, and sexual abuse share some basic goals that are then applied to the specific concern. For example, many programs call upon the child to think independently, resist peer pressure, while developing skills such as decision making, assertiveness, and effective communication skills. Essential to healthy, independent development, these tools will be used by the child in a variety of academic and nonschool related situations. Prevention curricula designed to address these more general concerns, concentrating primarily on promoting mental health and empowering individuals, and secondarily applying these skills to specific circumstances, may afford a more comprehensive, stable, and unified approach to "prevention."

Sexual Abuse Prevention: An Ongoing Process

Available research indicates that most children can successfully learn much of the content that we believe helps prevent sexual abuse, that this learning may decay over relatively short periods of time after training, and that periodic posttraining booster sessions may maintain levels of learning. There is also preliminary evidence that skill learning is more difficult, but it can take place when modeling and behavioral rehearsal teaching strategies are employed.

While the nature of the risk for sexual abuse may change over development (e.g., teenagers are more at risk for acquaintance assault than younger children), it seems clear that effective prevention training will require ongoing lessons and booster sessions over time. Communities that implement prevention programs will have to recognize that the content and training will need to be made available at various points throughout the time children are in school.

Innovations Should Be Sought

While the field of sexual abuse prevention has witnessed many innovations and an impressive beginning body of research knowledge, many areas remain for innovation and research. Space does not permit a full discussion of the numerous areas where such work might be profitable. However, several seem especially important to us. First, we need to understand more about the *victimization process*. Are some children at greater risk than others? Second, little is understood about *children's evaluations of prevention materials*. Children are consumers of prevention material along with adults who care for them. Few data are currently available that describe children's reactions to and evaluation of the programs directed toward them. Such information, along with information from the children about how they were able or not able to use the prevention knowledge after training, could be of considerable importance in improving current prevention efforts. Programs to *encourage disclosure versus preventing abuse* need to be developed. As Conte and colleagues (1986) have indicated, there is an inherent ambivalence in many programs about whether encouraging disclosure from child victims or helping children prevent abuse are more important goals. Additional research and programmatic work might well help the field understand how to encourage disclosure more effectively. It is not clear to us that both goals can be as successfully met in a single program than they might in separate programs.

Working with the Weakest Link Is Only Part of the Solution

Many prevention professionals recognize that working with children is working with the weakest link. Children are smaller, less powerful, and inherently vulnerable to attack by adults. If we knew how to prevent older persons from having sex with children, we would do so. Since we currently do not, we try to teach children concepts and skills that we hope will prevent their own abuse. Efforts to understand the causes and associated conditions of sexual use of children should be encouraged. Programs in schools that teach older children beliefs (e.g., just because one person is more powerful does not mean that person has a right to use another person), or skills (e.g., how to negotiate for shared activities), or how to identify risk factors for sexual aggression (e.g., sexual fantasies that involve younger age persons) may, in time, become effective strategies to help prevent older persons from developing sexual interest in children.

REFERENCES

Abel, G. G.; Becker, J. V.; Cunningham-Rathner, J.; et al. (1988). Multiple paraphilic diagnoses among sex offenders. *Bulletin of the American Academy of Psychiatry and the Law* 16(2): 153–168.

American Psychiatric Association (1987). *Diagnostic and Statistical Manual of Mental Disorders—Revised*. 3rd ed. Washington, D.C.: The Association.

Anderson, C. (1986). A history of the touch continuum. In M. Nelson & K. Clark (eds.), *The Educator's Guide to Preventing Child Sexual Abuse*. Pp. 15–25. Santa Cruz, Calif.: Network Publications.

Berliner, L., & Conte, J.R. (1989). What victims tell us about prevention. Unpublished manuscript.

Better Safe than Sorry II (1980). Film. Studio City, Calif.: Film Fair Communications.

Binder, R.L., & McNiel, D.E. (1987). Evaluation of a school-based sexual abuse prevention program: cognitive and emotional effects. *Child Abuse and Neglect* 11:497–506.

Blumberg, E.,; Chadwick, M.W.; Fogarty, L.A.; et al. (1988). The good touch/bad touch component of a sexual abuse prevention program: unanticipated positive consequences. Unpublished manuscript.

Borkin, J., & Frank, L. "Bubbylonian Encounter." A play. For information, contact Bubbylonian Productions, 7204 West 80th St., Overland Park, KS 66204.

Borkin, J., & Frank, L. (1986). Sexual abuse prevention for preschoolers: a pilot program. *Child Welfare* 65(1): 75–82.

Budin L.E., & Johnson C.F. (1989). Sex abuse prevention programs: offenders' attitudes about their efficacy. *Child Abuse and Neglect* 13: 77–87.

Chadwick, M.W. (1988). A comparison of two approaches to child sexual abuse prevention training. Unpublished doctoral dissertation, University of California, Irvine.

Committee for Children. (1983). *Talking about Touching: A Personal Safety Curriculum*. For information, contact Committee for Children, P.O. Box 15190, Seattle, WA, 98115.

Conte, J.R. (1985). Clinical dimensions of adult sexual abuse of children. *Behavioral Sciences and the Law* 3(4):341–354.

Conte, J.R. (1986). Sexual abuse and the family: a critical analysis. In T. Tepper & M.J. Barrett (eds.), *Treating Incest: A Multiple Systems Perspective*. New York: Haworth Press.

Conte, J.R.; Rosen, C.; Saperstein, L.; & Shermack, R. (1985). An evaluation of a program to prevent the sexual victimization of young children. *Child Abuse and Neglect* 9:319–328.

Conte, J.R.; Wolf, S.; & Smith, T. (1989). *What Sexual Offenders Tell Us About Prevention Strategies*. Unpublished manuscript.

de Young, M. (1988) The good touch/bad touch dilemma. *Child Welfare* 67 (1):60–68.

Downer, A.E. (1984). The development and testing of an evaluation instrument for assessing the effectiveness of a child sexual abuse prevention curriculum. Unpublished thesis, University of Washington, Seattle.

Earls, C.M., & Marshall, W.L. (1983). The current state of technology in the laboratory assessment of sexual arousal patterns. In S.G. Green & J.R. Stuart (eds.), *The Sexual Aggressor: Current Perspectives on Treatment*. Pp. 336–362. New York: Van Nostrand Reinhold.

Finkelhor, D., & Baron, W. (1986). Risk factors for childhood sexual abuse: A review of the evidence. In D. Finkelhor (ed.), *Sourcebook on Child Sexual Abuse*. Newbury Park, Calif.: Sage.

Finkelhor, D., & Strapko, N. (1987). Sexual abuse prevention education: a review of evaluation studies. In D.J. Willis, W. Holder, & M. Rosenberg (eds.), *Child Abuse Prevention*. New York: Wiley.

Fryer, G.E.; Kraizer, S.K.; & Miyoshi, T. (1987). Measuring actual reduction of risk to child abuse: a new approach. *Child Abuse and Neglect* 11:173–179.

Garbarino, J. (1987). Children's response to a sexual abuse prevention program: a study of the "Spiderman" comic. *Child Abuse and Neglect* 11:143–148.

Gilbert, N. (1988). Teaching children to prevent sexual abuse. *Public Interest* 93:3–15.

Gilbert, N.; Daro, D.; Duerr, J.; et al. (1988). Child sexual abuse prevention: evaluation of educational materials for pre-school programs. Family Welfare Research Group, School of Social Welfare, University of California at Berkeley, for the Department of Health and Human Services, National Center on Child Abuse and Neglect, Grant #90-CA-1163.

Harvey, P.; Forehand, R.; Brown, C.; & Holmes, T. (1988). The prevention of sexual abuse: examination of a program with kindergarten-age children. *Behavior Therapy* 19:429–435.

Hill, J.L., & Jason, L.A. (1988). An evaluation of a school-based child sexual abuse primary prevention program. *Community Psychologist* 10:36–38.

Illusion Theater Company & Media Ventures (Co-producers) (1984). *Touch*. Film. Deerfield, Ill.: MTI Tele-Programs.

Kenning, M.; Gallmeier, T.; Jackson, T.L.; & Plemons, S. (1987). Evaluation of child sexual abuse prevention programs: a summary of two studies. Paper presented at the National Conference on Family Violence, Durham, NH. July.

Kleemeier, C.; Webb, C.; Hazzard, A.; & Pohl, J. (1988). Child sexual abuse prevention: evaluation of a teacher training model. *Child Abuse and Neglect* 12:555–561.

Kolko, D.J. (1988). Educational programs to promote awareness and prevention of child sexual victimization: a review and methodological critique. *Clinical Psychology Review* 8:195–209.

Kolko, D.J.; Moser, J.T.; Litz, J.; & Hughes, J. (1987). Promoting awareness and prevention of child sexual victimization using the red flag/green flag program: an evaluation with follow-up. *Journal of Family Violence* 2 (1):11–35.

Kraizer, S.K.; Fryer, G.E.; & Miller, M. (1988). Programming for preventing sexual abuse and abduction: what does it mean when it works? *Child Welfare* 67 (1):69–78.

Miltenberger, R.G., & Thiesse-Duffy, E. (1988). Evaluation of home-based programs for teaching personal safety skills to children. *Journal of Applied Behavior Analysis* 21 (1):81–87.

Peters, S.D.; Wyatt, G.D.; & Finkelhor, D. (1986). Prevalence. In D. Finkelhor (ed.), *Sourcebook on Child Sexual Abuse*. Newbury Park, Calif.: Sage.

Piaget, J. (1963). *The Moral Judgment of the Child*. New York: Free Press.

Plummer, C. (1984). Preventing sexual abuse: what in-school programs teach children. National Conference for Family Violence Researchers. Available from Carol Plummer, Box 421, Kalamazoo, MI 49005.

Quinsey, V.L. (1986). Men who have sex with children. In D. Weisstub (ed.), *Law and Mental Health: International Perspectives*. Vol. 2. New York: Pergamon.

Quinsey, V.L. (1984). Sexual aggression: studies of offenders against women. In D. Weisstub (ed.), *Law and Mental Health: International Perspectives*. Vol. 1. New York: Pergamon.

Quinsey, V.L.; & Chaplin, T.C. (1988). Penile responses of child molesters and normals to descriptions of encounters with children involving sex and violence. *Journal of Interpersonal Violence* 3 (3): 259–274.

Rape & Abuse Crisis Center. (1986). *Red Flag, Green Flag Prevention Book.* Fargo, N.D.: The Center.

Ray, J., & Dietzel, M. (1984). Teaching child sexual abuse prevention. Unpublished manuscript. Available from authors at Rape Crisis Network, N1226 Howard St., Spokane, WA 98201.

Saslawsky, S., & Wurtele, S.K. (1986). Educating children about sexual abuse: implications for pediatric intervention and possible prevention. *Journal of Pediatric Psychology* 11: 225–245.

Spungen, L.A.; Jensen, S.E.; Finkelstein, N.W.; & Satinsky, F.A. (1989). Child personal safety: model program for prevention of child sexual abuse. *Social Work.* 34 (2): 127–131.

Swan, H.L.; Press, A.N.; & Briggs, S.C. (1985). Child sexual abuse prevention: does it work? *Child Welfare* 64 (4): 395–405.

Tharinger, D.J.; Krivacska, J.J.; Laye-McDonough, M.; et al. (1988). Prevention of child sexual abuse: An analysis of issues, education programs and research findings. *School Psychology Review* 17 (4): 614–634.

Thiesse-Duffy, E.; Miltenberger, R.; Kozak, C.; & Suda, K. (1987). Assessment of third graders' knowledge of personal safety skills and initial program evaluation. Paper presented at the thirteenth annual American Bar Association convention, Nashville, May.

Trudell, B., & Whatley, M. (1988). School sexual abuse prevention: unintended consequences and dilemmas. *Child Abuse and Neglect* 12:103–113.

Wolfe, D.A.; MacPherson, T.; Blount, R.; & Wolfe, V.V. (1986). Evaluation of a brief intervention for educating school children in awareness of physical and sexual abuse. *Child Abuse and Neglect* 10:85–92.

Wurtele, S.K. (1987). School-based sexual abuse prevention programs: a review. *Child Abuse and Neglect* 11:483–495.

Wurtele, S.K.; Kast, L.C.; Miller-Perrin, C.L.; & Kondrick, P.A. (1989). A comparison of programs for teaching personal safety skills to pre-schoolers. *Journal of Consulting and Clinical Psychology* 57.

Wurtele, S.K.; Marrs, S.R.; & Miller-Perrin, C.L. (1987). Practice makes perfect? The role of participant modeling in sexual abuse prevention programs. *Journal of Consulting and Clinical Psychology* 55:599–602.

Wurtele, S.K., & Miller-Perrin, C.L. (1987). An evaluation of side effects associated with participation in a child sexual abuse prevention program. *Journal of School Health* 57(6):228–231.

Developing a Child Sexual Abuse Curriculum

Thomas F. Curran

INTRODUCTION

The years since 1975 have witnessed an unprecedented explosion of professional literature and research on the sexual abuse of children. More has been written, studied, and learned about this very complex and sensitive problem since the late 1970s than ever before in history. This knowledge has been made available to child sexual abuse professionals and the general public in a variety of ways. Dozens of very good books on various aspects or intervention skills related to sexual abuse are easily obtainable today. Several professional, peer-reviewed journals devote a great deal of their publication space to sexual abuse. Increasingly, many multidisciplinary and discipline–specific conferences are held each year throughout the country. Some of these conferences are devoted exclusively to child sexual abuse. In addition, various national organizations and societies committed to enhancing professional practices, advocacy, and awareness of child maltreatment have formed.

All such efforts for disseminating knowledge about sexual abuse, however, are directed primarily at very busy professionals. It is assumed that these professionals have the time and financial resources to take advantage of education and training opportunities. Unfortunately, relatively few professionals who work with sexually abused children have the time, financial backing, or energy to stay abreast of developments in the field through the above means. In addition, relatively few professionals receive sufficient or updated on-the-job training on any aspect of sexual abuse. Given the myriad job requirements and time demands placed on such professionals, it is illogical to assume that they or their employers can effectively stay current with developments in a field advancing as rapidly as child sexual abuse. Exacerbating this problem is the fact that alarmingly few medical, psychology, nursing, or social work schools offer even an elective course on child sexual abuse.

In an effort to meet this training and education need, this chapter will present guidelines for developing a child sexual abuse educational curriculum. Key curriculum organizational and planning considerations will be reviewed, along with suggestions for implementing content material and learning activities.

THE NEED FOR A CHILD SEXUAL ABUSE CURRICULUM

The Incidence Rates and Prevalence of Child Sexual Abuse

It is difficult to determine precisely how widespread child sexual abuse is in our society today. Nonetheless, two kinds of data are used in research in an attempt to analyze the extent of child sexual abuse: actual reports of cases to government agencies that are mandated by law to investigate abuse and studies of various random populations that may contain victims or former victims.

The first kind of data, incidence rates, are taken from the number of sexual abuse cases reported during a given time period, usually a year. Incidence rates, then, are calculated by taking the number of abuse reports received during that specified time period and by comparing that number with the total number of children in the geographic population being studied. In 1986, for example, the American Humane Association calculated 132,000 reported cases of child sexual abuse nationwide (American Association for Protecting Children, 1986). This figure represented 15% of all child maltreatment cases received that year.

A major and potentially dangerous limitation of incidence rates is that they represent only reported cases of sexual abuse. Reported cases, it is reasonable to assume, comprise a minority of the actual number of sexual abuse cases. Child sexual abuse, it must be remembered, is a crime whose victims are forced to live with secrecy, fear, and tremendous personal guilt. Children usually are abused by a relative or other familiar adult who maintains the secret of the sexual activity through bribes, threats, or tricks for which the intellectually inferior young victims are no match. In addition, child sexual abuse victims quickly learn that society's most common response to their victimization is to minimize or totally deny its existence. Maintaining the secret sexual relationship with one individual often is perceived by victims as less problematic than trying to convince their families and others that it really happened. Thus, it is quite logical to assume that present incidence rates of child sexual abuse severely underestimate the true extent of the problem.

Much more trustworthy estimates of the extent of the problem are achieved by conducting prevalence studies, which are the other kind of data used to study the extent of sexual abuse. Generally, prevalence studies are conducted by collecting data from adults who are asked to recount any sexually abusive experiences they had as children. Data for prevalence studies can be gathered from a variety of samples, including random samples of the general population, volunteers, and very select populations, such as college students.

Several prevalence studies have concluded that child sexual abuse is one of the most widespread social and health-related problems in American society. More than a decade ago, for example, Finkelhor (1979) conducted the first major prevalence study. With a total sample of over 900 men and women from six New England colleges and universities, his results showed that 19.2% of the women and 8.9% of the men were sexually abused as children. In 1983 Russell used a very narrow definition of sexual abuse in her study of 930 women from the San Francisco area. Russell's study revealed that a staggering 38% of the women in her sample reported a childhood sexual abuse experience. In a 1985 study of 248 women in the Los Angeles area conducted by Wyatt, 62% reported a sexual abuse experience during childhood, with 45% having been subjected to contact sexual abuse. By far the largest prevalence study of child sexual abuse was a 1985 telephone survey conducted by the *Los Angeles Times* (Crewdson, 1988: 28). Of the total sample of over 2,600 men and women interviewed in that study, 22% said they were sexually abused as children. More specifically, over 27% of the women and 16% of the male respondents reported being sexually abused as children. If the percentages from this particular study were extrapolated and applied to the current population, it would mean that over 38 million American adults were sexually abused as children, which is several hundred thousand more than voted for Walter Mondale in the 1984 Presidential election (Crewdson, 1988: 28).

These prevalence study findings reveal that child sexual abuse is so widespread that, arguably, it qualifies as an epidemic. Any physical disease, for example, that medical research indicated affected anywhere from 19.2% to 45% of the nation's female child population unquestionably would be regarded as an epidemic, if not a national crisis. At the very least, therefore, such prevalence studies offer irrefutable evidence of the need for specialized training and formal educational curricula on child sexual abuse. In light of these prevalence rates, the growing number of very complex and bizarre multiple victim–multiple perpetrator cases (Burgess, 1984; Hollingsworth, 1986; Kelley, 1988), and the swift pace with which new research developments are being made, an educational curriculum on child sexual abuse should be required in all health, mental health, and human services schools throughout the country.

MORE PROOF OF THE NEED FOR A CHILD SEXUAL ABUSE EDUCATIONAL CURRICULUM

Curriculum Planning

Thorough and meticulous planning is essential to the success of any educational curriculum. This is especially true when considering a topic as highly specialized, controversial, and emotionally charged as child sexual abuse. Issues such as curriculum goals and objectives and content and learning activities are but a few of the many aspects of curriculum planning that must be carefully considered.

How Adults Learn

Planning a child sexual abuse educational curriculum, like any adult education activity, must be based upon an understanding of how adults learn. It is now widely recognized that adults do not learn in the same way or under the same conditions as children. Differences between child and adult learning were articulate as far back as the 1920s. Lindeman (1926), for example, noted a few major assumptions about adult learners and adult education. He observed the following about adult learning:

1. Adults are motivated to learn as they experience needs and interests that learning will satisfy.

2. Experience is the single richest source for adult learning; therefore, the core methodology of adult education should be the analysis of experience.

3. Adults have a deep need to be self-directing.

Andragogy vs. Pedagogy

The difference between how adults and children learn has been clarified and elaborated upon since 1970, primarily because of the work of Malcolm Knowles. The terms andragogy and pedagogy were popularized by Knowles to explain the difference between child and adult learning.

The term "pedagogy" is derived from the Greek *paid* (meaning "child") and *agogos* (meaning "learning"), and literally it is defined as the art and science of teaching children (Knowles, 1970). Knowles (1984a: 52) characterizes pedagogy as involuntary and teacher-directed education that leaves to the learner only the submissive role of following the teacher's instructions. The following are other assumptions Knowles (1984b: 9) makes about the pedagogical model of learning:

1. The learner is totally dependent upon the teacher.

2. The learner's life experiences are irrelevant; only the teacher's experiences are valued.

3. Readiness to learn is a function of age.

4. The orientation to learning is purely "subject-centered"; learning is limited to acquiring prescribed subject matter content.

5. The motivation to learn is primarily from external forces, such as parents, desire for good grades, or teacher pressure.

For several reasons, Knowles regards pedagogy as having failed and inappropriate for adult learners. First, adults are almost always voluntary learners and will leave learning experiences that do not satisfy their needs. Second, pedagogy is premised on the archaic notion that education's purpose is the transmittal of knowledge. Finally, adult learners are very likely to possess strong internal motivations to learn, but pedagogy does not consider such self-directed behavior. In some ways, in fact, self-directed behavior is regarded as antithetical to the purpose and goals of pedagogy.

Concluding that such a learning model could not meet the unique needs of adult learners, Knowles promulgated the term "andragogy," which comes from the Greek *Aner* (meaning "man") and *Agogs* (meaning "learning"). Translated literally, Knowles (1970) defines andragogy as the art and science of helping adults learn. Andragogy represented Knowles's attempt to formulate a theory of adult learning that included and highlighted the characteristics unique to adult learners.

Unlike pedagogy, the andragogical model is premised on several major assumptions about adults and adult learners. First, the andragogical model regards the learner as being self-directed (Knowles 1984b: 9). Much more than children, adults have a psychological need to be perceived and treated by others as being capable of taking responsibility for themselves. Knowles theorized that, because of their need to feel responsible for their own decisions, adults naturally will resent and resist learning situations in which they feel something is being imposed against their will. Adult learners need to know and should be told why they need to learn something before undertaking to learn it. Without this personal control, the ultimate value of the learning experience is questionable.

Second, the andragogical model values the learner's life experiences (Knowles 1984b: 10). Realizing that as people develop into adulthood they accumulate a ever growing reservoir of experiences, Knowles determined that, consequently, adults are the best and richest resource for one another in adult learning situations. Life experience is also important for adult learners because as adults grow older their experiences tend to shape their self-identities. To children, experience is something that happens to them; to adults, however, experience is who they are (Knowles, 1984a: 58). The obvious implication of this fact for any adult education experience is that in a situation in which adult experiences are ignored or minimized, they can be expected to perceive this as not just rejecting their experience, but also as rejecting them as people.

A third assumption that characterizes andragogy is that adults learn best and most effectively when they experience or perceive a personal need to know or do something in order to cope effectively with their real-life situations. Very often this "readiness to learn" is associated with an adult's job requirements or employment goals. A new job or a desired promotion, for example, often inspires a readiness to learn. For some adults, on the other hand, this readiness is a natural state that requires no external stimulus to activate.

Another assumption about adult learners included in the andragogical model is that adults' orientation to learning is different from children's. The orientation of formal learning for children is subject-centered. In contrast, adults' orientation to learning is life-centered (or task-centered or problem-centered). Adults are motivated to learn something to the extent that they perceive that it will help them solve real-life problems (Knowles, 1984a: 59). Content for adult learning experiences, then, is most effective when presented in the context of application to situations in adult learners' lives.

The final assumption that distinguishes child learners from adult learners is that the latter respond to and experience different motivations to learn. Unlike pedagogy, which assumes that learners can be motivated to learn only by external motivators such as grades or parental pressure, the andragogical model assumes that the strongest and most enduring motivators are internal. Some external motivators, such as higher salaries or job promotions, can motivate some adult learners, but they do not appear to have the strength of internal motivators such as self-esteem and the desire for a better quality of life.

It should be noted that the pedagogical model and its concomitant assumptions are not inherently inappropriate for all adults in all adult learning situations, nor is the andragogical model naturally appropriate. Knowles has clarified the very important distinctions and potential uses of the two models. Pedagogy, according to Knowles, is an ideological model that excludes the aforementioned andragogical assumptions. The andragogical model, on the other hand, he classifies as a system of assumptions that include the pedagogical assumptions (Knowles, 1984a: 62).

In real life this means that educators, trainers, and even curriculum designers should evaluate carefully which assumptions are realistic in a given learning situation. There may be situations, for example, in which a pedagogical strategy is appropriate for an adult learning situation. It would not be inappropriate for adult learners to be taught by the pedagogical model, for instance, in a learning situation where the subject matter is totally foreign (which would make the adult learners naturally dependent), when they did not initially understand the relevance of the subject matter to their life tasks, when they need to accumulate a given body of subject matter in order to accomplish a required task, or when they feel no internal need to learn vital or job-related course material (Knowles, 1984a: 62). To illustrate this possibility, imagine a medical student who participates in a child sexual abuse course. Despite the student's advanced academic training, she probably would need to have a didactic instructor teach her the course content, how to organize it, what its special terminology was, and what the resources were for learning about it before she would be able to take initiative for learning the course. When, however, the medical student reached the point in the child sexual abuse course where she no longer needed to be dependent on the instructor, the instructor's pedagogical assumptions must yield to andragogical assumptions of learning. At that point it will be the instructor's responsibility to do everything possible to help the medical student take more responsibility for her own learning.

The first step in planning a curriculum on child sexual abuse or any subject in which adults will be the anticipated learners, then, is to review carefully which learning assumptions, pedagogical or andragogical, initially are realistic for the target student population. The course content, teaching style, course organization, assignments, and resources to be used should be planned and developed to accommodate that learning assumption.

TRAINING VS. COLLEGE-BASED CURRICULUM

A second major curriculum planning step is to determine whether the curriculum will be job-related training or a college-based course. College curricula usually intend a broader knowledge base than job-related training. College-based curricula can be complicated, especially with nontraditional courses such as child sexual abuse, and long-range planning is usually necessary to get a program accepted for and actually included in a department or a school's course selection. The following approaches are offered merely as considerations when planning or attempting to introduce a new curriculum into an existing college program.

1. *The Problem/Theme Approach.* Start by defining the problem to be addressed by the proposed curriculum. Select a theme for the proposed curriculum and introduce it to the existing faculty through workshops, seminars, or other demonstrations. At the end of the demonstration, the faculty will determine the im portance of the problem/theme and make a decision regarding its integration into the existing course selections. The importance of curriculum organization, clarity of content, goals, and learning activities during such presentations cannot be overstated.

2. *The Emerging Field Approach.* Another approach to organizing a curriculum for introduction into a college program is what is referred to as "emerging field." Simply stated, emerging field focuses on such questions as, Have conventional learning ap proaches to this problem been successful? If not, present pos sible reasons why. Is a new professor emerging to address this problem? Why should a particular college department address this problem?

3. *The Discovery Approach.* In the "discovery approach" everybody agrees on the type of learning needed. The focus, therefore, is on curriculum design approaches that will result in the agreed-upon type of learning. A multidisciplinary approach, for example, may not lend itself to certain classroom lectures but may be very well suited for students from different disciplines to work on a case presentation.

Unlike college-based curricula, training curricula are usually job-related and provide students with specific skills needed to perform their jobs. The following suggestions are offered for consideration when planning a job training curriculum.

1. *Know the Target Population.* Knowing the training audience is a essential prerequisite for deciding upon an adult learning model. As noted, having a group of adult trainees does not automatically imply the application of an andragogical model of adult learning. Whether a pedagogical or andragogical assumption is realistic will depend on many characteristics of the population targeted to receive the training.

2. *Analyze the Job to Be Performed.* When analyzing the job to be performed, it is also important to provide a brief operational description of the individual duties and conditions under which the job is to be performed.

3. *Clearly Specify All Job Tasks.* In the process of providing the details of the job, the skills, knowledge, and attitude required to do the job will become clear.

4. *Identify Individual Characteristics.* The human and job-specific attributes necessary to do the job should be outlined as clearly as possible.

5. *Develop Written Behavioral Objectives.* Specify what the trainee should be able to accomplish after successfully completing the program, under what conditions and according to what performance standards.

6. *Design the Learning Environment.* Using principals and assumptions of adult learning, determine how the training curriculum content can be taught most effectively to the target audience.

7. *Evaluation.* Establish specific measures of success (criteria) and use experimental and nonexperimental designs to determine what changes have occurred during training and, later, on the job.

Student Motivation to Learn

In planning any educational or training curriculum, but especially one as specialized as a child sexual abuse curriculum, one must remember at all times that all people are not alike. While this notion may sound trite, if not insulting, it is a vitally important key to understanding the concept of motivation. Adult human learning could not occur without motivation (Ribler, 1983: 4). Many different motivation theories have developed to explain why people seem to have different motivations under similar circumstances. It is particularly important to consider such theories when planning a curriculum as emotionally charged as one on child sexual abuse. The curriculum planner and instructor must realize and accept that people are different and, therefore, cannot be expected to have the same motivations.

Motivation is an individual internal force. What motivates one person may have absolutely no meaning to another. When planning or conducting an education curriculum, for example, it is important to know what motivation to learn the students bring to the class. Not all adult learners are voluntary learners. This is especially true in many job training or in-service programs. Adult learners enrolled in a college-based course, on the other hand, usually will be voluntary learners. Regardless of the students' motivation, it is important when planning any curriculum to remember that adult learners will be much more receptive to training or course material that is perceived as being important to them. Having some knowledge of the learning audience, therefore, may be one way to capture the attention, if not the motivation, of some involuntary learners. It is also important to consider carefully the role of curriculum content and methods of instruction in student motivation.

CURRICULUM DEVELOPMENT

The process of actually developing an educational curriculum should be approached after very careful thought has been given to the various planning considerations. Curriculum development, then, usually involves the orderly completion of several tasks. Regardless of curriculum subject matter, it is recommended that these development tasks always be outlined in clear and precise behavioral terms. The importance of narrowly defining tasks when developing a child sexual abuse curriculum cannot be overstated. Because child sexual abuse is such a complex problem with a rapidly growing research and knowledge base in the fields of law, medicine, psychiatry and psychology, nursing, social work, sociology, and law enforcement, an educational curriculum must be narrowly focused with very specific developmental tasks to be performed. Any attempt at developing or implementing a sexual abuse curriculum with broad developmental tasks will seriously dilute the planned educational activity.

The following are tasks that must be specifically and clearly outlined when developing a child sexual abuse curriculum.

Develop Major Curriculum Goals

The curriculum goals should describe outcomes or ends desired. Most curricula have several goals, all of which should describe the various fundamental competencies to be expected upon completion. Curriculum goals may be stated in general terms, but it is strongly recommended that they be classified and ranked in order of importance. The following are examples of goals for a rather narrowly focused child sexual abuse curriculum:

1. To introduce students to the problem of child sexual abuse from the victim's perspective so the students can better understand its serious effects.

2. To enable students to explore their own attitudes about child sexual abuse and to consider the impact of those attitudes on their ability to respond appropriately to suspected cases.

3. To provide information on definitions and indicators of child sexual abuse.

One way to develop curriculum goals effectively is to conduct a needs assessment, which can be very elaborate and formal or informal. Such an instrument can be very useful in developing a curriculum on child sexual abuse because it draws from many different professional disciplines and involves a very wide range of skills, conceptual frameworks, and constantly emerging research findings. Because it would give adult learners some control over their leaning experience, a needs assessment would constitute one element of an andragogical model. A needs assessment is recommended particularly when planning and developing a sexual abuse curriculum for very experienced professionals.

Develop Curriculum Objectives

Curriculum objectives should express the intended student outcomes or performances expected of students upon completion of the program. Objectives should be stated in terms of specific observable behavior or performance and not simply describe what the students have learned (Ribler, 1983: 23). In addition, curriculum objectives should be measurable.

In a highly specialized curriculum, such as child sexual abuse, it is advisable to package objectives into stratified units. The total time allotted for the curriculum, for example, can be divided into sections or modules. These can represent different topics or subject areas of the curriculum.

The following are examples of objectives for a narrowly focused child sexual abuse curriculum that has been divided into units. At the conclusion of the unit, students will be able to

1. Give a general definition of child sexual abuse.

2. List four physical and four behavioral indicators of child sexual abuse.

3. Describe two ways in which the legal and child protective systems actually can increase emotional trauma for a victim of child sexual abuse.

Notice the specificity, clarity, and provision for measuring each of these curriculum objectives. It is important, too, for objectives to be practical and actually attainable by the students. Unrealistic or unattainable objectives can defeat the very purpose of a curriculum.

Identify Prerequisite Courses or Training

Because child sexual abuse is such a complex, multifaceted and emotionally charged topic, any educational curriculum must consider perquisite experience or course work to be completed before a student can participate. Identified curriculum prerequisites, of course, will depend upon the depth or complexity of the curriculum content being offered.

This, however, is not always the case. While most prerequisites are determined by the relevant skills or knowledge base necessary for students to participate effectively in a given course, prerequisites for a child sexual abuse curriculum should take other factors into consideration. If, for example, the curriculum content is very skill-intensive or -centered on advanced theoretical or research material, then only students with advanced child sexual abuse education or training backgrounds or with extensive work experience should be enrolled. It is virtually impossible to implement a curriculum effectively, particularly a specialized curriculum, when the target audience is simply unprepared or over-prepared to comprehend the content material.

In addition, students who enroll in a child sexual abuse curriculum undoubtedly do so with varied assumptions and expectations. Some may be adult survivors of child sexual abuse and expect the curriculum to address and remedy issues related to their own experience. Some may be very interested in the subject but have preconceived and simplistic ideas about sexual abuse that are incorrect. Still, other students may regard child sexual abuse to be a cause or issue for certain groups. These assumptions and expectations are not necessarily bad. When, however, a class contains students with vastly different levels of formal education or training, such assumptions and expectations can seriously obstruct learning opportunities in even the most organized curriculum.

It is strongly recommended, therefore, that prerequisite courses or direct practice experience be required for a sexual abuse curriculum. Developing a beginning or introductory course that covers very basic information about child sexual abuse could satisfy at least one of the prerequisites. Such an introductory course could be three to four hours in length and present information aimed at the following: sensitizing students about sexual abuse and their own attitudes and responses, conveying general information or definitions, possible indicators of abuse and characteristics, conveying general information about victims and offenders, and providing a general examination of some of the conceptual frameworks that have been developed to explain sexual abuse.

Develop Curriculum Criterion Test Measures

Curriculum criterion test measures assess whether, or to what extent, a curriculum satisfied its stated objectives. For a child sexual abuse curriculum, such test measurers should be designed to assess students' knowledge and performance. It is very important to develop a test in which the students can show knowledge they acquired from the curriculum. In a sexual abuse curriculum, however, it is necessary to design a test measure that asks students to preform or demonstrate what they have learned. This additional measure, of course, will depend on the curriculum purpose and concomitant learning activities. Regardless of the curriculum content or level of sophistication, demonstrating the application of knowledge through actual performance is the most accurate and meaningful measure of learning. Where a performance test measure is required, however, the curriculum developer or planner must outline precisely what performance will be tested, how and why.

Develop an Implementation Plan

The curriculum implementation plan should detail how the curriculum material will be presented to achieve most effectively the stated goals and learning objectives. An instructional model for the curriculum should be established as part of the implementation plan. This involves deciding how the curriculum material will be presented to the students. Presentation formats can be self-instructional, lecture, or seminar. Sometimes, particularly in college-based programs, the instructional model used will be determined by the class size.

Determine Class Size

The size of the class for a child sexual abuse curriculum is a very important consideration. Regardless of the mode of instruction chosen or the advanced level of the curriculum content, class size should be kept very small. The ideal size for such a specialized curriculum is 20 to 30 students. This number will prove very manageable, especially when the class works on small group exercises. A small class size also will provide for more orderly classroom discussion and exchange of ideas.

A child sexual abuse curriculum probably will be a very exciting and attractive selection at any level of a college-based program. It is highly recommended, however, that registration be closed at 30 students and that such a cap be rigidly followed. Large class sizes, especially with students from different educational backgrounds, will prove very problematic to a child sexual abuse curriculum.

Develop Curriculum Content

Because the focus of this chapter is on microlevel or classroom curriculum development, the selected content, like the learning activities, can and should be very specific. When first planning and developing the curriculum content, it may be useful to view it as a "road map" for reaching the promulgated goals and objectives. If the curriculum goals and learning objectives are clearly and specifically outlined, then the task of developing content material should be relatively easy. Keep in mind, however, that adult learners tend to be "problem-centered" in their orientation to learning. Because of this orientation, curriculum content should focus on problem areas relevant to the adult learners instead of purely academic subject areas.

When developing curriculum content, particularly for adult learners, it is important to make the material flow in a logical and practical sequence. Content material show flow, for example, from simple concepts and learning activities to the more complex and from the general to increasingly more specific. Depending upon the nature and objectives of the curriculum, it may be very useful to develop content that follows the sequence of the learners' actual job tasks. A curriculum developed for a course on the initial assessment, intervention, and management of child sexual abuse cases, for example, will contain skill-centered content material developed with a child protective services or law enforcement investigators' actual job duties in mind.

In addition to considering the curriculum goals and objectives, and how to make the material flow logically, the choice of content also must comport with the intended use of the curriculum. Content developers must ask themselves if the intended use of the curriculum is as an orientation to the topic and subject matter, to develop knowledge and skill, or to increase knowledge and skill. The answer to this question should help structure and formulate the curriculum content.

Timing is a very important consideration in the development of curriculum content. Because of the complex and controversial nature of so many areas of child sexual abuse, it is strongly suggested that the general curriculum subject matter be divided into smaller units or modules. Each unit or module, in turn, should have a specified time limit that should be closely followed. Without dividing the curriculum into smaller, more specific units and adhering to set time schedules, confusion and chaos will develop and valuable learning opportunities will be lost.

Select Instructional Method

After the curriculum content has been developed, how that content can be implemented most effectively must be decided. Very little controversy should surround the choice of instructional method for a child sexual abuse curriculum. While much of the instructional method will be didactic in nature, it is essential that a child sexual abuse curriculum also include experiential learning activities. Using methods such as case studies, role plays, and group problem assignments are very effective learning activities and instructional methods.

The Curriculum Instructor

Who should teach a curriculum on child sexual abuse? What background and qualities, both personal and professional, should this individual possess? These questions are very important to the overall success and effectiveness of the learning experience and should not be dismissed without careful consideration.

The following qualities are some of the more important ones that the curriculum instructor should possess:

1. Knowledge of child sexual abuse and current literature and research

2. Skill as a group leader

3. Organization

4. Self-awareness

5. A sense of humor

Of all these qualities, it is particularly important that the instructor know child sexual abuse and be familiar with the current literature and research. In addition, the instructor must be comfortable with him/herself and with discussing very sensitive and emotional material. If the instructor is not personally comfortable discussing these issues, the class will not be either.

CONCLUSIONS

In developing a sexual abuse curriculum, whether for a college-based or job training program, it is important to identify on what premise the curriculum is based. More specifically, it is helpful to articulate what premise about child sexual abuse and the most appropriate way of interviewing or managing cases is reflected in a particular curriculum.

A child sexual abuse curriculum, for example, can be based on the premise that individuals involved in the initial assessment and intervention of sexual abuse cases must have a very comprehensive understanding of the problem. A curriculum also can be based on the premise that personal comfort and self-awareness regarding sexual abuse, sexuality, and other emotional issues must at least accompany, if not supersede, all other formal training and education.

A premise can be compared to a theory of a curriculum. The developer's feelings about child sexual abuse, what component parts are particularly important, and how the problem should be managed all are reflected in the content of the curriculum. Pay very close attention, therefore, to the curriculum title. It will be far more effective and educational to limit the scope of any child sexual abuse curriculum content. The problem is far too vast and complex to address every aspect adequately in one course or curriculum. Except for a general introductory curriculum, it is much more practical to address small, separate aspects of child sexual abuse in a series of courses. Any attempt to do otherwise will weaken drastically the curriculum premise or theory.

Remember, too that a child sexual abuse curriculum's ultimate effectiveness will depend, in large part, on how well it is wedded to the specific needs of the community in which it is taught. A curriculum that dismisses or diminishes the community's needs regarding child sexual abuse will be of only minimal value to the students. During the planning and development stages of any type of child sexual abuse curriculum, the unique training and educational needs of the community, both lay and professional, should be surveyed. If a curriculum is viewed as a tool for developing greater sensitivity, knowledge and skill on the part of individuals who handle child sexual abuse cases, then that tool should be used to mend what is of particular concern to the community in which it is available.

REFERENCES

American Association for Protecting Children. (1986). *Highlights of Official Child Neglect and Abuse Reporting.* Denver: American Humane Association.

Burgess, A.W. (ed). (1984). *Child Pornography and Sex Rings.* Lexington, Mass.: Lexington Books.

Crewdson, J. (1988). *By Silence Betrayed.* P. 28. New York: Harper & Row.

Finkelhor, D. (1979). *Sexually Victimized Children.* New York: Free Press.

Hollingsworth, J. (1986). *Unspeakable Acts.* New York: Congdon & Weed.

Kelley, S. J. (1988). "Ritualistic abuse of children: dynamics and impact. *Cult Studies Journal* 5 (2): 228–236.

Knowles, M.S. (1984a). *The Adult Learner: A Neglected Species.* 3rd ed. P. 52. Houston: Gulf Publishing.

Knowles, M.S. (1984b). *Andragogy in Action.* San Francisco: Jossey-Bass.

Knowles, M.S. (1970). *The Modern Practice of Adult Education: Andragogy vs. Pedagogy.* New York: Associated Press.

Lindeman, E.C. (1926). *The Meaning of Adult Education.* P. 166. New York: New Republic.

Ribler, R.I. (1983). *Training Development Guide.* Reston, Va.: Reston Publishing.

Russell, D. (1983). The incidence and prevalence of intrafamilial and extrafamilial sexual abuse of female children. *Child Abuse and Neglect* 7: 133–146.

Wyatt, G. (1985). The sexual abuse of Afro-American and white American women in childhood. *Child Abuse and Neglect* 9: 507–519.

PART IV

THE AGGRESSORS

Research on Adolescent Sex Offenders

Judith V. Becker
Meg S. Kaplan

INTRODUCTION

Until recently, the adolescent sexual offender has been neglected in the clinical and research literature. This is surprising given that 20% of forcible rapes in this country are committed by adolescents and that adolescents are responsible for a considerable number of child sexual molestations.

This chapter will discuss our clinical research experience with a male adolescent sex offender population. Specifically, topics to be covered are characteristics of adolescent sex offenders, assessment, prior victimization, family variables, treatment and ethical issues.

Characteristics—Description of Population

Sexual aggression by adolescents is a serious and widespread problem in our society yet only recently have research efforts focused on this population of adolescent perpetrators. Several researchers have found that a significant number of adult offenders had the onset of their deviant sexual interest patterns soon after puberty (Brecker, 1978; Groth & Birnbaum, 1979; Longo & Groth, 1983).

Results from a study by Abel, Mittelman, and Becker (1985) indicate that of 411 adult sex offenders seen voluntarily at an outpatient clinic, 58.4% reported that the onset of their deviant sexual arousal occurred prior to the age of 18. Recent surveys of adolescent offenders have also found indications that a significant number had committed their first sexual offenses between the ages of 12 and 15 years (Awad, Saunders, & Levene, 1979; Longo, 1982)

Several researchers have suggested that the early onset of deviant sexual behavior in male adolescents may have simply been a matter of innocent sex play, experimentation, or that the sexual offenses were due to the normal aggressiveness of sexually maturing adolescents (Finkelhor, 1979; Gagnon, 1965; Reiss, 1960; Roberts, Abrams, & Finch, 1973). Research has suggested elsewise (Groth, 1977). Thus, although research efforts in the area of adolescent sexual aggression have begun, much further research needs to be conducted.

Becker, Cunningham-Rathner, and Kaplan (1986) conducted a study to provide data regarding the characteristics of adolescents who had been identified as sexual offenders and had been permitted to remain in the community under supervision rather then being incarcerated. Participating in the study were 67 adolescent males between the ages of 13 and 19 (mean, 15.47 years), the majority of whom had been charged with or convicted of a sexual crime. All subjects were referred either from the criminal justice system or from social service agencies to the Sexual Behavior Clinic (SBC), an outpatient evaluation and treatment clinic for sexual offenders. All subjects were nonpsychotic and able to give informed consent. Of the subjects, 12% were Caucasian, 63% were black, and 25% were Hispanic.

The majority of subjects were referred by probation officers (31.3%). Other referral sources included courts (22.4%), Division for Youth (17.9%), Legal Aid lawyers (9%), parole officers (3%), district attorneys (1.5%), and other sources (14.9%), which included social service agencies and special services for children.

The legal status of subjects at the time of referral was as follows: 43.3% on probation, 25.4% presentence, 11.9% in Division for Youth facilities, 6% on parole, 4.5% PINS (persons in need of supervision) petitions, 3% adjudicated contemplating dismissal (ACD), and 6% other (not officially charged with a sexual crime).

At the time of evaluation, 35.8% were residing with their mothers only, 32.4% with both parents, 11.9% in a group home, 4.5% with a legal guardian, 4.5% with a grandmother, 1.5% with a father only,

1.5% with foster parents, 1.5% in detention centers, 1.5% lived alone, 1.5% with a sibling; and 3% in homes for runaways.

Of the adolescents, 97% reported that they had never been hospitalized for a psychiatric illness; 88% reported that immediate family members had never been hospitalized for a psychiatric illness; 4.5% reported that at least one family member had been hospitalized for a psychiatric illness; and 7.5% reported that they did not have any knowledge of any family psychiatric hospitalizations.

Prior Arrests for Nonsexual Crimes

Subjects' self-reported arrests for nonsexual crimes were: never committed (71.6%), once (11.9%), twice (6%), three times (4.5%), and more than three arrests for nonsexual crimes (6%). Of the subjects, 3% reported using a weapon during these crimes. The most recent type of nonsexual crimes committed were robbery (9%) and burglary (6%). Although subjects reported using alcohol or marijuana on occasion, only 3% had been arrested for a drug-related crime.

Prior Arrests for Sexual Crimes

Of the subjects, 10.4% reported never having been arrested for a sexual crime, 79.1% reported being arrested once, 7.5% twice, and 3% three times or more. Of those arrested for a sexual crime, 49.3% did not spend any time incarcerated for the offense, 25.4% spent less than one week incarcerated, 6% less than one month, 7.5% less than six months, 1.5% between six months and one year, and 10.4% more than one year.

Types of Self-reported Sexual Crimes Committed

For the purpose of the study, the following categorical definitions were used:

1. Offenders whose victims were more than 5 years younger than themselves were defined as pedophiles. Pedophiles were then divided into groups on the basis of (a) age of victim (child 9 to 12 years of age or child age 8 or under); (b) sex of victim (female pedophile indicates that the offender had engaged in "hands-on" sexual behavior with a female child and male pedophile indicates an adolescent had engaged in "hands-on" sexual behavior with a male child); and (c) relationship of offender to the victim (female

incest pedophile indicates an adolescent who had engaged in "hands-on" sexual behavior with a female child relative and male incest pedophile indicates an adolescent who had engaged in "hands-on" sexual behavior with a male child relative).

2. Offenders whose victims were less than five years younger than themselves were defined as rapists. Rapists were then subdivided by (a) age of victim (adult, peer, or 9 to 12 years of age), (b) sex of victim (female rape was defined as forced sexual contact or sexual penetration against a nonrelative female, and male rape was defined as forced sexual contact or penetration of a nonrelative male), and (c) relationship of offender to the victim (female rape incest was defined as forced sexual contact or penetration of a female relative and male rape incest was defined as forced sexual contact or penetration of a male relative).

3. Consensual incest was defined as offenders who committed sexual acts with consenting relatives. (Again these offenders were subdivided by age and sex of the consenting relative.)

4. Offenders who rubbed (with their sexual body parts) or touched (with their hands) the genitals or buttocks of a clothed victim, usually in a crowd, were labeled as frotteurs. (Again these offenders were subdivided by age and sex of the victim.)

5. Offenders who looked at other people (usually through windows) for the express purpose of obtaining sexual excitement were labeled as voyeurs. (These were also subdivided by age and sex of the person at whom they were looking.)

6. Offenders who exposed their buttocks in public were labeled as mooners. (These offenders were also subdivided by age and sex of target.)

Of the subjects, 41 (63%) were categorized as pedophiles (24 female pedophiles and 17 male pedophiles). The majority of victims were unrelated to the offender and were younger than 8 years of age. *It was reported to the SBC or the pedophiles self-reported, that in total the 41 had completed 63 deviant sexual acts against 53 victims. However, for the majority of subjects, the official records noted only 1 offense per adolescent.* In addition, it was reported to the SBC or self-reported that the pedophiles had attempted 9 further deviant sexual acts against 9 victims. The aggression rating indicates the amount of force used against the victim in the commission of the crime. Rating is on a scale from 0 (not applicable), 1 (noncoercion), 2 (verbal coercion), 3 (physical coercion), to 4 (excessive physical coercion).

The average amount of force, either reported to the SBC or self-reported, that was used against these victims was a rating of 2.9, indicating that the adolescents used physical coercion to commit the crime.

The next largest category of offenders evaluated were rapists. Seventeen adolescents had committed rape (12 had raped females, 5 had raped males). It was reported to the SBC or self-reported that these 17 adolescents had committed 39 rapes against 13 victims, and had also attempted a total of 10 rapes against 10 victims. The average amount of force used against the female victims was 3.16 (more than enough physical coercion in order to commit the crime) and 2.88 (enough physical coercion in order to commit the crime) against male victims.

Two subjects had engaged in consensual incest with females aged 9 to 12. There was no coercion, as the sexual interest was mutual. The behavior involved a total of 155 sexual acts with 2 consenting female relatives. The remaining 7 subjects included 4 who had engaged in frottage against females aged 9 to adult. They had aggression ratings of 1 (noncoercion) and 2 (verbal coercion) since they rubbed against their victims without holding them or they said something to them and then ran. Two subjects had engaged in voyeurism and had committed 50 acts. Their aggression ratings were 1 (noncoercion) since their victims were unaware of their behavior. One subject had engaged in mooning against 2 female adults. His aggression rating was 1 (noncoercion) since he did not touch or speak to the targets.

It is important to note that these data likely reflect an underreporting of deviant sexual behaviors since most sexual offenders (both adolescent and adult) tend to minimize the extent of their arousal. Some subjects only reported the crimes for which they had been referred (even though official reports indicated that they had been involved in additional deviant sexual behavior). Other subjects' reports agreed totally with the official records (even though they may have committed other sexual crimes), and still other subjects admitted to engaging in additional deviant sexual behaviors that were unknown to the authorities. Therefore, the data includes what was self-reported to us by the subjects (behaviors both known and unknown to the authorities) as well as what was reported to us by the authorities (when the subjects denied any involvement in deviant sexual behaviors). In addition, the data reflect the highest aggression rating used during any of the deviant sexual behaviors for each individual subject. The aggression ratings may reflect higher levels of force than were actually used with any one victim; however, the data were reported in this manner since the highest aggression actually perpetrated against an individual shows the offender's potential dangerousness toward victims in our society.

Subjects were asked about the extent to which they agreed with the criminal justice records or referral sources's statements of their offense(s). The majority of subjects (41.8%) admitted in part to the reported offenses. The remaining subjects either admitted to the total extent of the reported act(s) (26.9%) or denied completely any involvement (31.3%). These findings are not surprising, since we know that subjects tend to minimize their deviant sexual interests, especially during an initial clinical interview.

Nondeviant Sexual Histories

For the purpose of this study, nondeviant sex was defined as a noncoercive sexual interaction with a nonrelative peer. Nondeviant sexual experiences were divided into two categories (1) nongenital (kissing, breast fondling, and hugging) and (2) genital (oral or manual stimulation, vaginal or anal stimulation of the genitals, or penetration). Of the 67 subjects, 82% had engaged in nondeviant, nongenital sexual behavior and 58% had engaged in nondeviant genital sexual behaviors.

Using the Kinsey Rating Scale, a self-report of sexual preference where 0 indicates exclusive heterosexual arousal and 6 indicates exclusive homosexual arousal, 88.1% of subjects rated themselves as Kinsey 0, 9% as 1, 1.5% as 2, and 1.5% as 3 (bisexual). No subjects reported exclusive homosexual arousal. Thus the deviant sexual behavior of the majority of adolescents in this study was not the only or the first sexual contact. Most of the subjects had previously engaged in nondeviant sexual behaviors. These findings support the notion that adolescents who engage in deviant sexual behavior are not merely experimenting but may be developing patterns of deviant sexual interest similar to those found in adult sexual offenders.

Discussion

We have described a population of male adolescents who have been identified by the criminal justice system as sexual offenders and allowed to remain in the community to receive evaluation and treatment. These data should not be generalized to all adolescent sexual offenders since (1) differences exist between those adolescents the criminal justice system allows to remain in the community and those who are incarcerated and (2) this sample was mostly inner-city adolescents from minority groups.

CHARACTERISTICS OF ADOLESCENT INCEST PERPETRATORS

A similar study was conducted with adolescent incest perpetrators (Becker, Kaplan, Cunningham-Rathner, & Kavoussi, 1986). Subjects were 22 adolescent males between the ages of 13 and 18 (X = 14.8) who had been charged or convicted of a sexual crime against a family member. For the purpose of this study, incest is defined as sexual contact between any family members, biological or individuals living in a family environment and recognized as a family member (e.g., stepbrothers). Of the subjects, 54% were black, 32% Hispanic, and 14% Caucasian.

Psychiatric Disorders

A psychiatrist interviewed 19 subjects to determine the presence of any psychiatric disorders; 5 of these subjects (26.3%) had no DSM-III disorders. The remaining 14 subjects (73.7%) had some type of psychiatric diagnosis. Some in the group had more than one disorder: 12 had conduct disorders (9 socialized, 3 aggressive), 5 had attention-deficit disorders, for alcohol and marijuana abuse, 2 adjustment disorders, 2 social phobias, 1 dysthymia, and 1 posttraumatic stress disorder.

Regarding history of significant medical disease or trauma, 77.3% reported no such history and 22.7% reported that they had some prior physical trauma.

Nondeviant Sexual Experiences

For the purpose of this study, nondeviant sex was defined as noncoercive sexual interaction with a peer. A prior nondeviant, nongenital sexual experience was reported by 95% of subjects. The mean age for first experience was 10.3 years. The range was from ages 7 to 15. Using the Kinsey Rating Scale, all subjects rated themselves as exclusively heterosexual.

Incest Diagnoses

Of the 22 subjects, 17 (77.3%) were defined as pedophiles. Of these pedophiles, 64.7% had female victims and 35.3% had male victims. The pedophiles had committed 37 acts against 18 victims.

Incest rapes (3) had been committed by 13.6% of the subjects. One subject had completed 24 rapes of 1 male victim. The 2 subjects who targeted females had 1 attempted rape against 1 victim and 1 completed rape against 1 victim. There were 2 cases (9.1%) of consensual incest where subjects had attempted 6 acts against 1 victim and completed 229 acts against 2 victims.

Total Deviant Sexual Attempts and Completions

In addition to their primary incest diagnoses, the 22 subjects also reported 6 additional incest diagnoses. These included 1 case of incest pedophilia with a female child age 9–12 (1 victim, 5 completions); 3 incest rapes; 1 female age 9–12 (1 victim, 1 attempt); 1 female age 13–17 (12 victims, 116 completions; and 1 victim, 4 attempts); and 1 female over age 18 (1 victim, 1 completion); and 1 case of voyeurism to a female age 13–17 (1 victim, 1 completion).

Nonincest Sexual Offenses

In addition to the incest diagnosis, the 22 subjects had committed an additional 6 types of nonincest sexual offenses. Two of these subjects had committed nonincest pedophilic acts (1 each against 1 male and 1 female); 1 had committed a rape of an adult female; 1 had committed 6 acts (against 6 victims) of frottage; 2 subjects had committed 50 acts of voyeurism against 10 victims; 2 had exposed buttocks to 3 victims; 1 had made 78 obscene phone calls to 39 victims. The mean age at the onset of these crimes was 13.4 years.

Discussion

These results cannot be compared to other studies because, to our knowledge, there are no published investigations surveying adolescent incest sexual perpetrators who volunteered to undergo evaluation and treatment on an outpatient basis. Caution must also be taken in generalizing to other adolescents charged with incest. The adolescents in this study were for the most part, inner-city minority youngsters from lower socioeconomic strata.

These findings challenge the assumption that incest perpetrators are different from other paraphiliacs. This is due to the fact that 9 out of 22 adolescents (41%) had engaged in other (nonincest) paraphiliac behaviors, thus indicating that they are similar to other paraphiliacs. It is important to note that these behaviors were self-reported and unknown to the referral source.

A unitary profile of an adolescent sexual perpetrator does not emerge from these preliminary findings. This may be related, in part, to the small sample size. However, the subjects in this study can be placed into four distinct categories: (1) adolescents who engage in consensual sexual behavior with a peer-age relative; (2) adolescents who initially engaged in consensual sexual behavior with a peer-age relative but then turned to coercive sex when the relative no longer consented; (3) adolescents who have developed a deviant sexual interest pattern and meet DSM-III diagnosis for paraphilia; and (4) adolescents who engage in nondeviant sexual behavior and have incidental occurrence of deviant sexual behavior.

In conclusion, these data suggest that adolescent sex offenses need to be taken seriously. They must not be ignored or treated as sexual experimentation. Additional investigative efforts need to focus on an explanatory theory concerning the development of deviant sexual interest patterns.

ASSESSMENT

The assessment of adult sexual offenders has been described in detail (Becker & Kaplan, 1988). We have proposed a model by which deviant or atypical sexual behaviors committed by adolescents can be explained. The model incorporates individual characteristics, family variables, and social-environmental variables as possible precursors to the adolescents engaging in atypical sexual behavior. Our assessment battery is based on that model.

At our clinic we obtain a signed consent from both the adolescent and the parent or guardian prior to conducting an assessment. The consent outlines exactly what the evaluation will consist of. The assessment is divided into three categories: a clinical interview, psychometric testing, and a penile plethysmograph evaluation.

The clinical interview begins by the evaluator asking nonthreatening questions, such as about family, school, and demographics. Once rapport has been established, the topic of sexuality is discussed. The interviewer begins by asking the adolescent about nondeviant sexual behavior with peers, such questions include ages of first nongenital and genital sexual experiences, number of sexual partners, Kinsey rating of sexual orientation, frequency of masturbation, sexual fantasies, and the effect of alcohol, drugs or sexually explicit material on sexual behavior.

The interviewer then asks about deviant sexual activity. The evaluator should always attempt to obtain from the referral source a copy of the charges and the victim's statement. Since adolescents find it difficult to discuss the nature of these atypical sexual behaviors, they may deny or minimize what occurred. Therefore, it is useful to have at hand the victim's statement and when necessary to read it to the perpetrator.

The interviewer then questions the adolescent as to whether he has engaged in any form of paraphilic behavior (each paraphilia is mentioned). The adolescent's paraphilia(s) are listed and a chronological sexually deviant lifeline is constructed.

It is important to assess family variables by interviewing the adolescent's parents. The parents are questioned as to the extent of their knowledge about the sex offense committed by their child as well as to what factors they feel may have contributed to his acting out sexually. It is also important to obtain information about developmental history and any family life events such as psychiatric illness, etc.

It is also important to conduct a psychiatric evaluation of the adolescent to determine if there are any psychiatric disorders. Kavoussi, Kaplan, and Becker (1988) reported on the psychiatric characteristics of a sample of adolescent sex offenders. Each adolescent was interviewed using two semistructured interviews. The SCID (Structured Clinical Interview for DSM-III) was used to diagnose affective disorders, psychotic disorders, anxiety disorders, and substance abuse. The KIDDIE SADS-E (Children's Schedule for Affective Disorders and Schizophrenia—Epidemiologic version) was used to diagnose conduct disorder and attention-deficit disorder.

The most common diagnosis was conduct disorder (48%). The majority of boys who met criteria for this diagnosis could be classified as socialized, nonaggressive. Substance abuse (marijuana, alcohol) was the only other diagnosis found in more than 10% of the sample. None of the boys met full criteria for major affective disorder, dysthymia, or psychotic disorder. There was no DSM-III diagnosis for 19% of the adolescents.

The assessment instruments used to evaluate the adolescent were

The Adolescent Sexual Interest Cardsort—a 64-item self-report measure of sexual interest.

The Adolescent Cognitions Scale—a 32-item true/false test developed at our clinic to determine if the adolescent has any distorted cognitions regarding his behavior.

The Math Tech Sex Test—to assure the adolescents sexual knowledge, attitudes and values.

The MATSON Evaluation of social skills in youngsters—to assess social skills.

Psychophysiologic assessment of sexual arousal—to evaluate objectively the sexual interest patterns of adolescent sex offenders. This procedure consists of the presentation of sexual stimuli (2 minute audio tape descriptions of paraphilic and non-paraphilic interactions) while the adolescents degree of penile tumescence is measured with a penile plethysmograph (see Becker and Kaplan, 1988 for a complete description of the procedure).

In a 1989 study (Becker, Hunter, Stein, & Kaplan, 1989) on the factors associated with erectile responding to age-inappropriate stimuli in an adolescent sex offender population, the factors that were studied included (1) admit/deny, (2) history of physical and/or sexual abuse, (3) history of nonsexual arrests, and (4) incest/nonincest. Results indicated adolescent sex offenders with a history of sexual victimization, who in turn had sexually abused male children, showed a more deviant erectile pattern than those adolescents who had not been sexually abused.

ABUSE REACTIVE ADOLESCENT PERPETRATORS

There is increasing evidence that a relationship exists between a history of sexual victimization and the development of an atypical sexual interest pattern.

Various percentages of prior sexual victimization of sexual offenders have been reported in the literature. The following sample will describe several samples of sexually victimized boys who committed sexual offenses (Becker, 1988).

Characteristics of Juvenile Sex Offenders with a History of Prior Victimization

The Sexual Behavior Clinic at the New York State Psychiatric Institute provides evaluation and treatment of adolescents who have been accused of committing sexual crimes. Of 139 adolescent sexual offenders seen at the clinic, 27 (19%) indicated on initial interview that they were victims of sexual abuse. The mean age of the abused adolescents was 15 years and 6 months. Ages ranged from 12 to 19 years. In total, 56% were black, 26% Hispanic, and 18% Caucasian. Clearly, for some of the adolescents (33%) the sexual crime was part of a pattern of delinquent behavior. We consider our sample to be biased in that it overrepresents minorities. Minority adolescents are no more at risk than any other adolescents in the population.

Victimization Profile

Of the 27 adolescents who were sexually abused, 3 (11.1%) were abused by strangers and 24 (88.9%) by people they knew. These data are consistent with those reported by Rogers and Terry (1984) in that the majority of boys were abused by nonfamily members, but people known to the victim or his family.

In total, 16 (59.2%) adolescents were sexually abused by nonrelative adults, most of whom were known to them. The second highest category was nonrelative adolescents (6 or 22% male and 1 or 4% female). It is of particular interest that 40.7% of the offenders were female. This finding may be related to how the adolescents were questioned as to abuse history. It has been our clinical experience that if adolescents are asked, "Were you sexually victimized?" they tend to answer in the negative. For many, that question is a direct threat to their masculinity. We have also observed that if the offender was a female, the adolescents are inclined to describe the experience as "learning about sex" even though there was a considerable age difference and the adolescent experienced anxiety about the behavior.

Consequently, we asked the adolescent about every person he had a sexual encounter with, the age and sex of the person, and whether the behavior was initiated or wanted by the adolescent. By posing the question in this manner, one can obtain a much more accurate account of abusive behavior.

Our clinical experience has also indicated that a number of adolescents did not recall their own abuse until they were involved in our therapy. We will reinterview our sample when they complete therapy about sexual abuse history, and we anticipate having a higher than 19% reported abuse history.

In total, 9 (33%) of the adolescents indicated that they were verbally coerced into engaging in the sexual behavior, 8 (29.6%) were physically coerced, 3 (11.1%) were the victims of excessive physical coercion (aggression beyond what was necessary to complete the sexual crime), and 7 (25.9%) indicated no coercion was used to gain compliance. Of the adolescents, 4% required medical attention for assault-related injuries.

COMFORT WITH GENDER

A problem associated with sensitive topics, such as sexual behavior, is accurate reporting. In reliable data collection characteristics of the interviewer have been a concern, since response effects can distort findings. There has been much speculation on how the gender of the interviewer can affect responses of subjects; however, little empirical data has been collected on the subject. Data that are available, for the most part, show either no significant differences in responses for male versus female interviewers (Darrow, Jaffe, Thomas, et al., 1986; Johnson & Delamater, 1976; Reiss, 1967) or a more reliable response for female interviewers (Conners, Watson, & Maisto, 1985).

In a recent study (Kaplan, Becker & Tenke, 1991), 264 inner-city adolescent males undergoing an evaluation at the Sexual Behavior Clinic for sex offenders were questioned as to their preference and comfort in talking about sex with a male versus female interviewer. Overall, these adolescents were significantly more comfortable with a female interviewer (p < .05). Of the 135 nonabused subjects, 53% did not express a preference. However, those adolescents who had themselves been victims of sexual and/or physical abuse (49%) preferred a female interviewer (p < .02). Individuals victimized by males showed the greatest preference, although those abused by females also preferred a female interviewer. These results indicate that self-disclosure about sexual material may be facilitated when interviewers of both genders are available.

DEPRESSIVE SYMPTOMATOLOGY

Since the presence of depression has been cited as a possible diagnosis in the assessment of adolescent offenders (Becker & Kaplan, 1988), we decided to assess depressive symptomatology systematically in an outpatient adolescent sex offender population using the Beck Depression Inventory (Becker, Kaplan, Tenke, & Tartaglini, in press). Of 246 male adolescent sex offenders, the racial composition was black, 147; Hispanic, 62; Caucasian, 34. Subjects were divided according to their self-reports of having been sexually or physically abused.

The mean Beck score across all subjects was 14.3, a value markedly higher than published norms and indicative of mild depression. Scores indicative of appreciable depressive symptomatology were attained by 42% of subjects. A history of sexual or physical abuse was significantly related to high Beck scores; abused subjects have a mean Beck score of 16.4, as contrasted to 12.3 for nonabused subjects (Wilcoxon test: $Z = 2.82$; $p <. 005$). This relationship was apparent across all racial groups. While Hispanic subjects tended to have higher Beck scores and Caucasians lower scores, racial differences were not statistically significant.

The results of the present study indicate that adolescent sex offenders have an appreciably higher level of depressive symptomatology than would be expected of a random sample of adolescents (Kaplan, Hong, & Weinhold, 1984). In the study by Kaplan only 8.6% of subjects had BDI scores indicative of major depression. Almost half (41.9%) of our subjects scored in this range.

These results indicate that adolescents who have committed sexual crimes, particularly those with a history of abuse, should be evaluated for depression.

FAMILY VARIABLES

Previous research with adolescents has focused on the family and hypothesized that family environment may be one of a number of variables that impact on an adolescent who commits a sexual crime. In a review of the literature (Kaplan, Becker, & Cunningham-Rathner, 1988) found the following. Family environment has been linked to the development of aggression (Bandura & Walters, 1959; Farrington, 1978) and delinquency (Loeber & Dishion, 1983, Patterson & Stouthamer-Loeber, 1984). Several other researchers have suggested a relationship between family characteristics and sexually delinquent behavior, such as (1) exposure to family violence or physical abuse (Glaser, 1978; Lewis, Shankok, & Pinkus, 1979; VanNess, 1984), (2) neglect and abuse (Davis & Leitenberg, 1987), and (3) the absence of a strong marital bond (Mrazek, 1981).

In their review of the literature Davis and Leitenberg (1987) postulate how the family may influence the adolescent to commit a sexual crime and point out a number of plausible explanations: (1) when physical aggression and marital violence are tolerated, the adolescent learns that this is acceptable behavior; (2) neglect and abuse may predispose the adolescent to seek revenge on substitute targets; (3) parental abuse may lower self-esteem, and the sexual offense may be a way of restoring self-worth; (4) parental abuse may sensitize the child concerning intimate relationships with peers, and, consequently, he may socialize and then sexualize relation-ships with much younger children.

In an attempt to evaluate the family environment of the adolescent sex offenders seen at our outpatient clinic in New York City, we described the characteristics of parents of adolescent incest perpetrators (Kaplan, Becker, & Cunningham-Rathner, 1988). In this study we presented data on 27 parents of adolescent incest perpetrators; 70% (19) of those interviewed were mothers. Results indicated that (1) parents underreport physical and sexual abuse of their sons, (2) there is a high incidence of prior sexual abuse in the parents themselves, (3) there is a high rate of denial of the incestuous behavior committed by their sons, (4) these parents fail to educate their children about sex. Although we cannot definitively determine why incest has occurred in these families, factors that may play a significant role in the adolescent committing incest include (1) lack of appropriate sex information or education, (2) parental cover-up or denial of abuse, and (3) a cycle of abuse (modeling). These factors, in combination with individual and environmental characteristics, may place an adolescent at risk for engaging in incest.

This study was limited by the lack of a comparison group. In a follow-up study conducted by Kaplan, Becker, and Martinez (1990), one hundred and thirty mothers of adolescent sexual perpetrators were interviewed.

The present study was designed to compare mothers of incest perpetrators to mothers of nonincest perpetrators (n = 82) on several variables. It was hypothesized that the mothers of incest perpetrators would have a higher degree of abuse themselves and less denial than nonincest perpetrators.

The following results were obtained. Regarding *prior sexual and physical victimization of mothers*, significantly more mothers of incest perpetrators (43.8%, n = 21; total n = 48) admitted to being physically abused than mothers of nonincest perpetrators (24.7%, n = 20; total n = 81; p = .04; chi square =　4.2).

Similarly, significantly more mothers of incest perpetrators (34.0%, n = 16; total n = 47) admitted to being sexually abused than mothers of nonincest perpetrators (13.6%, n = 11; total n = 81; p = .01, chi square = 6.30).

Regarding *sexual dysfunction*, our mothers of incest perpetrators (31.3%, n = 15; total n = 48) were more likely to self-report a sexual dysfunction than mothers of nonincest perpetrators (11.3%, n = 9; total n = 80; p = .01, chi square = 6.61). Regarding this finding, research has indicated that women who have been abused have a higher incidence of sexual dysfunctions that nonabused women (Becker, et al., 1986).

In addition, mothers of incest offenders reported that they had been in therapy significantly more than mothers of nonincest offenders (p = .004). Regarding mothers self-report about their sons, a higher percentage of mothers of incest perpetrators reported that they believed their son had committed the sexual offense, was in need of treatment, and had a history of being physically abused. Additionally, a significantly lower percentage of incest perpetrators had involvement with the juvenile justice system. Since more of the mothers of incest perpetrators had a prior history of therapy, this may have facilitated disclosure.

In conclusion, in this study, mothers of incest perpetrators either (1) tend to disclose more about themselves in areas such as prior therapy, history of sexual and physical abuse, and sex dysfunction or (2) have experienced more of the above. In addition, given that mothers of incest versus nonincest perpetrators differ on a number of factors, further research needs to focus on how and if their sons' behavior has been due to parental influence, and what role familial variables play in the development of atypical sexual interests in adolescents.

TREATMENT

While there is a paucity of controlled therapy outcome studies on the treatment of adolescent sex offenders, treatment issues have been discussed (Becker, 1990; Becker, Kaplan, and Kavoussi, 1988; Becker & Kavoussi, 1989).

There has been a recent growth in adolescent sex offender programs in this country. In response to this, a National Adolescent Perpetrator Network was established in 1983. The network has published a preliminary report that describes basic "assumptions" upon which treatment is based (National Adolescent Perpetrator Network, 1988).

Becker, Kaplan, and Kavoussi (1988) describe a cognitive behavioral treatment program for adolescent sexual offenders. This multicomponent treatment program consists of verbal satiation, cognitive restructuring, covert sensitization, social skills training, anger control training, sex education, and relapse prevention sessions. In their 1985 paper the researchers present data on 24 adolescents who completed treatment. Those adolescents who had victimized males (n = 11) significantly decreased deviant sexual arousal pre- and posttreatment as measured by penile plethysmography. For those who molested female victims (n = 13), a decrease in deviant arousal was also evidenced, although not statistically significant.

More recently, Becker (1990) presented one-year follow-up data on a sample of adolescents treated on an outpatient basis. Follow-up data was available on 52 adolescents who had completed treatment. On the basis of referral source reports and self-reports 5 adolescents had recommitted sexual crimes.

ETHICAL ISSUES

There are a number of ethical issues that must be addressed in the assessment and treatment of adolescent sex offenders. Becker and Abel (1985) and Becker (in press) have outlined these issues. The first issue is confidentiality; since every state has sexual abuse reporting laws, it is important that both the adolescent and his parents be informed prior to any interview being conducted that if the specifics of past sexual offenses are reported, then the therapist is obliged to report this information. A second issue involves disclosure of detailed and specific information provided by the adolescent that is unknown to the parents but that they may wish to access. This issue can be addressed by having the adolescent and his parents sign a consent form before the treatment and evaluation are initiated. The consent form would specify what, if any, information the adolescent wants to share.

It is also recommended that the therapist ascertain what the adolescent's fears and concerns are relative to disclosing information to the parents. With the adolescent's permission an attempt can be made to discuss his fears and concerns with the parents. If the parents are able and willing to assure the therapist and the adolescent that his fears will not be realized, then the adolescent may give permission for total disclosure. If, however, the adolescent does not give permission for total disclosure, total disclosure is not advised.

A third issue relates to those adolescents who are under mandate to receive treatment or who are unmotivated to receive treatment.

It is advisable for the therapist to develop a contract with the adolescent or with the adolescent and his parents. The contract would establish what behaviors are expected of the adolescent and what the therapist's function will be. In this manner the patient and his family will know exactly what treatment will involve. The contract would also specify how reports to the criminal justice system will be handled. If therapists are required to send progress reports to the court, it is recommended that the contents of those reports be shared with the adolescent.

In conclusion, more clinical research studies on adolescent sex offenders are needed. Studies should focus on a typology and controlled therapy outcome studies.

REFERENCES

Abel, G.G., Mittelman, M; & Becker, J.V. (1985). Sex offenders: results of assessment and recommendations for treatment. In H.H. Ben-Aron, S.I. Hucker, and C.D. Webster (eds.), *Clinical Criminology: Assessment and Treatment of Criminal Behavior*. Toronto: M & M Graphics.

Awad, G.A.; Saunders, E.; and Levine, J. (1979). A clinical study of male adolescent sex offenders. *International Journal of Offenders Therapy and Comparative Criminology* 28 (2): 105–116.

Bandura, A., & Walters, R.H. (1959). *Adolescent Aggression*. New York. Ronald Press.

Beck, A.; Ward, C.; Mendelson, M.; et al. (1961). An inventory for measuring depression. *Archives of General Psychiatry* 4: 53–63.

Becker, J.V.(1988). The effects of child sexual abuse on adolescent sexual offenders. In G. Wyatt and G. Powell (eds.), The *Lasting Effects on Child Sexual Abuse*. Pp. 193–207. Newbury Park, Calif.: Sage.

Becker, J.V. (1990). Treating adolescent sexual offenders. *Professional Psychology: Research and Practice* 21.

Becker, J.V., & Abel, G. (1985). Methodological and ethical issues in evaluating and treating adolescent sexual offenders. In *Adolescent Sex Offenders: Issues in Research and Treatment*. Washington, D.C.: U.S. Department of Health and Human Services, No. (ADM) 85-1396.

Becker, J.V.; Cunningham-Rathner, J.; and Kaplan, M.S. (1986). Adolescent sexual offenders: Demographics, criminal and sexual histories, and recommendations for reducing future offenses. *Journal of Interpersonal Violence* 1 (4):431–445.

Becker, J.V.; Hunter, J.; Stein, R.; & Kaplan, M. (1989). Factors associated with erection in adolescent sex offenders. *Journal of Psychopathology and Behavioral Assessment* 2 (4): 353–362.

Becker, J.V., & Kaplan, M.S. (1988). The assessment of adolescent sexual offenders. In R. Prinz (ed.), *Advances in Behavioral Assessment of Children and Families*. Vol. 4, pp. 97–118. Greenwich, Conn.: JAI Press.

Becker, J.V.; Kaplan, M.S.; & Kavoussi, R. (1988). Measuring the effectiveness of treatment for the aggressive adolescent sexual offender. In R.A. Prentky & V.L. Quinsey (eds.), *Human Sexual Aggression: Current Perspectives*. Pp. 215–222. New York: New York Academy of Science.

Becker, J.V.; Kaplan, M.S.; Tenke, C.; & Tartaglini, A. (in press). The incidence of depressive symptomatology in juvenile sex offenders with a history of abuse. Child *Abuse and Neglect*.

Becker, J.V., & Kavoussi, R. (1989). Diagnosis and treatment of juvenile sex offenders. In R. Rosner and H. Schwartz (eds.), *Juvenile Psychiatry and the Law*. Pp. 133–143. New York: Plenum Press.

Brecker, E. (1989). *Treatment Program for Sex Offenders*. Washington, D.C.: U.S. Department of Justice.

Conners, G.J.; Watson, D.W.; & Maistro, S.A. (1985). Influence of subject and interviewer characteristics on the reliability of young adults' self reports of drinking. *Journal of Psychopathology and Behavioral Assessment* 7 (4): 365–374.

Cooper, I., & Cormier, B. (1982). Inter-generational transmission of incest. *Canadian Journal of Psychiatry* 27: 231–235.

Darrow, W.D.; Jaffe, H.W.; Thomas, P.A.; et al. (1986). Sex of interviewer, place of interview, and responses of homosexual men to sensitive questions. *Archives of Sexual Behavior* 15 (1): 79–88.

Davis, G.E., & Leitenberg, H. (1987). Adolescent sex offenders. *Psychology Bulletin* 101: 417–427.

Farrington, D.P. (1978). The family backgrounds of aggressive youths. In L.A. Hersov, M. Berger, & D. Shaffer (eds.), *Aggression and Anti-Social Behavior in Childhood and Adolescence*. New York: Pergamon.

Finkelhor, D. (1974). *Sexually Victimized Children*. New York: Free Press.

Gagon, J.H. (1965). Sexuality and sexual learning in the child. *Psychiatry* 28 (3): 212–228.

Glaser, D. (1978). Evaluation of sex offender treatment programs. In E. Brecher, (ed.), *Treatment Programs for Sex Offenders*. Washington, D.C.: National Institute of Law Enforcement and Criminal Justice.

Groth, A.N. (1977). The adolescent sex offender and his prey. *International Journal of Offenbders Therapy and Comparative Criminology*.

Groth, A.N., and Birnbaum. (1979). *Men Who Rape*. New York: Plenum.

Johnson, W.T., & Delamater, J.D. (1976). Response effects in sex surveys. *Public Opinion Quarterly* 40: 165–181.

Kaplan, M.S.; Becker, J.V.; & Cunningham-Rathner, J. (1988). Characteristics of parents of adolescent incest perpetrators: preliminary findings. Journal *of Family Violence* 3 (3): 183–191.

Kaplan, M.S.; Becker, J.V.; & Martinez, D. (1990). A comparison of mothers of adolescent incest vs. non-incest perpetrators. *Journal of Family Violence* 5 (3): 209–214.

Kaplan, M.S.; Becker, J.V.; & Tenke, C.E. (1991). Influence of abuse history on adolescent self-reported comfort with interviewer gender. *Journal of Interpersonal Violence* 6: in press.

Kaplan, M.S., Hong, G.; & Weinhold, C. (1984). Epidemiology of depressive symptomatology in adolescents. *Journal of the Academy of Child Psychiatry* 23: 91–98.

Kavoussi, R.; Kaplan, M.; & Becker, J. (1988). Psychiatric diagnosis in juvenile sex offenders. *Journal of the American Academy of Child and Adolescent Psychiatry* 27: 241–243.

Lewis, A.N.; Shankok, S.S.; & Pincus, J.H. (1979). Juvenile male sexual assaulters. *American Journal of Psychiatry* 136: 1194–1196.

Loeber, R., & Dishion, T. (1983). Early predictors of male delinquency: a review. *Psychology Bulletin* 94: 68–99.

Longo, R.E., and Groth, A.N. (1983). Juvenile sex offenses in the history of adult rapists and child molesters. *International Journal of Offender Therapy and Comparative Criminology* 27 (2): 150–155.

Mrazek, P. (1981). The nature of incest: a review of contributing factors. In P. Mrazek & H. Kempe (eds.), *Sexually Abused Children and Their Families*. New York: Pergamon.

Patterson, G.R., & Stouthamer-Loeber, J. (1984). The correlation of family management practices and delinquency. *Child Development* 55: 1299–1307.

Reiss, A.J. (1960). Sex Offenses: The marginal status of the adolescent. *Law and Contemporary Problems* 25 (2).

Reiss, I.L. (1967). *The Social Context of Premarital Sexual Permissiveness*. New York: Holt, Rinehart and Winston.

Roberts, R.E.; Abrams, L.; and Finch, J.R. (1973). Delinquent sexual behavior among adolescents. *Medical Aspects of Human Sexuality* 7 (1): 162–183.

VanNess, S.R. (1984). *Rape as Instrumental Violence: A Study of Youth Offenders*. New York: Haworth Press.

An Exploration of Incest in the Childhood Development of Serial Rapists

Arlene McCormack

Frances E. Rokous

Robert R. Hazelwood

Ann Wolbert Burgess

Data collection and analysis were supported by a
U.S. Department of Justice, Office of Juvenile
Justice and Delinquency Prevention grant (84-JN-
K010). Reprinted with permission of the *Journal
of Family Violence*.

INTRODUCTION

This chapter explores the phenomenon of male incest in a sample
of 41 incarcerated serial rapists. Of 31 men who reported childhood
sexual abuse (penetration, exploitation, and/or witnessing), just over
half were victims of incest. All incestuous experiences occurred before
puberty, and the majority of the experiences were protracted in
nature. When compared to nonincest victims of sexual abuse, incest
victims were more likely to report parental physical abuse and to
describe their childhood family structure at 16 years of age as reconstituted (step-parent present). In all cases in which the step-
father was implicated in the abuse, the abuse was of the witnessing
variety, i.e., the boy witnessed sexual activity that he found disturbing. Incest victims were significantly more likely than were nonincest

victims to reenact sexually abusive behavior within the family. This finding suggests that clinical discoveries of sibling sexual activity should alert clinicians that other incestuous activities may be occurring or have occurred.

In the last several years, there has been growing interest in the childhood sexual abuse experiences of males (Bell & Weinberg, 1978; Carmen, Reiker, & Mills, 1984; Fritz, Stoll, & Wagner, 1981; Janus, Burgess, & McCormack, 1987; Janus, Scanlon, & Price, 1984; Kaslow, Haupt, Arce, & Werblowsky, 1981; Kercher & McShane, 1984; McCord, 1984; McCormack, Janus, & Burgess, 1986; Petrovich & Templar, 1984; Rogers & Terry, 1984; Sarrel & Masters, 1982). Although studies of sexual abuse in the histories of adult male sexual offenders are not abundant, the presence of sexual abuse in this population has been fairly well established (Abel, 1982; Burgess, Hartman, Ressler, et al., 1986; Ressler, Burgess, Hartman, et al., 1986; Seghorn, Prentky & Boucher, in press; U.S. Department of Justice, 1985).

A 1987 study (Burgess, Hazelwood, Roukas, et al., 1987) shows that convicted serial rapists are much more likely to report sexual abuse in childhood (76%) than are males from the general population (16%) (*Los Angeles Times*, 1985) and those from normal college populations (7%) (Risin & Koss, in press). Using the same categories of sexual abuse as did Risin and Koss in their study of college males, Burgess, Hazelwood, Roukas, et al. (1987) also demonstrate that the abusive experiences are more likely to involve members of the rapist's family. This high incidence of incest in the childhood development of rapists is also substantiated by Seghorn, Prentky, Boucher, et al., (in press), who found that rapists were three times more likely to be victimized by a family member than were child molesters. The present study takes advantage of the high degree of incest in the childhood development of rapists to explore further the phenomenon of male incest in the same sample of 41 serial rapists studied by Burgess, Hazelwood, Roukas, et al. (1987). Incestuous experiences are analyzed in terms of age of victim at first experience, length of first experience, sex of perpetrator, and type of abuse.

The literature on sexual abuse of offenders, in general, relates this abuse to such family environmental and structural factors as child physical abuse, violence between parents, parental misuse of alcohol and drugs, and parental criminal and psychiatric histories. Also noted is the absence of the biological father from the family home (Feldman, Mallouh, & Lewis, 1986; U.S. Department of Justice, 1985). In the present study we compare incest victims with nonincest victims of sexual abuse to provide additional knowledge of incestuous family environments and structures.

Reenactment, a trauma response to victimization, is the direct replication of the abuse experience and has been noted most clearly in the play of very young children (Hartman & Burgess, 1986; Pynoos & Eth, 1985; Terr, 1981). Evidence of reenactment includes sexual activity and assertive behaviors with family members, acquaintances, and/or strangers. In the present study we assess the tendency of incest victims to reenact incestuous activities.

METHOD

Sample

The sample consists of 41 serial rapists who were incarcerated in 12 states at the time of the interview (Maryland, Kentucky, Oklahoma, New Mexico, Utah, Arizona, Colorado, Idaho, California, Oregon, Michigan, and Montana). In order to be included, each rapist committed 10 rapes, exhausted all forms of appeal, and voluntarily participated in this study through signing a human subject's consent form. All of the men who met the criteria for inclusion in this study consented to participate.

The ages of the 41 men in the sample range from 23 to 55 years with a mean of 35.2 years. The majority are white (86%); 12% are black; and 2% are Hispanic. The educational level ranges from 5 years of schooling to 17 years with an average of 11.3 years. Questions about preadult institutionalization history reveal that 41% of the men had spent time in a detention center, 26% in a mental health facility, 15% in a state home or orphanage, 8% in a foster home, and 4% in a boarding or military school.

The 41 serial rapists reported 837 rapes and 401 attempted rapes of strangers. Of this number, there were 200 convictions. The hidden rape statistics from these subjects' early and mid-adolescent age period account for an additional 100 known victims (e.g., siblings, cousins, neighborhood girls, and dates). The number of rapes of strangers committed by those in the sample range from 10 to 59 with a mean of 30 per offender.

Data Collection

Data collection consisted of face-to-face interviewing with two special agents from the Behavior Science Unit of the Federal Bureau of Investigation. Thirty-seven of the interviews were taped and transcribed; the shortest interview requiring 4 1/2 hours and the longest 12 1/2 hours. In addition, a 79-page questionnaire containing both closed- and open-ended questions was completed by the agents from the review of interview data and pre- and postsentencing records. This information included offender background information, chronic behavior patterns noted in records, family structure and environment, offense data, victimization history, and assault history as well as victim data and characteristics of the assaultive encounter. The protocol is a revised version of an instrument used in a study of 36 sexual murderers (Ressler, Burgess, Hartman, et al., 1986; U.S. Department of Justice, 1985).

Measurement

Acknowledging that investigators have questioned the validity of self-reported sexual behavior and speculating that most boy sexual abuse would not be documented in records, the researchers determined that additional methods would have to be taken to ascertain the presence of sexual trauma in the childhood histories. Thus, the procedure was routinely to ask subjects if they had ever been sexually abused. They were also asked their memories of childhood sexual experiences. A panel of special agents and clinicians determined if the sexual experiences met the criteria for sexual abuse and then classified the experience according to a level of abuse.

The experience was defined as sexual abuse if one of the following three criteria, recommended by Finkelhor and Hotaling (1984), was present: (1) some form of force or coercion was used to obtain the participation of the victim (i.e., gifts or money, threats to hurt or punish, use of power over victim, actual physical force); (2) there was an age discrepancy of at least five years between the child and the other person; and (3) the other person was a caregiver or an authority figure (i.e., parent, teacher, coach, babysitter, family member, step-parent).

Those experiences deemed sexually abusive were categorized by level of abuse using a classification system adapted from Burgess and Holmstrom (1974). The three mutually exclusive classes of sexual abuse include (1) penetration, (2) exploitive sex, and (3) the witnessing of sexual events deemed stressful.

> *Forced or penetration* experiences are ones in which oral or anal intercourse, attempted or completed, is achieved; ejaculation is not necessary. The legal term of rape is often used to characterize the experience.

> *Exploitive* situations are ones in which another person sexually fondles the boy or the boy is requested to touch or stroke another person's sex organs; the exploiter uses a variety of methods to lure, entice, or seduce the child into sexual activity.

> *Witnessing* disturbing sexual situations are ones in which the boy views sexual activity or another person's sex organs, was requested to do something sexual, or exhibited sex organs at another person's request and reports it confusing or disturbing.

Five raters examined the rapists' experiences of sexual abuse and decided whether each experience would be classified as either penetration, exploitive sex, or the witnessing of sexual events deemed stressful. Agreement was 90%. Consensus was reached for the remaining 10%. Total agreement was 100%.

When asked if sexually abused as a boy, most offenders said no. When asked their earliest sexual memories, 56.1% (23 of 41) of the rapists had one or more sexually abusive experiences of either a forced (n = 15) or exploitive (n = 8) nature. An additional 8 (19.5%) reported the most serious level of abuse as witnessing disturbing sexual activity. Only 10 of the rapists (24.4%) could not recall any sexually abusive events.

Information on who perpetrated the sexual abuse was available for 29 of the 31 victims. Of these, 15 rapists experienced sexual abuse that we classified as incest (abuse by an immediate family member living in the home and, in one case, a maternal grand-mother who was living in the home at the time of the abuse).

Analysis

Descriptive statistics and cross-tabular analysis are used to explore personal and family characteristics related to male incestuous experiences. Examples drawn from interview transcriptions are used to illustrate major study findings.

Findings

The first incest experiences occurred when the men were prepubescent (5 to 10 years of age; mean = 7 years), and the experiences tended to be protracted in nature, i.e., the majority lasting from one year to nine years with an average of five years. The perpetrator(s) were just as likely to be either female (n = 5), or male (n = 5), or male and female (n = 5). These experiences were about equally likely to be of a forced (n = 6) or witnessing nature (n = 7).

In order to explore characteristics of the families of incest victims, the 15 incest victims were compared to the 14 nonincest victims on the basis of family environment and family structure.

Family Environment

Findings showed that incest victims were no more likely to report parental or sibling criminal, psychiatric, alcohol, and drug histories than were nonincest victims. Both populations reported a high level of parental alcoholism (33% and 38%). The males in incestuous families were, however, more likely to report parental physical abuse than were males in nonincestuous families (60% vs. 29%). The physically abusing parent also tended to be the perpetrator of incestuous sexual abuse. And, as the following example illustrates, the physical abuse was usually of a very serious nature.

> *"I got to the point where discipline didn't bother*
> *me anymore. I realized that his main objective was to*
> *see me cry, see me hurt. So I wouldn't show hurt*
> *anymore, and sometimes he'd get to the point where*
> *he'd break out sweating and screaming, and my*
> *mother would have to jump in to stop him because he*

> *wouldn't stop unless I showed tears. I wouldn't stop*
> *fighting him. I'd laugh at him. . . . Sometimes he*
> *would jump on my mother when she intervened."*

This offender went on to relate how his father drilled holes in a ping pong paddle to spank him. Afterwards, the father forced the boy into a bathtub filled with hot water and alcohol, hoping that the welts raised by the paddle would rupture and the alcohol water would burn.

Family Structure

One interesting finding is that incest victims were significantly more likely to report reconstituted families (step-parent present) at 16 years of age than were nonincest victims (60% vs. 8%) ($X2 = 8.30$, df = 1, p < .005). One might speculate that the sexual abuse may have itself served as a stimulus to divorce in these families or it might be speculated that the step-parent was implicated in the abuse. Our results from further exploring this finding support the latter interpretation. Only two of the incestuous experiences in reconstituted families occurred prior to the step-parent (in all cases step-fathers) joining the family. In one of these cases the mother forced sex with the child, age 6 years, soon after she was divorced but not yet re-married, and in the other case the natural father anally assaulted the child prior to being divorced by the mother. In the majority of the remaining instances of incest in reconstituted families (5/7), the step-father was implicated. However, in all of these cases the sexual abuse was of the witnessing variety, i.e., the child is disturbed because he witnessed sexual activity between the step-father and his natural mother.

In contrast to the incestuous experiences in reconstituted families, only two of the six incestuous experiences in intact families (both natural parents present) involved witnessing sexually disturbing activity.

The Reenactment of Incestuous Activity

Sexual activity between siblings is often considered as more experimentation than preoccupation, although the relationship between adult-child incest and the child's repeating of this activity has been noted (Cantwell, 1981). Just over half of the 41 offenders (51.6%)

had direct examples of reenactment, usually with younger children, when they themselves were preadolescent. The most common pattern was for the subjects to molest children in their neighborhood (50%), or in their family (25%), or "girlfriends" (25%).

To ascertain the degree to which the incestuous activity is reenacted by the victims, we compared incest victims with younger siblings (n = 12) to nonincest victims with younger siblings (n = 12). The findings showed that half (50%) of the incest victims reenacted the incestuous activity with younger siblings compared to none of the nonincest victims ($X2 = 8.00$, df = 1, $p < .005$). All of the victimized siblings were younger sisters. In one case the boy victimized all four of his younger sisters. In another the boy victimized two younger sisters, impregnating one of them. Further, of the six incest victims who did not victimize younger siblings, two reported that they fantasized about engaging in this activity. One subject who was forced to perform fellatio on his older brother when he was 6 years old recalls such fantasizing.

> *"All of my first sexual fantasies were about my sister. . . . I know it was around the age of 11 to 13. . . . I masturbated to them a lot. I used her underwear and masturbated into them and put them right back into her drawer."*

Incest victims at all three levels of abuse were just as likely to reenact abusive sexual activity.

DISCUSSION

This study looked at sexual abuse in the childhood development of 41 serial rapists in order to explore the experiences of male incest victims. We found that just over half of the men who were sexually abused (n = 31) recalled an incestuous experience as their first sexual experience. All experiences occurred before puberty, and the majority were protracted in nature. These prepubertal and protracted experiences are also overwhelmingly noted in studies of female incest victims (Berliner, 1977; Burgess, Holmstrom, & McCausland, 1977).

In their 1986 study of incest Van der Mey and Neff note characteristics of incest families, and they highlight violent and alcoholic fathers. Our findings substantiate a high level of parental alcoholism in incestuous families, although this level does not differ significantly from that found in nonincestuous families. Also, both groups were just as likely to report parental and sibling criminal, psychiatric, and drug histories. These results substantiate other studies whose findings note the chaotic early family life of sexual offenders and argue that these family lifestyles exist whether or not the sexual abuse is intra- or extrafamilial.

Parental violence as measured by parental physical abuse was found to be much higher in incestuous families. This finding substantiates the generally held belief that familial sexual abuse and familial physical abuse tend to go "hand in hand."

The nature of the sexual abuse for males in reconstituted families was found to differ from that commonly reported for female victims. While female incest victims are more likely to suffer forced or exploitive sexual experiences with their stepfathers, our findings suggest that male victims are more likely to be subjected to witnessing parental sexual activity. As Brenner (1984) points out, while sexual tensions in reconstituted households are seldom discussed, it is believed that even the child's sensing of the parents' strong mutual attraction can prove distressing to the child. Thus, it is not surprising that these young boys are disturbed to witness actual sexual activity between their natural mother and their stepfather. With the departure of the natural father from the son's everyday life, the son may come to view himself in the traditional male role of "head of the house." The entrance of the stepfather may threaten the son's territory, i.e., his perceived control over his mother and, perhaps, his younger siblings. Witnessing of the new male intruder's sexual activity with the mother may strengthen the young boy's feelings of helplessness and powerlessness to control his everyday environment. This perception of lack of control has been noted to heighten the probability that victims of familial abuse will develop symptomatology consistent with the diagnosis of posttraumatic stress disorder (McCormack, Burgess, & Hartman, 1988).

Study findings showed that young male incest victims reenacted the sexually abusive behavior within the family. In all cases the victims were younger female siblings. The data suggest that early sexual abuse is responded to by reenactment behavior as an attempt to manage the confusion and stress generated by the sexual activities. That intrafamily sexual abuse is perpetuated reflects the effect of early socialization to nonnormative sexual activity and argues that the direction of such activities are shaped by childhood experiences.

The results of our study of male incest in serial rapists indicate that more attention must be paid to clinical discoveries of sibling incest. Such discoveries should serve as a "red flag" that other incestuous activities are occurring or have occurred. The clinician should further probe sexual activities within the family, perhaps by involving each member of the child's family in counseling. Each child must be helped to acknowledge sexual abuse within (or outside of) the family without creating overwhelming anxiety for the child. It is important that the clinician be careful not to blame anyone without having all of the facts. Once the abuse is validated, the overall goal of intervention is to create a safe environment for the child, which, more often than not, involves the removal of the child from the family or the relocation of the abusing parent. Further information on validation of sexual abuse during clinical interviews and subsequent treatment implications can be found in Sgroi (1982).

REFERENCES

Abel, G. (1982). Who is going to protect our children? *Sexual Medicine Today* 6: 32.

Bell, A., & Weinberg, M. (1978). *Homosexualities*. New York: Simon & Schuster.

Berliner, L. (1977). Child sexual abuse: what happens next? *Victimology: An International Journal* 2:327–331.

Brenner, A. (1984). *Helping Children Cope with Stress*. Lexington, Mass.: Lexington Books.

Burgess, A.W.; Hartman, C.; Ressler, R.K.; et al. (1986). Sexual homicide: a motivational model. *Journal of Interpersonal Violence* 1 (3): 251–271.

Burgess, A.W.; Hazelwood, R. R.; Roukas, F.E.; et al. (1987). Serial rapists and their victims: reenactment and repetition. Paper presented at the New York Academy of Sciences Conference on Human Sexual Aggression: Current Perspectives, New York City, January 9.

Burgess, A.W., & Holmstrom, L.L. (1974). *Rape: Victims of Crisis*. Bowie, Md.: Brady.

Burgess, A.W.; Holmstrom, L.L.; & McCausland, M.P. (1977). Child sexual assault by a family member: decisions after disclosure. *Victimology: An International Journal* 2:236–250.

Cantwell, H.B. (1981). Sexual abuse of children in Denver, 1979: reviewed with implications for pediatric intervention and possible prevention. *Child Abuse and Neglect* 8:75–85.

Carmen, E.; Reiker, P.; and Mills, T. (1984). Victims of violence and psychiatric illness. *American Journal of Psychiatry* 141 (3):378–383.

Feldman, M.A.; Mallouh, K.; & Lewis, D. (1986). Filicidal abuse in the histories of 15 condemned murderers. *Bulletin of American Academy of Psychiatry Law* 14 (4): 345–352.

Finklehor, D., & Hotaling, G.T. (1984). Sexual abuse in the national incidence study of child abuse and neglect: an appraisal. *Child Abuse and Neglect* (8):22–23.

Fritz, G.; Stoll, K.; and Wagner, N. (1981). A comparison of males and females who were sexually molested as children. *Journal of Sex and Marital Therapy* 7 (1): 54–59.

Hartman, C.R., & Burgess, A.W. (1986). Child sexual abuse: generic roots of the victim experience. *Journal of Psychotherapy and the Family* 2 (2): 77–87.

Janus, M.; Burgess, A.W.; and McCormack, A. (1987). Sexual abuse in life histories of adolescent male runaways. *Adolescence* 22: 405–417.

Janus, M.; Scanlon, B.; & Price, V. (1984). Youth prostitution. In A.W. Burgess (ed.), *Child Pornography and Prostitution*. Lexington, Mass.: Lexington Books.

Kaslow, F.; Haupt, D.; Arce, A.; & Werblowsky, J. (1981). Homosexual incest. *Psychiatric Quarterly* 53 (3):184–193.

Kercher, G., & McShane, M. (1984). The prevalence of child sexual victimization in an adult sample of Texas residents. *Child Abuse and Neglect* 8 (4):495–501.

Los Angeles Times (1985). 22% in survey were child abuse victims. August 25:33–34.

McCord, J. (1984). A forty-year perspective on the effects of child abuse and neglect. *Child Abuse and Neglect* 8 (4):295–501.

McCormack, A.; Burgess, A.W.; & Hartman, C. (1988). Familial abuse and posttraumatic stress disorder. *Journal of Traumatic Stress* 1 (2): 231–242.

McCormack, A.; Janus, M.; & Burgess, A.W. (1986). Runaway youths and sexual victimization: gender differences in an adolescent runaway population. *Child Abuse and Neglect* 10: 387–395.

Petrovitch, M.; & Templar, D. (1984). Heterosexual molestation of children who later became rapists. *Psychological Reports* 54:810.

Pynoos, R.S., & Eth S. (1985). Children traumatized by witnessing acts of personal violence: homicide, rape, or suicide behavior. In S. Eth & R.S. Pynoos (eds.), *Post-Traumatic Stress Disorder in Children*. Washington, D.C.: American Psychiatric Press.

Ressler, R.K.; Burgess, A.W.; Hartman, C.R.; et al. (1986). Murderers who rape and mutilate. *Journal of Interpersonal Violence* 1 (3): 273–287.

Risin, L.I., & Koss, M.P. (1988). The sexual abuse of boys: frequency and descriptive characteristics of the childhood victimizations reported by a national sample of male postsecondary students. In A.W. Burgess (ed.), *Rape and Sexual Assault II: A Research Handbook*. New York: Garland.

Rogers, C., & Terry, T. (1984). Clinical intervention with boy victims of sexual abuse. In I. Stuart & J. Greer (eds.), *Victims of Sexual Aggression: Treatment of Children, Women and Men*. New York: Van Nostrand Reinhold.

Sarrel, P., & Master, W. (1982). Sexual molestation of men by women. *Archives of Sexual Behavior* 2 (2): 117–131.

Seghorn, T.K.; Prentky, R.A.; & Boucher, R.J. (1986). Childhood sexual abuse in the lives of sexually aggressive offenders. *Journal of the American Academy of Child Psychiatry* 26: 262–267.

Sgroi, S.M. (1982). *Handbook of Clinical Intervention in Child Sexual Abuse*. Lexington, Mass.: Lexington Books.

Terr, L. (1981). Forbidden games: post-traumatic child's play. *Journal of American Academy of Child Psychiatry* 20:741–760.

U.S. Department of Justice. (1985). *Violent Crime*. Pp. 8, 54. F.B.I. law enforcement bulletin. Washington, D.C.: The Department.

Van der Mey, B.J., & Neff, R.L. (1986). *Incest As Child Abuse*. New York: Praeger.

CHAPTER

19

Rehabilitation of Child Molesters: A Cost-Benefit Analysis

Robert Prentky

Ann Wolbert Burgess

Preparation of this manuscript was supported by the National Institute of Justice (82-IJ-CX-0058), the National Institute of Mental Health (MH32309). the Office of Juvenile Justice and Delinquency Prevention (84-JW-AX-JO10) and the Commonwealth of Massachusetts. We would like to gratefully acknowledge our colleagues who made valuable contributions to this project, including Austin Lee, Ruth Rosenberg, William Pithers, Daniel Carter, Raymond Knight and Vernon Quinsey. In addition, we are most grateful to the numerous members of the criminal justice and human service communities who provided the data used in this study. This article is reprinted with permission of the *American Journal of Orthopsychiatry* (1990) 60 (1): 108–177.

INTRODUCTION

Over the past several decades the escalation of sexual aggression has become an increasingly acute problem, manifested in costs to both victims and society at large. The long-term psychological impact of sexual assault on adult and child victims has been documented many times (Burgess & Holmstrom, 1974; Burgess & Lazare, 1976; Finkelhor, 1984; Finkelhor, 1979; Geiser, 1979; Jaffe, Dynneson, & ten Bensel, 1975; Jones, Jenstrom, & McFarlane, 1980; Norris & Feldman-Summers, 1981; Peters, 1976). The costs incurred by society include a network of medical and psychological services provided to aid victim recovery, the investigation, trial and incarceration of offenders—often in segregated units or special facilities—and the invisible blanket of fear that forces potential victims to schedule normal daily activities around issues of safety. Simple questions for parents—such as choosing day care or babysitters or permitting unsupervised outside play, or equally common questions for adult women, such as when to leave work in the evening, what mode of transportation to use, where to park the car, where it is safe to walk or jog, and whether to use your first name on your mail box or in the phone book—become major concerns, especially in larger cities.

Although it is impossible to estimate with any accuracy what the base rates are for sexual offenses, it is commonly reported that sex offenders account for a large number of victims. Abel, Becker, Cunningham-Rathner, et al. (1984) concluded that the "average adolescent sex offender" may commit 380 sex crimes over his lifetime. Finkelhor (1984) has estimated that somewhere between 46,000 and 92,000 boys are victimized each year, and the number of girls victimized may be three times higher. If even a fraction of these estimates are accurate, the magnitude of the problem is enormous.

It would thus seem reasonable to explore what strategies can reduce effectively victimization rates. A secondary intervention strategy that may be efficacious is offender treatment. That is, if an offender presents with a certain base expectancy rate of violence expressed in terms of "risk," how much does the risk decrease as a function of treatment? And is the cost of treatment offset by the cost to society incurred by those presumptively avoidable crimes? How much "risk" must decrease in order to justify the added cost of treatment is essentially a social policy question. While we cannot answer the question, "Is it worth it?" we can tentatively address the questions does treatment decrease likelihood of reoffending and what are the relative monetary costs associated with sexual victimization. If treatment is effective in reducing victimization rates, the potential "savings" (human as well as monetary), given the crude estimates of victimization rates, would be incalculable.

The application of benefit-cost analysis to juvenile justice and correctional programs is, of course, not new. Mahoney and Blozan (1968) discussed such issues at the end of the 1960s. Blumstein (1971) did a cost-effectiveness analysis of the allocation of police resources, and Holahan (1973) devised a benefit-cost model for correctional programs and applied it to a pretrial diversion program (Holahan, 1970a) and a drug addiction program (Holahan, 1970b). In general, writers have encouraged the use of benefit-cost analysis as a potentially informative evaluation procedure for correctional programs (Adams, 1975; Glaser, 1973). In an excellent review of this literature, Weimer and Friedman (1979) recommended the judicious use of benefit-cost analysis while underscoring the need for attention to the methodological shortcomings of previous research efforts.

Of all of the applications of benefit-cost analysis to rehabilitation or resource allocation in the correctional sphere, one noteworthy omission has been to sex offenders. In fact, the only study we are aware of that looked at the monetary cost to society of sexual victimization was Frisbie's (1969) study of 887 sex offenders in California. Chapter 4 in Frisbie's monograph, entitled "Society Pays and Pays," delineated the lengthy and expensive process once a sex offender has been charged with a crime. Frisbie (1969) concluded, "The magnitude of measurable and hidden costs implicit in processing a sex offender's case from apprehension, through trial, jail, institutionalization at Atascadero or prison or both, and final discharge from probation or parole, cannot but jar society into more vigorous concern over the tax dollars which are channeled into financing the present system" (Frisbie, 1969: 99).

Despite the rather affirmative statement by Marshall, Abel, and Quinsey (1983) that "of all the men convicted of crimes and sent to prison for their offenses, none are more likely to benefit from treatment than those who commit acts of sexual assault" (p. 43). It is quite apparent that the primary motive for legislating alternative dispositions for sex offenders has been, as Pacht (1976) noted, preventive detention and not rehabilitation. Given the unabating controversy over what to do with sex offenders in general and child molesters in particular, it is all the more remarkable that there have been no concerted efforts to subject treatment programs for these offenders to benefit-cost evaluations. Indeed, as West (1983) stated, outcome evaluations for sex offender treatment programs have been conducted so rarely with any scientific rigor that issues of cost effectiveness have been moot.

Decisions regarding the disposition of sex offenders will ultimately reflect a complex set of factors, including prevailing societal attitudes.

Those decisions should be based, however, on informed judgments that consider the approximate costs and potential benefits of whatever disposition is chosen. It is the intention of this chapter to address the issue of the cost effectiveness of rehabilitation through the use of reoffense and program data derived from the Massachusetts Treatment Center and costs derived from averaged figures obtained through state agencies.

METHOD

The Massachusetts Treatment Center

The Massachusetts Treatment Center was established in 1959 as a maximum-security residential facility to provide for the evaluation, treatment, and safe release of repetitive and/or violent sex offenders. The facility is operated jointly by the Departments of Correction and Mental Health. Over 5,000 sex offenders have been screened since 1959. Of these, approximately 1,790 were judged to be possible candidates for commitment and were referred to the center for an intensive 60-day observation. Of those observed at the center, 600 have been committed. Of the committed residents, 315 have been discharged, about 40 through legal technicality or death. Of these released residents, detailed criminal follow-up data was available on 129 child molesters and 111 rapists.

The rehabilitation program at the Treatment Center is discussed in detail by Carter and Prentky (1988) and will not be elaborated upon here.

Subjects

All 129 released child molesters were used for estimating reoffense rates of *treated* offenders. They are characterized by the following demographic variables. The sample is 94% Caucasian and 6% black with an average IQ of 96.8 (SD = 15.4) and an average school-grade level of 8 (SD = 2.3; range = 2–16). The average achieved skill level on a scale of 0 (unskilled)–4 (professional) was 1.10 (SD = 1.23), and about one-half the sample had been married (48%). Approximately one-third of the sample (31.5%) had a juvenile penal record, and close to 90% had an adult penal history prior to commitment.

More detailed discussion of the offender population at the Treatment Center may be found elsewhere (Bard, Carter, Cerce, et al., 1987).

Criminal Follow-up Investigation

Grants from the National Institute of Justice and the National Institute of Mental Health supported the follow-up of all men discharged from the Massachusetts Treatment Center between 1960 and 1985. In obtaining a chronology of postrelease criminal activity, the incidence of criminal *charges* was summed over the *entire postrelease* period for each discharged resident of the Treatment Center, as well as matched and random samples of sex offenders who were observed but not committed to the center. Postrelease criminal activity was obtained from five sources: (1) Massachusetts Department of Correction Research Department records, (2) Massachusetts Treatment Center outpatient and Gradual Release Program records, (3) Massachusetts Board of Probation, (4) Department of Public Safety, Massachusetts State Police, and (5) Federal Bureau of Investigation. Although they were somewhat redundant in terms of the information provided, multiple sources allowed for cross-checking of information.

Recidivism is typically operationalized as a "failure rate" or reoffense rate over time. The procedure for calculating failure rate, however, varies widely, as well as the definition of failure itself (Barton & Turnbull, 1981; Harris, Kaylan, & Maltz, 1981; Harris & Moitra, 1978; Maltz, 1984; Maltz & McCleary, 1977; Schmidt & Witte, 1980; Witte & Schmidt, 1977). Failure can be defined as (1) a charge, (2) an arrest, (3) a conviction, (4) any reincarceration, (5) reincarceration for a specified period of time (e.g., 30 days or longer as in the Commonwealth of Massachusetts), or (6) a parole violation. Each will yield different failure rates, with studies using charges or parole violations producing the highest failure rates and studies using reincarceration producing the lowest failure rates. The Treatment Center recidivism figures reported in this study are based entirely on charges. The intention was to provide the most reliable estimate of recidivism possible.

Not only is it essential to define recidivism in dispositional terms, recidivism must also be defined in criminal terms (i.e., precisely what criminal conduct falls within the reoffense domain). A Commission of Probation handbook and an FBI handbook were used to identify 174 criminal charge options, which were then assigned to seven main categories of offenses (traffic/automobile, property, substance abuse, rule breaking, behavior-related, victim-involved, other illegal activities). Of the 178 criminal charges that were identified, 78 appeared for coding in our sample. We chose to adopt the most inclusive approach by using the widest possible criminal domain, which is to say all of the possible charges that fell within the discrete category we were examining. For the purposes of this study, we are reporting charges for *all* victim-involved sexual offenses. This domain includes 15 charges (carnal abuse, abuse of female child, accosting, unnatural acts, indecent assault, assault with intent to rape, rape, sodomy, indecent assault and battery on a child under 16, rape of a child under 16, assault to rape a child under 16, unnatural acts on a child under 16, statutory rape, incest, abominable and detestable crimes against nature). Nuisance sexual charges (e.g., open and gross lewdness, voyeurism, obscene language) were not included since there was no physical contact with a victim. There were only 10 individuals with nuisance sexual charges (7.8%).

Recidivism Rates

For Treated Offenders

Over a period of 5 years there was a total of 32 men out of the sample of 129 that had a serious sexual charge filed against them. According to the way that we have defined recidivism, the failure (or reoffense) rate for all sexual charges over 5 years would be 25%. A 5-year follow-up period is being used for purposes of comparability with Marshall and Barbaree (1988) over the ensuing 20 years of the follow-up (i.e., year 6 to year 25), only an additional 7 men recidivated, yielding a 25-year recidivisim rate of 30%.

For Nontreated Child Molesters

Determination of a reliable, relatively accurate estimate of recidivism for child molesters—treated or untreated—is the weakest component of this analysis. In their lengthy review of the literature, Furby. Weinrott, and Blackshaw (1988) clearly indicated that methodological variability and ambiguity precludes any meaningful conclusions about recidivism rates for sex offenders. The precise criminal domain used for determining reoffense, length of follow-up, how the crime was disposed of (e.g., arrest, conviction, imprisonment, etc.) and what comprised the sample (e.g., offenders against only children, children and adolescents, boys only, girls only, etc.) are among the considerations that vary across studies. For the purposes of this study, the ideal comparison group would have been a group of child molesters determined to be "sexually dangerous" but randomly assigned to a no-treatment group. For obvious legal and ethical reasons this was not possible. Consequently, to obtain a useful recidivism figure for this study we elected to use the results from a carefully executed, methodologically rigorous treatment program for child molesters conducted by Marshal and Barbaree (1988). Marshall and Barbaree reported on a four-year follow-up of 53 untreated and 64 treated child molesters, finding that the recidivism rates were 32% and 14%, respectively. These groups included incest-only offenders, and Marshall (1988) indicated that the recidivism rate for the untreated group, if incest offenders were dropped, would be 40–42%. Because the Treatment Center sample does not include any incest-only offenders, we decided to use the figure of 40% as the recidivism estimate for untreated child molesters. This figure happens to be reasonably consistent with other reports. Christiansen, Elers-Nielson, Le Maire, and Sturup (1965), for instance, followed 2,934 sexual offenders for periods of 12 to 24 years. Of this sample, 714 (24.3%) were *sentenced* for a new offense during the observation period. Of this same sample 37.1% of the men between the ages of 26–50 had a prior history of only sexual offenses. Within this same age group 44.2% had a prior history of sexual and nonsexual offenses. Soothill and Gibbens (1978) estimated through the use of a life table that 48% of their sample of sex offenders would be reconvicted by the end of the 22 year at risk.

Cost per Offense

A detailed delineation of offender-related and victim-related costs for an offense is provided in the Appendix to this chapter.

Cost of Treatment

The cost of treatment was determined as the combined budgets for custodial supervision (Department of Correction—DOC) and rehabilitation (Department of Mental Health—DMH). This amount for fiscal year 1988 was $6,023,140, which translates to $23,166 per man. The cost for rehabilitation *alone* (i.e., the total DMH component) was $2,747,140, or $10, 566 per man. The total costs were divided by a constant population of approximately 260 men. There were an additional 20–25 observation cases at the center. These cases were *not* included, though doing so would have further reduced the per man cost. The duration of rehabilitation was determined as the median length of commitment for all 129 child molesters discharged from the facility over a 25-year period (5.1 years). The cost of treatment alone (DMH component) would be $53,886. The total cost (including DOC component) would be $118,146 (5.1 x $23,166).

Cost of Incarceration

The cost of incarceration was determined by averaging the annual inmate cost at seven different penal facilities in Massachusetts (one maximum security; three moderate security; three minimum security) The average for these seven prisons in fiscal year 1987 was $22,662 per year. Thus, the cost of incarceration would be $158,635 ($22,662 x 7 years).

Duration of Treatment vs. Length of Incarceration

In this study the duration of treatment was set at 5.1 years and the duration of incarceration 7 years for purposes of estimating costs.[1] It may not typically—or necessarily—be the case that a prison sentence will detain an offender longer than a civil sentence to a treatment facility. Length of sentence and amount of time served on a given sentence are highly variable. For this study we relied on the guidance of five assistant district attorneys, who concurred that a 10–15-year sentence was likely for a repeat rape offense against a child. There was less agreement as to the likely amount of time served, with the consensus being that the offender would at least serve the minimum sentence of 10 years. We opted for a more conservative cost estimate by using the first parole eligibility date of 7 years.

As indicated, the length of treatment was set at 5.1 years, which was the median length of time at the Treatment Center for the 129 discharged offenders. On occasion men have been cleared of "sexual dangerousness" only to be returned to prison. In practice this rarely happens with child molesters, who typically choose to remain at the center until their criminal sentence has been served and/or they are parole eligible. Thus, for most of the sample examined here, 5 years is a reasonably accurate estimate of "time detained" and hence a reasonably accurate estimate of cost.

Estimation of Costs Associated with a Single Offense

In order to determine the cost of a single offense a prototype case was created. The case is that of a 34-year-old child molester who is released from prison and re-offends within the first year while on parole. The offense is a sexual assault on a child in an urban location. There is a single victim who is unknown to the offender, and there is a single encounter. The offender is indigent. He is convicted and receives a 10–15 year sentence. He remains in prison until his parole eligibility (7 years) and is paroled. He is discharged from parole after 5 years.

The authors delineated the offender and victim-related cost categories (c.f. Appendix) that comprise the model. After the categories were established, a minimum of three and a maximum of five individuals representing each cost category were asked how long it would take to perform their service given the above mentioned hypothetical case. The responses for each category were then averaged. The salaries of the respondents were then averaged and the costs associated with "service delivery" for that category determined. Since most of the respondents were state employees, it was easy to determine salary levels. As an example, five police detectives from varying locations in the state were asked to estimate how long it would take to investigate the above case. There responses were averaged, and a cost determined using an average salary for detectives. The same procedure was followed for each category.

Results

The data that were entered into the cost-benefit model are as follows:

A) Total Cost Per Offense:

Offender-Related Costs (note Appendix)	$169,029
Victim-Related Costs (note Appendix)	<u>$14,304</u>
TOTAL	$183,333

B) Cost of Incarceration:	$158,635
C) Cost of Treatment:	$118,146
D) Recidivism: Treated	25%
Not Treated	40%

The model proposes in the first case (Treated) that a convicted child molester is committed to the Treatment Center. He spends 5.1 years at the Center at a cost of $118,146. He is released to the street with a .25 risk of re-offending within the first five years. The cost of re-offense is $183,333. Thus, the expected cost in the Treated case would be: $118,146 + ($183,333 x .25) = *$163,979.25*.

The model proposes in the second case (Not Treated) that a convicted child molester is sent to prison. He serves 2/3 of his minimum sentence (7 years) at a cost of $158,635. He is released to the street with a .40 risk of re-offending within the first five years. The cost of re-offense is $183,333. Thus the expected cost in the Not Treated case would be: $158,635 + (183,333 x .40) = *$231,968.20*.

The difference between $231,968.20 and $163,979.25 ($67,988.05) represents the additional cost of one victim in the event of a re-offense by one offender.

Cost of Multiple Victims by the Same Offender

If the same child molester had more than one victim, the overall cost would be increased primarily by victim-related expenses ($14,304). Although other costs might increase as well (e.g., length of investigation and/or trial), the major source of added expenses would be related to the second victim. The expected cost of a second victim of a *non*treated child molester may be determined as: $14,304 x (.40), or $5,722. The expected cost of a second victim of a treated child molester would be $14,304 x .25, or about $3,576. Thus, the increase in expected cost with nontreated child molesters will be about $2,100 (i.e., $5,722 - $3,576) as the number of victims is increased by one. This analysis assumes that the risk of re-offense remains constant. That is, the risk after one victim is the same as the risk after the second victim, and so forth. In reality, of course, the coefficient of risk would not remain the same.

Cost of Multiple Offenders

As noted above, the difference of $68,000 represents the additional cost of one victim in the event of a re-offense by one offender. Hypothetically, if 1,000 untreated child molesters were released from prison, the actual cost incurred by society over a period of five years would be $68,000 x 1,000, or about $68,000,000: ($231,968.20 x 1,000) – ($163,979.25 x 1,000).

Cost Parity Analysis

The reliability of probability estimates of re-offense is critically dependent on the accuracy of available data. Given that there are no truly reliable probabilities or risks associated with re-offense, it makes sense to ask what the minimal difference in re-offense rates between treated and nontreated groups would be for the cost difference to be negligible.

If we hold constant the recidivism rate of .40 for *non*treated child molesters, the recidivism rate for *treated* child molesters would have to be approximately .62 for there to be *no* difference in cost:

Treated Case: $118,146 + (183,333 x .62) = $231,812

$231,968 - $231,812 = $156

Stated alternatively, if the recidivism rate for nontreated child molesters is .40, there will be no difference in cost if the recidivism rate for treated child molesters is .62 or greater.

If we hold constant the recidivism rate of .25 for treated child molesters, the recidivism rate for *non*treated child molesters would have to be approximately .03 for there to be no difference in cost:

Nontreated case: $158,635 + (183,333 x .03) = $164,135

$164,135 - $163,979 = $156

That is, if the recidivism rate for treated child molesters is .25, there will be no difference in cost if the recidivism rate for nontreated child molesters is 3% or lower.

A Theoretical Approach to the Cost Parity Question

If we set R1 equal to the risk of recidivism for treated child molesters, and R2 equal to the risk of recidivism for nontreated child molesters, we can solve the following equation:

$$\$118,146 + (\$183,333 \times R1) = \$158,633 + (\$183,333 \times R2) \text{ as}$$
$$R2 = R1 - .22.$$
$$\text{Thus, if } R1 = .22, \text{ than } R2 = 0.$$

From the above solution, we can derive a table of comparative risks. With the use of such a table, one can plug in any recidivism estimate for a treated or untreated child molester and obtain the "needed" or "required" recidivism estimate for the cost to be negligible. For instance, if the known recidivism rate for a sample of treated child molesters was 37%, the rate for nontreated offenders would have to be 15% for there to be no difference in cost.

R1	R2
(Recidivism Risk for Treated)	(Recidivism Risk for Nontreated)
.22	.0
.25	.03
.30	.08
.37	.15
.42	.20
.47	.25
.52	.30
.57	.35
.62	.40

Controlling for Cost Differences Between Treatment and Nontreatment Conditions

In deriving costs for this model, one area of disparity is the time of incarceration (7 years) versus the time of treatment (5.1 years).

Although these two figures were independently and objectively derived, they nevertheless represent a major cost difference. If we control for this difference, by setting treatment time equal to 7 years, then the principal cost difference must be attributable to re-offense risk.

By multiplying the original annual cost per resident at the Treatment Center ($23,166) by 7 years, a revised cost of treatment is obtained ($162,162).

If we then take this new figure and substitute it for the $118,146 figure, the revised expected cost in the treated case would be:

$$\$162,162 + (\$183,333 \times .25) = \$207,995.25.$$

The "time adjusted" difference between the treated case ($207,995.25) and the untreated case ($231,968.20) is now $23,972.95. Thus, the additional cost of one victim in the event of a re-offense by one offender would now be about $24,000. If we hold constant the incarceration and treatment times, then our hypothetical sample of 1,000 untreated child molesters would incur and additional cost over five years of approximately $24,000,000, rather than the previously derived figure of $68,000,000.

Discussion

We set out to design a stringent model, one that would be as "blind" to preconceptions and bias as possible and one that would, if anything, underestimate costs. We did not, and realistically could not, assess and quantify the long-term psychological "costs" of victimization. Such costs inevitably take their toll not only on the child who was victimized, but also on society as a whole. Indeed, it may be argued that these emotional costs far outweigh the monetary costs in their impact on society. Nevertheless, we found that we could demonstrate through conservative estimates of monetary costs the benefit of rehabilitation. When the added "cost" of a given offense (about $68,000 or $24,000 if one wishes to use the revised estimate) is multiplied times an estimate of the number of offenses within a given time period, the magnitude of the potential "savings" becomes evident.

In addition, based on only "in-house" treatment and recidivism data gathered on 129 child molesters at the Treatment Center, we may tentatively conclude that rehabilitation can reduce the likelihood of committing a new sexual offense. It should be kept in mind that our assessment of recidivism was intentionally as stringent as possible. That is, we considered *all* charges for a large domain of criminal conduct, regardless of arrest or conviction, to be evidence of recidivism. Moreover, the population that we followed can reasonably be considered as the most "dangerous" (i.e., at high risk to reoffend sexually) of the child molesters in the Massachusetts penal system. This point may be illustrated by examining a sample of 67 child molesters who were observed at the Treatment Center but determined to be "not sexually dangerous" and returned to the prison system to serve their sentence. For this untreated group of men who presented with comparatively minor histories of sexual offending (e.g., a single relatively nonviolent offense), the recidivism rate was 13%. Hence, among the multitude of critical issues that *must* be addressed when discussing treatment efficacy and recidivism is the nature of the sample that is being examined. Child molesters comprise such a heterogeneous group that it makes little sense to derive a single model for all such offenders. There is ample evidence to suggest, for instance, that risk rates for reoffense may vary considerably among different "types" of child molesters (e.g., Abel & Mittelman, 1988; Groth, Hobson, & Gary, 1982; Quinsey, 1986). Consequently, it will be necessary to consider important typological discriminators when designing future benefit-cost models for this population.

Importantly, this study should *not* be regarded as an evaluation of treatment. As Quinsey (1983) noted, there is a paucity of treatment evaluation studies and those that do exist are, for the most part, poorly done. A rigorous examination of the efficacy of different treatment modalities with different types of child molesters is clearly needed. Ideally, such studies should employ random assignment of cases to a number of different treatment conditions as well as a no-treatment condition. While we are still a long way from the point where we can draw reliable conclusions about the impact of treatment on recidivism for different types of offenders, we are making progress (e.g., Abel, Mittelman, Becker, et al., 1988; Becker, Kaplan, & Kavoussi, 1988; Laws ,1986; Marques, 1988; Marshall & Barbaree, 1988; Marshall, Earls, Segal, & Darke, 1983; Pithers, Kashima, Cumming, et al., 1988). The results of well-designed and competently executed treatment programs provide little support for the nihilistic belief that sexually aggressive behavior is irremediable.

Finally, we wish to emphasize that the conceptual framework for a benefit-cost model presented in this chapter is of greater importance than the actual figures that were plugged into the model. Costs will vary considerably between counties, cities, and, of course, states. Although the figures are subject to much variation, within a given jurisdiction they provide a reasonably "hard" (i.e., accurate) reflection of the actual cost for that jurisdiction at a given point in time. Despite variation in estimated costs, the expense categories employed in this study[2] (cf. Appendix) should be fairly consistent across jurisdictions. Overall, offender- and victim-related costs, treatment costs, and incarceration costs can be determined with reasonable accuracy. Clearly, the weakest component in this model, from an empirical standpoint, is the assessment of recidivism, which is why we chose to adopt as stringent criteria as possible.

Social Policy Considerations

Given the apparent magnitude of the human and monetary costs incurred by society as a result of sexual victimization, the response has been remarkably ambivalent. The most rudimentary response to those who violate the canons of society appears in the Old Testament as *lex talionis* or the law of an eye for an eye.[3] The law proposes, from a seemingly rational perspective, that those who do bad things should pay in a way equal to the damage they wrought. Our language teems with colloquial expressions that convey this sentiment. The wrongdoer, for instance, should "get a taste of his own medicine," or get his "just deserts," or get his "comeuppance," or simply get "what's coming to him." The psychological underpinning of such sentiment can be understood, in part, as the need for retaliation (or punishment).[4] It is a fully understandable, rather instinctive, response to those who hurt us. The effectiveness of this response in redressing wrongdoing has its limitations, however. Those of us who have struggled with the joy and pain of developing an attachment to another human being realize the limited utility of punishment as a way to mitigate hurt or to achieve restitution. Those of us who have acquired some expertise in modifying behavior, whether we are parents, teachers, or therapists, appreciate the liabilities of wanton punishment in affecting long-term behavior change. Despite our common-sense appreciation of what impedes and what facilitates behavior change, our instinctive need is to exact our pound of flesh in response to wrongdoing, particularly when the perpetrator is a stranger and the act is as incomprehensible as child molestation is to most of us.

The struggle between the visceral desire to inflict punishment and the cerebral recognition of the potential shortcomings of punishment is evident in discretionary decisions involving sex offenders. This struggle is epitomized by the legislative ambivalence that created and then repealed sexual psychopath laws. Between 1937 and 1950, 12 states and the District of Columbia enacted such laws. Between 1950 and 1972, an additional 13 states enacted statutes governing sex offenders. Thus, over a period of about 40 years one-half of all the states adopted statutes that created a special category for sex offenders, and then repealed or modified those statutes. For the most part, the statutes served the singular purpose of preventive detention (Pacht, 1976) and thus were found to be unconstitutional. Indeed, it may be argued that the reactionary nature of the adoption of these special statutes suggests a primary intention to circumvent determinate sentencing for sex offenders.

The swinging of the pendulum between incarceration and rehabilitation is obviously a complex phenomenon and reflects an ever changing network of forensic, sociological, and psychological factors (cf. Wolfgang, 1988, for an interesting discussion). Rape law reform, the increased prominence and authority of the women's movement, the introduction of new treatment techniques, and changing attitudes about the efficacy of treatment and the reliability of prediction are among the contributing factors. The intention of this chapter was not to explore the enactment and repeal of legislation or to track the protean nature of the pendulum, but rather to look circumspectly at costs of victimization relative to the risk of reoffense associated with incarceration without treatment and incarceration with treatment.

In conclusion, we appear to resist treating child molesters because it is a "humane" response to egregious behavior. If the over-riding goal is reducing victimization rates, as well as the costs incurred by victimization, and if rehabilitation of offenders can be shown to reduce the likelihood of reoffense, then it is imperative that we overcome our resistance to treating child molesters—*not* for the sake of the offenders but for the sake of the victims.

NOTES

1. We wish to caution against drawing the parsimonious conclusion that cost is exclusively a function of length of treatment or length of imprisonment. Any reasonably accurate approximation of expenses must take into consideration differences in recidivism and the myriad monetary and emotional costs associated with re-offense. Furthermore, the actual lengths of time that we used (5.1 and 7 Years) are *not* standards and should not be construed as such. They were used for cost estimation in this study, but in practice they will vary widely.

2. Perhaps the most critical societal impact may be the cyclic perpetuation of child sexual abuse. A high percentage of child molesters were sexually victimized. We have reported elsewhere that 57% of a sample of 54 child molesters at the Treatment Center were themselves the victim of sexual assaults. Finkelhor has delineated a variety of maladaptive outcomes that may be associated with childhood sexual abuse, including delinquency in adolescence and low self-esteem, substance abuse, sexual dysfunction, prostitution and further victimization in adulthood.

3. The Old Testament law of an "eye for an eye" was tempered with more humane New Testament adages such as "love thy neighbor" and "turn the other cheek," suggesting that the seers and sages who composed the Bible may have experienced the same ambivalence that we feel today.

4. Punishment is *not* used here to imply the intentional, systematic administration of negative or aversive consequences to modify inappropriate behavior.

REFERENCES

Abel, G. (1982). Who is going to protect our children? *Sexual Medicine Today* 6: 32.

Abel, G.G.; Becker; J.V., Cunningham-Rathner, J.; et al. (1984). *The Treatment of Child Molesters*. Manual. Cited in J.V. Becker & G.G. Abel (1985), Methodological and ethical issues in evaluating and treating adolescent sexual offenders. *Research Monograph* No. 85-1396. Washington, D.C.: U.S. Department of Health and Human Services.

Abel, G.G.; Mittelman, M.; Becker, J.V.; et al. (1988). Predicting child molesters' response to treatment. In R.A. Prentky & V.L. Quinsey (eds.), *Human Sexual Aggression: Current Perspectives*. Annals of the New York Academy of Sciences. New York: The Academy.

Adams, S. (1975). *Evaluation Research in Corrections: A Practical Guide*. Washington, D.C.: National Institute of Law Enforcement and Criminal Justice, U.S. Department of Justice.

Bard, L.A.; Carter, D.L.; Cerce, D.D.; & et al. (1987). A descriptive study of rapists and child molesters: developmental, clinical and criminal characteristics. *Behavioral Sciences and the Law* 5 (2): 203–220.

Barton, R.R., & Turnbull, B.W. (1981). A failure rate regression model for the study of recidivism. In J.A. Fox (ed.), *Models in Quantitative Criminology*. New York: Academic Press.

Becker, J.V.; Kaplan, M.S.; & Kavoussi, R. (1988). Measuring the effectiveness of treatment for the aggressive adolescent sexual offender. In R.A. Prentky & V.L. Quinsey (eds.), *Human Sexual Aggression: Current Perspectives*. Annals of the New York Academy of Sciences. New York: The Academy.

Blumstein, A. (1971). Cost-effectiveness analysis in the allocation of police resources. In M.G. Kendall (ed.), *Cost-Benefit Analysis*. London: English University Press.

Burgess, A.W., & Holmstrom, L.L. (1974). Rape trauma syndrome. *American Journal of Psychiatry* 131: 981–986.

Burgess, A.W., & Lazare, A. (1976). The sexually abused. In A.W. Burgess & A.A. Lazare, *Community Mental Health: Target Populations*. Englewood Cliffs, N.J.: Prentice-Hall.

Carter, D.L., & Prentky, R.A. (1988). Overview of the program at the Massachusetts Treatment Center. In D. Weisstub (ed.), *Law and Mental Health: International Perspectives*. New York: Pergamon Press.

Christiansen, K.O.; Elers-Nielsen, M.; Le Maire, L.; & Sturup, G.K. (1965). *Recidivism Among Sexual Offenders. Scandinavian Studies in Criminology*. Vol. 1. London: Tavistock.

Finkelhor, D. (1984). *Child Sexual Abuse: New Theory and Research*. New York: Free Press.

Finkelhor, D. (1979). *Sexually Victimized Children*. New York: Free Press.

Frisbie, L.V. (1969). Another look at sex offenders in California. *California Mental Health Research Monograph*. No. 12. Sacramento: State of California Department of Mental Hygiene.

Furby, L.; Weinrott, M.R.; & Blackshaw, L. (1988). Sex offender recidivism: a review. *Psychological Bulletin* 105: 3–30.

Geiser, R.L. (1979). *Hidden Victims: The Sexual Abuse of Children.* Boston: Beacon Press.

Glaser, D. (1973). *Routinizing Evaluation: Getting Feedback on Effectiveness of Crime and Delinquency Programs.* Washington D.C.: National Institute of Mental Health, U.S. Department of Health, Education, and Welfare.

Harris, C.M.; Kaylan, A.R.; & Maltz, M.D. (1981). Recent advances in the statistics of recidivism measurement. In J.A. Fox (ed.), *Models in Quantitative Criminology.* New York: Academic Press.

Harris, C.M., & Moitra, S. (1978). Improved statistical techniques for the measurement of recidivism. *Journal of Research in Crime and Delinquency* 15: 194–213.

Holahan, J. (1970a). *A Benefit-Cost Analysis of Project Crossroads.* Prepared for the Manpower Administration. U.S. Department of Labor (contract No. 82-34-68-15). National Committee on Children and Youth. Washington, D.C.: Government Printing Office.

Holahan, J. (1970b). *The Economics of Drug Addiction and Control in Washington, D.C.: A Model for Estimation of Costs and Benefits of Rehabilitation.* Washington D.C.: Office of Planning and Research, District of Columbia Department of Correction.

Holahan, J. (1973). Measuring benefits from prison reform. In *Benefit-Cost and Policy Analysis 1973.* An Aldine annual on forecasting, decision-making, and evaluation. Chicago: Aldine.

Jaffe, A.C.; Dynneson, L.; & ten Bensel, R.W. (1975). Sexual abuse of children: an epidemiologic study. *American Journal of Diseases of Children* 129: 689–692.

Jones, B. McC.; Jenstrom, L.L.; & MacFarlane, K. (1980). *Sexual Abuse of Children: Selected Readings.* Pub. No. OHDS 78-30161. Washington, D.C.: U.S. Department of Health and Human Services.

Laws, D.R. (1986). *Prevention of Relapse in Sex Offenders.* Project No. 1 R01 MH42035. Washington, D.C.: National Institute of Mental Health.

Mahoney, M., & Blozan, C.F. (1968). *Cost-Benefit Evaluation of Welfare Demonstration Projects: A Test Application to Juvenile Rehabilitation.* Prepared by the Research Management Corporation for the U.S. Department of Health, Education, and Welfare.

Maltz, M.D. (1984). *Recidivism.* New York: Academic Press.

Maltz, M.D., & McCleary, R. (1977). The mathematics of behavioral change: recidivism and construct validity. *Evaluation Quarterly* 1: 421–438.

Marshall, W.L. (1988). Personal communication.

Marshall, W.L.; Abel, G.G.; & Quinsey, V.L. (1983). The assessment and treatment of sexual offenders. In S.S. Jones (ed.), *Sexual Aggression and the Law*. Burnaby, British Columbia: Criminology Research Centre, Simon Fraser University.

Marshall, W.L., & Barbaree, H.E. (1988). An outpatient treatment program for child molesters. In R.A. Prentky & V.L. Quinsey (eds.), *Human Sexual Aggression: Current Perspectives*. Annals of the New York Academy of Sciences. New York: The Academy.

Marshall, W.L.; Earls, C.M.; Segal, Z.; & Darke, J. (1983). A behavioral program for the assessment and treatment of sexual aggressors. In K. Craig & R. McMahon (eds.), *Advances in Clinical Behavior Therapy*. New York: Brunner/Mazel.

Marques, J.K. (1988). The sex offender treatment and evaluation project: California's new outcome study. In R.A. Prentky & V.L. Quinsey (eds.), *Human Sexual Aggression: Current Perspectives*. Annals of the New York Academy of Sciences. New York: The Academy.

Norris, J., & Feldman-Summers, S. (1981). Factors related to the psychological impacts of rape on the victim. *Journal of Abnormal Psychology* 90: 562–567.

Pacht, A.R. (1976). The rapist in treatment: professional myths and psychological realities. In M.J. Walker & S.L. Brodsky (eds.), *Sexual Assault: The Victim of the Rapist*. Lexington, Mass.: Lexington Books.

Peters, J.J. (1976). Children who are victims of sexual assault and the psychology of offenders. *American Journal of Psychotherapy* 30: 398–421.

Pithers, W.D.; Kashima, K.M.; Cumming, G.F.; et al. (1988). Relapse prevention of sexual aggression. In R.A. Prentky & V.L. Quinsey (eds.), *Human Sexual Aggression: Current Perspectives*. Annals of the New York Academy of Sciences. New York: The Academy.

Quinsey, V.L. (1983). Prediction of recidivism and the evaluation of treatment programs for sex offenders. In S.N. Verdun-Jones & A.A. Keltner (eds.), *Sexual Aggression and the Law*. Burnaby, British Columbia: Criminology Research Centre, Simon Fraser University.

Schmidt, P., & Witte, A.D. (1980). Evaluating correctional programs: models of criminal recidivism and an illustration of their use. *Evaluation Quarterly* 4: 585–600.

Seghorn, T.K.; Prentky, R.A.; & Boucher, R.J. (1987). Childhood sexual abuse in the lives of sexually aggressive offenders. *Journal of the American Academy of Child and Adolescent Psychiatry* 26 (2):262–267.

Soothill, K.L., & Gibbens, T.C.N. (1978). Recidivism of sexual offenders: a re-appraisal. *British Journal of Criminology* 18: 267–276.

Weimer, D.L., & Friedman, L.S. (1979). Efficiency considerations in criminal rehabilitation research: costs and consequences. In L. Sechrest & S. White (eds.), *The Rehabilitation of Criminal Offenders: Problems and Prospects*. Washington, D.C.: National Academy of Sciences.

West, D.J. (1983). Sex offenses and offending. In M. Tonry & N. Morris (eds.), *Crime and Justice: An Annual Review of Research*. Chicago: University of Chicago Press.

Witte, A.D., & Schmidt, P. (1977). An analysis of recidivism, using the truncated lognormal distribution. *Applied Statistics* 26: 302–311.

APPENDIX

Offender-Related Expenses

1. *Apprehension and Pretrial Investigation*

    police investigator

    defender's investigator

    presentence investigation

2. *Trial*

    superior court judge

    court officers

    court reporter

    clerk

    probation officer

    defense attorney

    prosecutor

12-member jury + 2 alternates

3. *Incarceration*

4. *Parole Supervision*

Victim-Related Expenses

1. *Department of Social Services*

2. *Hospital Medical Expenses*

3. *Victim Evaluation*

4. *Victim Witness Services*

5. *Victim Treatment*

Determination of Expenses

Expenses were determined by contacting appropriate state agencies. At least three independent estimates were obtained in each case and an average taken.

A. Offender-related Expenses

1.   *Apprehension and pretrial investigation*—based on annual salaries of $45,000 for detectives and $32,000 for police officers.

a. Initial response by uniformed officer 3 hrs. ($46.14)

b. Detective's investigation   20 hrs. ($432.60)

c. Pretrial preparation (police)   5 hrs. ($108.15)

d. Detective's court testimony   20 hrs. ($432.60)

Subtotal: *$1,020* (rounded)

2.   *Trial expenses*—estimates for trial length consistently ranged between three and five days. Thus, an intermediate figure of four days is used.

a.   Superior court judge: annual salary $75,000 or $205/day total: $820

b.   Court officers (2): annual salary $28,000 or $77/day total: $616

c.   Court reporter: annual salary $25,000 or $69/day total: $276

d.   Clerk: annual salary $35,000 or $96/day total: $384

e.   Probation officer: annual salary $25,000 or $69/day total: $276

f.   Defense attorney from public defender's office: annual salary $25,000 or $69/day total: $276

g.   Prosecutor from county D.A.'s office: annual salary $40,000 or $114/day   total: $456

h.   12-member jury + 2 alternates—employers pay jurors expenses for the first three days; calculation is based on one day.

i.   Jurors: $50/day x 14 members = $700

Subtotal: $3,804

3.   *Incarceration*—the cost of incarceration was determined by averaging the annual inmate cost at 7 penal facilities in Massachusetts (1 maximum security; 3 moderate security; 3 minimum security)

a.   7 prisons in fiscal year 1987; average $22,662/yr.
Subtotal: $158,635 ($22,662 x 7 years)

4.   *Parole Supervision*—the annual salary for an assistant chief Parole officer is $40,825 (or $20/hour). Assuming a sentence of 10–15 years and parole at the parole eligibility date of 7 years (2/3 minimum), the offender would owe the parole board 8 years. These calculations are based on the assumption that the offender is not followed for the full 8 years but is discharged from parole after 5 years.

a.

Supervision	Time	Total Hours
First year	1 hour/week	50
Second year	3 hours/month	36
Third year	2 hours/month	24
Fourth year	1 hour/month:	12
Fifth year	1 hour/3 months:	4

Subtotal: 126 hours x $20/hour = $2,520

b. Parole board hearing:

Institutional parole officer meets with offender prior to parole board hearing: 3 hours   ($60)

Parole board hearing + preparation time ~ report: 4 hours x 3 members of panel = 12 hours   ($240)

c. Postrelease treatment:

Assuming that postrelease treatment is a condition of pa role. the minimum expense of such treatment by a licensed therapist would be $2,750. This figure is based on one session/ week for 1 year $55/hour (the amount that a clinical psychologist is reimbursed by insurance).

Subtotal: $5,570

"A" TOTAL: $169.029

B. Victim-related Expenses

1.   *Department of Social Services*

Intake Investigation—An intake investigation on an unfounded case requires 15–18 hours at a cost that may range from $350 to $1.000. In a substantiated case of abuse the investigation will take anywhere from 20–30 hours. According to the Department of Social Services the average cost of an investigation is $406 and the average cost of an assessment is $812, for a total of about $1,200.

Case Management—The average cost of case management (developing service plans for the family, case reviews, etc.) is $242/ month. Cases are typically followed for 6 to 12 months. The cost of an eight month follow-up would be $1,936.

Subtotal: $3,136

2. *Hospital/Medical Expenses*

Emergency Room	$110
Examining Physician	$100
Laboratory Tests	$75

Subtotal: $285

3.   *Victim Evaluation*—A thorough evaluation by an experienced independent professional, including 4–5 sessions and a report, would cost about $1,000.

4.   *Victim Witness Services* (all figures based on $17/hour)

Initial Consultation with DSS & AOA: 2 hrs. = $34

Assessment/Evaluation of Case (interview/visits: with child/parents & consultation with ADA, DSS, & therapist)	6 hrs. = $102
Between Assessment & Initiation of Criminal Case (Grand Jury) (referral work, ongoing support, contact with DSS, police therapist)	3 hrs. = $51
Preparation for Grand Jury Appearance	3 hrs. = $51
Grand Jury Appearance	2 hrs. = $34
Between Grand Jury & Trial	8 hrs. = $136
Preparation for Trial	16 hrs. = $272
Trial (4 days)	32 hrs. = $544
Disposition (preparation for Victim Impact Statement, sentencing hearing)	4 hrs. = $68
Posttrial Follow-Up	3 hrs. = $51
Victim Witness Supporting Costs	
Advocate Training	50hrs./yr.=$4,000
Professional Reading	20 hrs./yr.= $340
Supervision Costs	24 hrs./yr.= $480
Supplies (toys, books, crayons, games)	$70
Anatomical Dolls (1 set)	$150

Subtotal: $6,383

5.   *Victim Treatment*—An average hourly rate charged by a licensed professional therapist who works with child victims is $70. Assuming one session per week, the cost of treatment would be $3,500/year. While the length of treatment obviously will vary considerably across victims, we chose, for present purposes, to use a more conservative estimate of one year. Given protracted victimization, treatment might well last for longer than one year. The estimate used here also does not include any treatment services provided to the family of the victim.

Subtotal: $3,500

"B" TOTAL: $14,304

Summary

A.			B.		
	1.	$1,020		1.	$3,136
	2.	3804		2.	285
	3.	158,635		3.	1,000
	4.	5,570		4.	6,383
		$169,029		5.	3, 500
					$14,304

Totals for A + B =$183,333

Serial Child Molesters and Abductors

Ann Wolbert Burgess, John Campbell, Theresa A. Delaney, Robert O. Heck, Raymond Knight, Kenneth V. Lanning, Robert A. Prentky, John B. Rabun, Jr., Robert K. Ressler

Serial child abductors and molesters pose one of the most dangerous threats to the safety of our children. Although the number of such offenders is unknown, each of these criminals typically has a very large number of victims and a long history of criminal behavior.

To date, little research has been done on the patterns and motivations of serial child molesters and abductors. One such effort, however, is ongoing at the Massachusetts Treatment Center (MTC) in Bridgewater, Massachusetts, which houses sex offenders. The MTC was established in 1959, under Section 123A of the Massachusetts General Laws, for the evaluation and treatment of "sexually dangerous persons." This law provides that a person found guilty of a sexual offense can be committed to the Massachusetts Treatment Center for a period of time from one day to life if he is judged to be sexually dangerous. The following study included 157 child molesters who met the MTC inclusion criteria. This chapter examines the two different types of child molesters studied at MTC.

In the MTC study a *child molester* is defined as someone whose sexual offenses are against victims under the age of 16. A sexual offense is defined as any sexually motivated assault involving physical contact with the victim. When the victim age criterion is not sufficient (for example, because the offender is young or because of multiple victims of varying ages), several additional guidelines are used. Age discrepancy between offender and victim is considered, as is the predominant ages of victims and any other victim age trends.

Note: For this study, the definition of *abduction* is not necessarily in accord with statutes nor stereotypes of "stranger danger." The determination of abduction in this study is made on the basis of detailed information in the offender's research file. Each offense is coded in terms of the place in which the offender initially encountered the victim and the place in which the offense actually took place. For cases in which the place of encounter and offense differed on 50% or more occasions for all known offenses, the offender was coded as an abductor. Offenders were coded as nonabductors when the place of encounter and offense matched for *all* known offenses.

The MTC study examined a number of descriptive aspects of the child molesters. This information is outlined in the Matrix of Abducting Child Molesters Compared to Non-Abducting Child Molesters. The matrix is provided as a useful tool in the work of both mental health clinicians and law enforcement officers in understanding the patterns of child molesters. The following case histories of three offenders represent the two different categories of child molesters in the MTC study. (*Note: All names and locations have been changed.*)

SPECIAL CASE HISTORY A: AN *ABDUCTING* CHILD MOLESTER

> *Charles Adler's most recent crime was only one in a series of many attempted as well as completed rapes of young girls. His abduction pattern consisted of luring preadolescent and adolescent girls—for whom he had a sexual preference—into the woods on the pretense of looking for animals and then attempting to rape them. His last known crime began when he met two children in a post office and asked if they would like to help him catch rabbits. He led them into the woods, and when the 12-year-old girl stated that she had to get home, he grabbed her from behind, pulled out a sheath knife, held it to her throat cutting her, forced her to undress, and attempted to rape her. The girl's 8-year-old brother watched the entire attack*

after running to hide in nearby bushes. Adler, as in many of his attempted rapes, was impotent. He was so infuriated by his inability to rape the girl that he had the urge to "do her in." Instead, Adler fled from the woods, leaving the injured victim and her brother to find their way to safety. The attempted rape and murder were committed while Charles Adler was on parole—having been incarcerated for nearly 10 years for the attempted rape of a 14-year-old girl.

Charles Adler was the oldest of three children. His parents were alcoholics, and when drinking, the father often beat Charles with his fists and a horsewhip. When he was 3 years old, his father knocked him out of his high chair and shattered his hip. Throughout childhood and adolescence, Adler was ridiculed by his peers because of a noticeable limp.

When his father beat him, Adler would run off into the swamps near his house ending up at his grandparents' farm. While staying on the farm, his grandfather taught Adler how to care for animals and how "to live off the land." At age 7 Adler's grandfather died, and his father would not let Charles go to the funeral. Adler states that he blames himself for his grandfather's death. On the day his grandfather died, Adler had split his head open jumping for a tree limb and believes that the news of his accident caused his grandfather's death.

A social loner, he was easily frustrated and angry. Adler beat up other children and got pleasure from torturing animals. The animal torture included tying up frogs in order to burn them alive and throwing cherry bombs at cats.

Feeling rejected by his family and peers, Charles Adler grew up mistrusting others and despising authority. He reports that he began drinking heavily in adolescence. His first sexual experience occurred at age 12 when he was sexually exploited by a cousin and her mother. Around age 13 Adler once again ran away from home. This time he lived in the swamps for eight to nine months. He states that it was like being Tarzan, claiming that he lived off the land with no one to tell him what to do or when to do it.

At age 14 Adler began to have rape fantasies that involved tying up young victims, raping, and then burning them. He reports tying up his sister at that time but claims that he did not actually rape her. His heroes during adolescence were Batman, Al Capone, and John Dillinger. Adler believed that his gangster heroes had the guts that he lacked. Adler dropped out of school in the ninth grade and was on his own at the age of 16. Adler's nonsexual offenses include three vagrancy charges and he spent two years in prison for a grand larceny conviction at the age of 17. After being released, Adler claims to have committed nine rapes before his first conviction for the attempted rape of a 14-year-old girl. He spent one year in a state hospital for that offense and was cleared of four charges of attempted rape due to lack of sufficient evidence.

Adler was married at the age of 21 for two years. His wife divorced him while he was in prison. Although Adler managed to marry, it is evident that he has remained socially isolated most of his life with few, if any, significant adult relationships. Moreover, his sporadic, menial work history further underscores his general low level of social competence. Rehabilitation attempts through therapy and incarceration seem to have little effect in subduing Charles Adler's intent to force sex on young girls. While in group therapy in prison, he admits fantasizing about rape using a gun or knife and he has stated that if he were let out of prison, he would do the same thing all over again.

Adler has few friends within the prison population and spends a great deal of time reading literature on wildlife and the occult. His therapists state that he has not made full use of therapy sessions, and he has not been recommended for release.

CRIME CLASSIFICATION*: Abducting Child Molester

SOCIAL COMPETENCE: low

Sᴇxᴜᴀʟ ᴘʀᴇᴏᴄᴄᴜᴘᴀᴛɪᴏɴ ᴡɪᴛʜ ᴄʜɪʟᴅʀᴇɴ: high

Nᴏɴᴏғғᴇɴsᴇ ᴄᴏɴᴛᴀᴄᴛ ᴡɪᴛʜ ᴄʜɪʟᴅʀᴇɴ: low

Pʜʏsɪᴄᴀʟ ɪɴᴊᴜʀʏ ᴛᴏ ᴄʜɪʟᴅ: high

Sᴀᴅɪsᴍ: high

*See Appendix at end of chapter.

SPECIAL CASE HISTORY B: AN *ABDUCTING* CHILD MOLESTER

At the time of his last arrest, Philip Brisio, a school bus driver, had raped and forced oral and anal sex on numerous children—both boys and girls—and had been incarcerated a number of times for sexual offenses. These offenses include lewd and lascivious behavior, contributing to the delinquency of a minor, indecent assault and battery on a child, sodomy, and unnatural acts. Yet, Brisio has claimed repeatedly that he has never hurt a child and that all of his victims were willing partners. Also, he believes that the children truly enjoyed being with him. For example, he would take the children to the movies, restaurants, playgrounds, and beaches without the permission or knowledge of their parents.

The events leading to Brisio's last arrest involve a child sex ring in which children were exchanged among adults for money, and nude photographs were taken of the children. Brisio victimized both male and female children and encouraged the boys to have sex with their sisters. The children involved in these activities ranged in age from 10 to 13 years.

Brisio is the seventh of twelve children. The family lived in a three-room apartment with sparse furnishings and little food. His father was a quiet, sickly man who worked all day, coming home in the evening to eat and go directly to bed. Brisio described his father as "a good guy," though passive and ineffectual. Brisio recalls, however, that his mother ran their home "like a tyrant" and says that he had a "miser-

able" childhood. He stated, "I didn't think anyone cared about me or loved me. I didn't feel like I belonged anywhere . . . like if I didn't come home one day nobody would even notice. I got along okay with my brothers and sisters, but my mother gave me really bad beatings almost every day." Frustrated and teased by other children, Brisio had frequent temper tantrums, was difficult to control, and often ran away from home.

At age 7 Brisio began taking female children into the cellar, disrobing them, and rubbing up against them. At the age of 11 Brisio was sexually assaulted and sodomized by an adult male. By the age of 12 he was engaging in sodomy with male peers, and by the age of 13 he had become involved in an ongoing sexual relationship with an adult male. At the age of 14 he began to sodomize 6- and 7-year-old boys. Brisio's victimization of children continued well beyond adolescence. At the age of 15 he ran away from home and began wandering. At the age of 17 he enlisted in the U.S. Marine Corps, but he was discharged after 6 months because of headaches he claims to have faked in order to be released from military duty. He then enlisted in the U.S. Air Force, but he was discharged after 15 months for fraudulent enlistment. His sporadic employment history includes jobs as a security guard, janitor, bus boy, grocery clerk, and school bus driver.

His criminal record begins at about the time he left home when he was arrested for gambling. Most of his nonsexual offenses were automobile-related, with the exception of charges for one count each of assault and battery and breaking and entering. His first arrest for a sexual offense occurred at the age of 22 when he tried to commit sodomy on a 10-year-old boy. He was committed to a state hospital for this offense, but he was discharged shortly thereafter.

Emotionally unstable, bitterly angry, and diagnosed as a sexual psychopath, Brisio has not stopped his criminal sexual behavior despite his many incarcerations for sexual offenses. Throughout his life, he has been in and out of jails and hospitals for repeated sexual crimes against children. At one time his parole was revoked because of new offenses against children.

Philip Brisio has mainly targeted young boys between the ages of 8 and 9 for abduction and sexual exploitation. He claims that he takes out his sexual urges on children because of inner pressures of anger and frustration. While in prison, Brisio denies any sexual fantasies of children. He manipulates the therapy group, has used treatment to avoid prison, and does not fully utilize treatment. Thus, therapists do not recommend his release.

CRIME CLASSIFICATION[*]: Abducting Child Molester

SOCIAL COMPETENCE: low

SEXUAL PREOCCUPATION WITH CHILDREN: high

NONOFFENSE CONTACT WITH CHILDREN: high

PHYSICAL INJURY TO CHILD: low

SADISM: low

*See Appendix at end of chapter.

SPECIAL CASE HISTORY C: A *NONABDUCTING* CHILD MOLESTER

Donald Wynn's sexual abuse of his daughter, which began immediately after her birth, was one of many instances of his repeated pattern of sexual victimization of young girls. He admits to dating women in order to be close either to their younger sisters or to their young daughters and is skillful in gaining employment that brings him into contact with children.

When Donald Wynn opened his music studio, at age 26, he was very excited about the prospect of being alone with children. He reports teaching half-hour music lessons to 70 students each week during which he often victimized his young female students while their parents were in the waiting room just next door. The offenses against young girls consisted of fondling the children—with and without their clothes on—and forcing the children to hold his penis. At times, he would perform oral sex on the girls while he masturbated himself to ejaculation. Involved with child pornography collectors, Wynn would take photographs of his students in the nude and then exchange them with other collectors. His sexual behavior with his students continued for 10 years before he was arrested.

Donald Wynn, the second of three siblings, reports being close to his mother while growing up, since his father was rarely home and drank heavily when he was with the family. The father often called his son by a girl's name and teased him for being effeminate. His father kept a collection of "girlie" magazines, which Donald discovered and read avidly. Wynn became sexually involved with his younger brother around the age of 6, and the involvement did not end until he was in his early 20s. This relationship left him feeling guilty and ashamed. As a teen, Wynn began to engage in oral sex with younger boys in his neighborhood to keep them quiet about the sexual activity with his brother.

Overweight, shy, and friendless, Wynn had an inferiority complex. He first became sexually involved with little girls at the age of 18. At that time he dated a girl in order to be close to her 5-year-old sister. Later he married a divorced mother with two young sons. After his marriage, Wynn repeatedly victimized the children's 14-year-old babysitter.

Donald Wynn's wife forced him to see a psychiatrist after he confessed to molesting the babysitter sexually. His doctor prescribed medication in an attempt to control Wynn's fear, anxiety, paranoid ideation, and erotic preoccupations. Wynn has been hospitalized a number of times for his sexual preoccupation with children and for depression.

Following his arrest for the sexual victimization of his music students, Wynn was examined by a psychiatrist at a mental health clinic. He was found competent to stand trial and no evidence of illness was found. While committed to the treatment center, however, Wynn continued his preoccupation with little girls, having been caught twice ordering child pornography through the mail using the names and addresses of other inmates.

The following excerpt is from a letter written by Wynn to another child pornographer. The letter, confiscated by postal agents, in an unrelated child pornography investigation, illustrates Wynn's motivation and refers to his sexual relationship with his daughter that began when she was 1 week old.

"After I was arrested, my wife was shown the photos I took of my daughter and informed of what had been going on. She was shocked and it's taken her a long time to forgive me, but it appears now she has finally accepted it and will stick with me. This has all happened within the last few weeks. Now that my wife has come around, I'll see my family on a regular basis. You know what helped? My wife had my daughter examined and interviewed both by a pediatrician and a psychologist, and both of them told my wife that my daughter has suffered no ill effects whatsoever from our relationship. That convinced her that I've always treated my daughter with love, gentleness, and tenderness, and I didn't harm her. Of course, in here I have to play their game, so I do, but we both know that the facts speak for themselves."

Cunning and manipulative, Donald Wynn's status at the treatment center is described in the following statement by his therapist. "Overall, Mr. Wynn . . . is lacking a sense of true pain on an emotional level...He tends to externalize blame quite often. There appears to be at this time little true motivation to change . . . It appears his current goal in therapy is to say the right things in order to be released in the near future."

CRIME CLASSIFICATION: Nonabducting Child Molester

SOCIAL COMPETENCE: high

SEXUAL PREOCCUPATION WITH CHILDREN: high

NONOFFENSE CONTACT WITH CHILDREN: high

PHYSICAL INJURY TO CHILD: low

SADISM: low

ABDUCTING CHILD MOLESTERS COMPARED TO NONABDUCTING CHILD MOLESTERS

Abduction may be understood as a strategy for achieving control over the victim and *not* necessarily as a sign of greater brutality or aggression. Child abductors, when compared to nonabducting child molesters, were found to be (1) *lower* in social competence, (2) *lower* in amount of nonoffense-related contact with children, and (3) *higher* in presence and use of weapons during offenses, but *not* higher in amount of aggression or victim injury.

This study suggests that for some offenders abduction may be a strategy for controlling the victim. Abductors, as compared to nonabducting child molesters, more frequently carry and use weapons to intimidate and control the children, not necessarily to hurt them. The greater need to control the children (through abduction and intimidation) may stem from their poor interpersonal and social skills. Offenders who do *not* typically abduct their victims may have a higher degree of social competence and a greater ability to gain control over their victims by verbally enticing or tricking them. All child abductors cannot, however, be subsumed under the motivational umbrella of control. Analysis of the data further indicates that abduction tends to be associated with the presence of sadism. This would seem to be a different motivation from control, suggesting fantasy-driven offenses in which abduction is a part of the fantasy. The descriptive characteristics of the abductors and nonabductors are reported in the following matrix. Both groups were predominantly Caucasian and were comparable with respect to IQ, educational achievement, and achieved skill level. There was a tendency for the nonabductors to have less post high school education (5% vs. 17%

for abductors). The nonabductors were more likely to have been married (58% vs. 35% for abductors). The average victim age was comparable for both groups. Nonabductors were more likely to have offended against children in their nuclear or extended family (26% vs. 8% for abductors) and the abductors were more likely to have offended against a child not known to them (33% vs. 20% for the nonabductors).

MATRIX
ABDUCTING CHILD MOLESTERS COMPARED TO
NONABDUCTING CHILD MOLESTERS

	Abductors	*Nonabductors*
Number	97	60
Race		
Caucasian	93%	95%
Noncaucasian	7%	5%
Achieved Skill Level		
Unskilled/semi-skilled	74%	71%
Skilled/lower management	25%	27%
Professional/upper management	1%	2%
Educational Achievement		
Elementary school (partial or completed)	23%	23%
High school (partial or completed)	60%	72%
Post High School	17%	5%
Marriage		
Never	65%	42%
Once	28%	46%
More than once	7%	12%
IQ		
Average	96.40	94.80
Standard deviation	15.20	15.00
Average Number of Victims While Offender Still a Juvenile		
Average	.52	.20
Standard deviation	1.19	.55
Range	0-6	0–3

Average Number of Victims in Offender's Adult Years

Average	3.63	2.92
Standard deviation	3.22	2.41
Range	1–16	0–16

Average Age of Victims

Average	10.28	9.69
Standard deviation	3.30	2.91

Relationship to Victims

Family member	8%	26%
Acquaintance	58%	54%
Not known by offender	33%	20%

Total Offenses with Weapon Present

Average	.59	.19
Standard deviation	.94	.44

Total Offenses With Weapon Used

Average	.55	.19
Standard deviation	.91	.44

Severity of Sexual Aggression

Average	1.35	1.24
Standard deviation	.96	1.12

Severity of Nonsexual Aggression

Average	1.85	1.88
Standard deviation	1.50	1.44

APPENDIX

The Crime Classification module is based on five elements: social competence, sexual preoccupation with children, nonoffense contact with children, physical injury to child, and sadism. Following are the criteria used to classify an offender within this module.

Social Competence

Five criteria twere used to determine *social competence*. If an offender fit two or more of the following criteria, then he was listed as having high social competence. If an offender fit less than two of the following criteria, then he was listed as having low social competence.

1. Maintained a single job for three or more years.

2. Involved in a sexual relationship with another adult that included marriage or cohabitation for at least one year.

3. Provided evidence of assuming responsibility for parenting a child for three or more years.

4. Actively involved in an adult-oriented organization (nonvocationally related) with frequent adult interpersonal contact for one or more years.

5. Maintained a friendship with an adult, not involving marriage or cohabitation, lasting at least one year and involving active contact and shared activities.

Sexual Preoccupation with Children

Three criteria were used to determine *sexual preoccupation with children*.

1. The offender is considered to have a low sexual preoccupation with children if he is over 20 years old and *all* of his sexual encounters with children (both charged and uncharged incidents) occurred within a six-month period of time. The offender is considered to have a high sexual preoccupation with children if he is over 20 years old and there is evidence of three or more sexual encounters with children in which the time period between the first and third-encounter is greater than six months. These encounters may be with a single victim over many incidents and should not be limited to charged offenses.

2. For the offender with a high sexual preoccupation with children there is evidence that he has had enduring relationships with children (excluding parental contact). This includes sexual and nonsexual and professional and nonprofessional contacts.

3. In addition, an offender with a high sexual preoccupation with children initiates contact with children in numerous situations over his lifetime.

Nonoffense Contact with Children

Many factors were taken into consideration when classifying *nonoffense contact with children*. In general, the amount of contact is a behavioral measure of the time spent with children. It includes both sexual and nonsexual situations but excludes contact resulting from parental responsibilities. This definition must be distinguished from sexual preoccupation with children, which attempts to assess the strength of an individual's pedophilic interest (i.e., the extent to which thoughts of children dominate his fantasy life).

A low amount of nonoffense contact with children is characterized by little or no contact with children in a job or recreational setting. In general, the only contact such a person has with children is in the context of sexual assault.

An offender with high nonoffense contact with children has regular contact with children in both sexual and nonsexual contexts. It is assumed that repeated sexual encounters with the same child implies the development of a relationship that goes beyond sexual involvement. For that reason, when there are three or more sexual encounters with the same victim, the offender is coded as having high nonoffense contact with children.

Physical Injury to Child

Low *physical injury to victim* is characterized by the absence of physical injury to the victim and the presence of only such acts as pushing, shoving, slapping, holding, or verbal threats—as long as these acts result in no lasting physical injury (e.g., cuts, bruises, or contusions). High physical injury to victim includes hitting, punching, choking, aggressive sodomy (i.e., any violence causing physical injury to the victim). High injury also includes forcing the victim to ingest urine or feces.

Sadism

In regards to *sadism* there must be evidence that the offender is sexually aroused or otherwise derives pleasure from placing the victim in pain or fear. In lieu of self-report of such arousal or sadistic fantasies, it is necessary to rely upon behavioral evidence—such as the use of violence to facilitate arousal or ritualized, bizarre acts—not usually seen as part of normal sexuality. Other examples of sadistic acts include aggressive sodomy, object insertion, or violence focused on breasts, genitals, or the anus. A presence of any of the above behaviors would qualify an offender to be rated high in sadism. The absence of the above factors would qualify an offender to be rated low in sadism.

Sexual Aggression

Sexual aggression is the amount of harm done to the victim in the context of an offense. It is based on a 5-point scale with 0 denoting no evidence of sexual aggression and 4 denoting evidence of extreme sexual aggression.

Nonsexual Aggression

The nonsexual aggression category is based on a 7-point scale with 0 denoting no evidence of aggression in a nonsexual context and 6 denoting evidence of extreme aggression in a nonsexual context.

CHAPTER
21

Juveniles Who Murder

Christine A. Grant, Ann Wolbert Burgess,
Carol R. Hartman, Allen G. Burgess,
Edward R. Shaw, Gloria MacFarland

This chapter is reprinted with permission from,
Juveniles who murder, *Journal of Psychosocial
Nursing 27* (12) 4–11. Preparation of this article
was supported, in part, by a Department of
Justice, Office of Juvenile Justice and Delin-
quency Prevention grant (#84-JN-K010).

> *A 15-year-old white youth is admitted to the
> adolescent inpatient unit of a psychiatric hospital
> following his arrest for the murder of a 13-year-old
> neighbor boy. Community response was one of shock
> and astonishment as the youth was reported to be a
> good student, quiet, and respectful. After a week on
> the unit, nursing observations concurred with the
> community, noting the youth was cooperative during
> interviews and interactions on the unit. It was
> difficult for the staff to believe he committed such an
> act. (Case 1.)*

Mental health clinicians assume a critical role in observing and
assessing patients in residential and inpatient settings. As crime and
violence continue to escalate in our society, psychiatric staff will
need forensic knowledge and skills as patients, especially juveniles,
are hospitalized for evaluation. How do they obtain critical information for planning inpatient treatment? How do they manage
their own beliefs and feelings about criminal behavior so that they
may be therapeutic? In the above case, if additional information

about the juvenile's thoughts and feelings are not obtained, therapeutic intervention will not occur and he will be at risk for repeating his actions.

While juveniles who murder stir a wide range of reaction from disbelief to public outcry and fear, aggressive behavior has long been a concern in the clinical management of children (Barlow, 1989), adolescents (Pond, 1988), adults in hospital settings (Jones, 1985), and in long-term settings (Winger, Schirm, & Stewart, 1987). Research on adolescents who murder has advanced from descriptive psychological case reports (Bender, 1959; Duncan & Duncan, 1971; King, 1974; Malmquist, 1971; Russell, 1979; Smith, 1965) to controlled studies that seek to design classification systems as a method of communication (Cornell, Benedek, & Benedek, 1987; Lewis, Shanok, Pincus, & Glaser, 1979; Sendi & Blomgren, 1975).

Disciplines have varied in their classification of violent criminal behavior. Psychiatric nursing includes categories of aggressive/violent behaviors toward the environment, others, and the self in the 1987 working draft of the American Nurses' Association's *Classification of Human Responses of Concern of Psychiatric Mental Health Nursing Practice* (Loomis, O'Toole, Pothier, et al., 1987). With the creation of the FBI's National Center for the Analysis of Violent Crime (NCAVC) at Quantico, Virginia, law enforcement research has contributed through its efforts to profile criminal behavior by motive (Ressler, Burgess, & Douglas, 1988). This chapter seeks to add to the taxonomy by applying this law enforcement homicide typology to a juvenile sample for insights regarding treatment interventions. It presents (1) descriptive research findings as to emerging profiles of juvenile murderers, (2) a crime classification typology, and (3) the use of crime scene drawings as a technique to assess memories related to the crime for planning treatment.

METHOD

Records of 85 juveniles who were convicted of murder were analyzed regarding background and crime scene characteristics. This sample represented a total sample of juveniles committed between 1978–1986 to a residential facility after the enactment of the 1978 New York State Juvenile Offender Act. The type of murder was classified from the statement of the crime by two of the authors using the FBI NCAVC homicide classification system (Douglas, Ressler, Burgess, & Hartman, 1986). The reader is to understand that this typology attempts to look at the most conscious level of violent acts and the modus operendi for carrying out these acts.

MURDER CLASSIFICATION

The murders were classified into one of two categories, criminal enterprise or cause-specific. In the criminal-enterprise category the individual is focused on the business of crime, and the crime represents an act performed as part of a group or having a social context. The intent has its origins in some type of personal gain for an individual or group. This gain could be money (i.e., burglary, robbery), an assignment for some transgression (i.e., assassination), or right of passage into a particular group. Criminal-enterprise murders may involve a solo offender or a group and include contract murders, gang murders, competition murders, and political murders (Douglas, Ressler, Burgess, & Hartman, 1986).

When the crime involves a self-intent motive, the classification is cause-specific. These homicides include a host of intentions that are idiosyncratic to the perpetrator. Individuals may kill for self-defense and compassion as in "mercy" killings. Family disputes/violence may lie behind matricide or sibling killings. Paranoid reactions may result in murder or the mentally disordered juvenile may commit a symbolic crime or have a psychotic outburst. In this category the murderer may kill as a result of or to engage in sexual activity, dismemberment, mutilation, or other activities that have sexual meaning only for the juvenile (Ressler, Burgess, & Douglas, 1988).

SAMPLE

At the time of the offense the 85 juveniles ranged in age from 13 to 16 years with a mean age of 14.7. The youths were racially divided with 49.4% black, 32.9% Hispanic, 12.9% white, 2.4% Asian, and 2.4% other.

Of the group, 68% lived with their mother and 3.5% with the father, a small number (10.6%) lived with both parents or foster parents, 7% lived with grandparents, and 2.4% lived in other arrangements. The marital status of the parents included 28.2% separated, 28.2% never married, 14% divorced, 10.6% married, and 18.8% of the records did not have the marital status of the parents recorded.

The youths, more likely than not, had siblings. There were 11.8% only children, 12.9% had one sibling, 61% had 2 to 4 siblings, and 14% had 5 or more siblings. In terms of education level, for the information recorded, eighth grade was the mean grade. Twenty-nine did not include last grade completed.

In examining for history of truancy, 57.6% had a history of truancy, 7.1% did not have a truancy history, and 35% of the records did not clarify if there was a history of truancy. A history of alcohol abuse was positive for 24 (27%), negative for 14 (17%), and 47 (56%) unknown. A history of drug abuse was positive for 48%, no history for 12%, and unknown for 40%. Twenty-one youths (25%) had a psychiatric history, 11 (13%) reported no psychiatric history, and it was not known for 53 (62%) of the youths. In terms of a history of delinquency, 5 (6%) had no record, 53 (62%) had a history noted, and 27 (32%) did not.

CRIME CHARACTERISTICS

In defining the nature of the contact between offender and victim, a category was devised between a confrontation of immediate surprise (blitz assault) and a confrontation characterized by a level of verbal interaction (confidence assault) prior to attacking the victim. Seventy-four (87%) assaults were blitz style, 10 (12%) were confidence style, and 1 could not be determined. The method of killing included 34 (40%) deaths by gun shot, 21 (25%) by stabbing, 6 (7%) by beating, 4 (5%) by strangulation, and the remainder (23%) by some other method.

The majority of these juveniles carried weapons (77.6%). Sixty-six youths brought weapons with them to the offense, 15 did not, and there were 4 without data. Of the 66 who brought weapons, 45 brought guns, 21 brought knives, 11 brought some other type of weapon.

Thirty one juveniles (36.5%) killed alone and almost two-thirds (63.5%) of the juveniles who killed had a codefendant. Over one-third (35%) had second or multiple charges.

There were 85 victims. Sixty-six (78%) were male, 18 (21%) were female and the sex of one victim was not recorded. Of the 85 victims, 22 (26%) were known to the offender, 56 (66%) were not known, and in 7 (8%) cases it could not be determined. In terms of relationships of age between victim and offender, 53% of the victims were older than the offender; 12% were younger, 1% was the same age, and 34% of the records did not have the age of the victim recorded.

RESULTS

Significant findings from the statistical tests applied included that those juveniles with a delinquent history tend to use a weapon ($p = .017$) and have a history of truancy ($p = .024$). Those juveniles who abuse drugs also abuse alcohol ($p = .0036$).

When juveniles commit a blitz style of attack, it is usually carried out in combination with a peer ($p = .015$). Weapons and a short time between meeting the victim approached significance ($p = .085$), thus indicating a type of impulsivity to homicidal acts when in possession of a weapon.

In terms of murder classification, 56 juveniles (67%) were classified as committing a criminal-enterprise homicide and 28 juveniles (33%) were classified as committing a cause-specific homicide. Juveniles committing a criminal-enterprise murder were more likely than those committing a cause-specific homicide to have a codefendant ($X = 28.294$, $p= .0000$), to kill an unknown victim ($X = 14.633$, $df = 1$, $p = .0001$) and a victim who was male ($X = 6.443$, $df = 1$, $p = .011$).

Males were more likely to be victims of a criminal-enterprise murder (74.2%), while females were more likely to be a victim of a cause-specific crime (61%). Familiarity with a victim was more likely to be in a cause-specific crime with 57.7% of the victims being known to the offenders, while the criminal-enterprise offenders knew only 13.5% of their victims. Additional people assisting in the crime, as expected, was found to occur most often in the criminal-enterprise group with 86% of the offenders having a codefendant while the cause-specific homicides were almost a complete opposite with 75% of the offenders killing alone. Background data when examined by type of crime suggests that the criminal-enterprise offender most often came from a single-parent (mother) family structure (79.2% of the criminal-enterprise offenders and 61.5% of the cause-specific offenders).

Other demographic data when cross-tabulated with the type of crime that approaches a level of significance was the relationship with race. More white offenders committed cause-specific crimes (63.6%) than criminal-enterprise crimes (36.4%). Black and Hispanic offenders were more likely to perpetrate a criminal-enterprise crime (71.4% and 75%, respectively; $X = 6.919$, $df = 3$, $p = 0.075$).

DISCUSSION AND CRIME SCENE DRAWINGS

As a total sample, this group of homicidal juveniles share the following characteristics. They are male and tend to come from a household of two or more siblings where the dominant caretaker is the mother who is alone in the process of child rearing. There is a high incidence of truancy and delinquency with this group, and there is a relationship between alcohol and drug abuse. These findings support the literature on characteristics of juvenile murderers (Cornell, Benedek, & Benedek, 1987; Lewis, Shanok, Pincus, & Glaser, 1979).

Two Emerging Profiles: Solo vs. Codefendant Murder

In addition, the data suggest two emerging profiles of male offenders between the ages of 13 and 16 who are involved in very serious crimes against other people. There is a split between young males who carry out these violent acts independently as opposed to being involved with a codefendant. Those involved in codefendant murder and violence most often are armed with guns and knives and assault male victims. The motive differs if the victim is known to the offender.

Case 2: Codefendant Murder

In the following codefendant murder, Case 2, two 15-year-olds inflicted numerous stab wounds to a 13-year-old youth and left him lying on the ground in an unconscious state.

The crime scene drawing has strong use of color and is drawn before the murder. The anxiety of the offenders is noted in the large-size victim, weapons, and lack of grounding for the figures.

Killing with a codefendant and/or in a group implies the youths have no compunction about killing. They usually are upset that they were caught. As in this case, the victim was left to die. The offenders often have a strong justification for violent acts and overpower the victim through numbers and weapons. By interview data, this case was premeditated. Intervention would focus on the belief system of the juvenile, i.e., how he believes he has the right to kill.

When data on the involvement with a codefendant is examined there is a peaking in this collaborative effort among youths around the 14-to-15-year age period. The use of weapons, the guns and knives, seems to be associated more with the fact that these offenders are engaging with other males in violent acts. The age of the victim appears less determinant of the weapon carrying nature of the attacks than the sex of the victim. An armed juvenile with a codefendant suggests a blitz encounter with lethal outcome.

In contrast to the codefendant murderer, the solo offender may or may not be armed with a knife or gun and tends to offend against both known and unknown victims as well as male and female. The crime scene drawing in Case 1 was a detailed illustration of the bedroom where the murder occurred. Information regarding the crime was obtained from a second victim of this youth. The incident occurred when the juvenile invited two neighbor boys to his house to see his gun collection and to play his electric guitar. He then asked the boys if they wanted to play roulette and loaded a shotgun with two dummy shells and two live bullets. He gave neither boy an opportunity to leave the room, placed the gun to his shoulder, and pulled the trigger killing one boy and wounding the other. There was no statement of motive made, merely a comment that the youth wondered what it would be like to shoot someone. The youth strongly identified with the father who had a gun collection. The youth owned many guns and collected literature that glorified destruction as a solution of world problems. He sought to initiate among his peers a club, the function of which was to eliminate enemies of the state.

Case 1: The Victimless Crime Scene

The precision and calculation of the Case 1 drawing suggest the absolute disregard for the victim (e.g., missing). It is important for staff to understand that this will be a youth who will conform, be somewhat distant but because of his intelligence be overlooked as to the underlying aggressive fantasies. The drawing is an impressive statement of denial and indicates that a long length of time will be necessary to elicit the basis of the underlying rage and to explore the lack of attachment. The monochromatic pencil quality and emptiness of the drawing indicates a lack of attachment of this youth to people. Objects, not people, are more important. The drawing suggests massive denial and avoidance.

Type of Murder: Criminal Enterprise vs. Cause-Specific

The second major study finding is the type of murder. The majority of juveniles committed a criminal-enterprise type of crime (Case 2) involving one or more co-defendants. The stranger aspect of the criminal enterprise coupled with a justification for violence, lack of family attachment, and the impersonal nature of the victim may be a reinforcement for continued violent acts.

The cause-specific type of crime finds youths committing individual violent acts within the family context or the immediate neighborhood. In this group there is a suggestion that the intensity of particular relationships triggers violence. Since most of the sexual homicide and the family violence came out of this group, one speculates that fantasy and preoccupation with particular individuals and acts becomes a central part of the release of violence (Burgess, Hartman, Ressler, et al., 1986; Prentky, Burgess, Rokous, et al., 1989). Both crime groups tend to arm themselves with knives and guns, with guns most frequently being found in the criminal-enterprise group. Also the victims of both groups tended to be older than the offender, suggesting anger and discontent toward authority. There is also an important counterpoint that both groups collectively were less likely to act impulsively to those younger suggesting some differential response and control.

An example of a cause-specific homicide with fantasy is Case 3, a 16-year-old Hispanic youth on five years probation for the separate rapes of two women, one being his best friend's mother, when he committed two murders of women ages 80 and 64. After pleading guilty, he admitted that he was "turned on" by helpless women.

Both victims were found with extensive stab wounds to the face, neck, and chest, and in one case, the eye. The juvenile described his initial motive for entering the victims' homes as robbery, but he then stated the victims threatened him physically, necessitating his violent response. After the victims were dead, he committed additional acts to their bodies, e.g., pouring oil on the body, inserting a flashlight into the vagina, stabbing at the eyes.

Treatment has revealed a strong suspicion of sexual abuse by the mother. Upon arrest, police discovered his obsession with guns and artwork depicting violence and destruction covering the walls of his apartment home. He is reported to have wired powder caps to telephone poles, blowing them out of the ground. Since residential treatment, he reports depression and sadistic fantasies of killing the detective by cutting him into thin pieces and the jury, one by one, by strangling, hanging, or tearing something out—their eyes, throat, or groin.

Case 3: Serial Sexual Killer

This crime scene is drawn after the murder and illustrates role reversal (victim larger than offender). Attention to the color red on the victim is apparent on the victim's body and the offender's knife. Arrows depict his departure from the room. There is no mention of guilt associated with his sexually offending and murderous behavior. It is important to be aware that this juvenile is very dangerous, has already repeated violent crimes, and incorporates people in the system into his violent fantasies.

TREATMENT IMPLICATIONS

The following principles, based on our clinical experience, are offered for the in-patient management of juvenile murderers.

Assessment for Dangerousness

Staff need official information on the juvenile's crime and history of aggression. A youth who has committed a major crime such as murder has made a statement that he is a dangerous person. It is important to assess the basis of the individual's self-control and assess for current dangerousness. This assessment is familiarization of the nature and type of murder that has occurred and all forensic information, e.g., autopsy and investigative reports, victim statements, crime scene photographs, probation reports, etc.

Suicidal potential needs to be assessed in all situations, but especially in situations where the murder is classified as non-premeditated or impulsive and in which the juvenile feels remorse after the realization that the individual has been killed. Juveniles who kill in the context of another crime, such as robbery, need to be evaluated in terms of the sense of remorse or anger over the act or the propensity to strike out violently whenever they feel their acts are justified.

Unit Status of the Juvenile

Murderous acts are sometimes held in awe by the general public, staff included. Thus, a second principle of intervention is not to treat the juvenile murderer as special. Staff behavior should not aggrandize the murder or make the murder event so special that it creates a secondary gain associated with the act. By the same token, staff are not to handle their own abhorrence or negative reaction by being oversolicitous and guillible with the youth. In essence, clinicians have to learn to appraise their own emotions and reactions to the criminal behavior of the youth and not try to compensate for these reactions by either being "conned" by the youth or becoming angry and cruel. Much of this is avoided by reviewing official records and reports of the crime and being able to deal in a factual way with the youth about all aspects of the criminal behavior.

Honest Disclosure

Juveniles need an environment in which they can honestly disclose and admit what they have done and what they are preoccupied with in doing to others. They may be limited in their capacity and awareness to do this because they do not believe in the value of social and personal control, they are ignorant of the rules of social and personal control, or they have extensive impairments in understanding the antecedents and consequences of behavioral acts. All of these areas become critical points for assessment and therapeutic intervention in any kind of residential program.

The counterpoint to this is the legal defense can interfere with honest recall and integration of the facts. Clinicians need to know what lawyers are advising their client to say and not say. Treatment cannot be conducted if juveniles cannot discuss their crime.

Family Assessment

Data from juveniles suggest that family structure as a single variable does not adequately describe the social network context that can contribute and interact with the youth's potential to act in a violent, assaultive manner. The crime typology suggests that some youths are more connected to group peer violence than other youths whose motivation for violence is idiosyncratic. This finding, while certainly tentative and influenced by the nature of the sample, suggests further research and that there need to be different interventions based on the nature of the violent acts themselves.

Substance Use Assessment

The fact that that almost 50% of the juveniles admitted to drug use implies careful assessment of substance abuse. Studies note that drugs are used to block feelings (e.g., heroin) or heighten feelings (amphetamines, LSD, PCP) or that have a differential effect (cocaine). Thus, it is critical to talk to the juvenile to understand the type of drug use and its primary intent as to whether the youth is trying to heighten or block feelings. For those numb in feeling, a strategy would try to break through the numb state. For those who are blocking feelings and on the verge of panic and unable to handle arousal, a strategy to neutralize emotions would be indicated.

Classifying the Murder

The murder classification indicates that intervention strategies will be different in the initial stages of working with these juveniles. Also, clinicians will probably see more cause-specific murderers in hospital settings than criminal-enterprise type with the latter more likely seen in juvenile detention settings.

The criminal-enterprise murder suggests much more socialization in crime than the cause-specific one and where there is some contextual rationalization for violent acts and behaving oneself. Those involved in criminal-enterprise crime also indicate some attachment to a peer. Efforts to have them work in groups and move toward attachment to potential victims or what blocks attachment toward potential victims would be a first step in increasing their sense of personal control. The next phase of treatment would certainly bring the juvenile closer to the emotions connected with disappointing relationships, i.e., the absent father, the neglecting or abusing caretaker.

In cause-specific murders, the juvenile will usually know the victim. The murder usually includes a personal dynamic reason for killing. In the juvenile's mind there is a set of circumstances that in some way justifies the act. Individual and group work would be indicated since isolation from others plays a role in maintaining deviant fantasies.

In both crime classification groups the older age of the victim gives some clue to the potential of the offender to attachment to the younger sense of self. This may be extremely important as a starting basis for empathy in that there is some respect for or caring for the younger self. In those cases where victims are younger than the offender, we suggest that one is dealing with a level of self-hatred that will be much more compromising of therapeutic efforts.

The pragmatic issue of judicial disposition of the serious habitual juvenile offender has been addressed (Heck, Pindur, & Wells, 1985) as well as lifestyle patterns (Vachss & Bakal, 1979). Both components are critical in multidisciplinary efforts toward converging those disciplines whose work brings them into contact with victim, offender or both. It is important in work with violent juveniles that mental health add its efforts to focus on an interruption of the factors that justify violence and support its repetition.

REFERENCES

Barlow, D.J. (1989). Therapeutic holding: effective intervention with the aggressive child. *Journal of Psychosocial Nursing and Mental Health Services* 27 (1):10–14.

Bender, L. (1959). Children and adolescents who have killed. *American Journal of Psychiatry* 116:510–513.

Burgess, A.W.; Hartman, C.R.; Ressler, R.K.; et al. (1986). Sexual homicide: a motivational model. *Journal of Interpersonal Violence* 1 (3):251–272.

Cornell, D.G.; Benedek, E.P.; & Benedek, D.M. (1987). Juvenile homicide: prior adjustment and a proposed typology. *American Journal of Orthopsychiatry* 57 (3):383–393.

Douglas, J. E.; Ressler, R.K.; Burgess, A.W.; & Hartman, C.R. (1986). Criminal profiling from crime scene analysis. *Behavioral Science and the Law* 4:401–421.

Duncan, J. W., & Duncan, G.M. (1971). Murder in the family: a study of some homicidal adolescents. *American Journal of Psychiatry* 127 (11):74–78.

Heck, R.O.; Pindur, W.; & Wells, D.K. (1985). The juvenile serious habitual offender/drug-involved program: a means to implement recommendations of the national council of juvenile and family court judges. *Juvenile and Family Services* (Summer): 27–37.

Jones, M.K. (1985). Patient violence. *Journal of Psychosocial Nursing and Mental Health Services* 23 (6):12–17.

King, C.H. (1974). The ego and the integration of violence in homicidal youth. *American Journal of Orthopsychiatry* 45 (1):134–145.

Lewis, D.O.; Shanok, S.S.; Pincus, J.H.; & Glaser, G.H. (1979). Violent juvenile delinquents. *American Academy of Child Psychiatry* 18:307–319.

Loomis, M.; O'Toole, A.; Pothier, P.; et al. (1987). Classification of human responses of concern for psychiatric mental health nursing practice. Kansas City, Kans.: American Nurses' Association, Phenomenon Task Force, 1987.

Malmquist, C.P. (1971). Premonitory signs of homicidal aggression in juveniles, *American Journal of Psychiatry* 128 (4):93–97.

Miller, D., & Looney, J. (1984). The prediction of adolescent homicide. *American Journal of Psychoanalysis* 34:187–198.

Pond, V.E. (1988). The angry adolescent. *Journal of Psychosocial Nursing and Mental Health Services* 26 (12):15–17.

Prentky, R.A.; Burgess, A.W.; Rokous, F.E.; et al. (1989). The presumptive role of fantasy in serial sexual murder. *American Journal of Psychiatry* 146 (7): 987–991.

Ressler, R.K.; Burgess, A.W.; & Douglas, J.E. (1988). *Sexual Homicide: Patterns and Motives*. Lexington, Mass.: Lexington Books.

Russell, D. H. (1979). Ingredients of juvenile murder. *International Journal of Offender Therapy and Comparative Criminology* 23 (1):65–72.

Sendi, I.B. (1975). A comparative study of predictive criteria in the predisposition of homicidal adolescents. *American Journal of Psychiatry* 132 (4):423–427.

Smith, S. (1965). The adolescent murderer. *Archives of General Psychiatry* 13: 310–319.

Vachss, A.H., & Bakal, Y. (1979). *The Lifestyle Violent Juvenile*. Lexington, Mass.: Lexington Books.

Winger, J.; Schirm, V.; & Stewart, D. (1987). Aggressive behavior in long-term care. *Journal of Psychosocial Nursing and Mental Health Services* 25 (4):28–33.

INDEX

Subject Index

Author Index